TO TREAT OR NOT TO TREAT

To: the NICU Nurses.

Thanks for the great work you do for the neonates & their families.

Peter [signature]

TO TREAT OR NOT TO TREAT

The Ethical Methodology of Richard A.
McCormick, S.J., as Applied to Treatment
Decisions for Handicapped Newborns

by

PETER A. CLARK, S.J.

CREIGHTON UNIVERSITY PRESS
Omaha, Nebraska
Association of Jesuit University Presses
©2003 by Creighton University Press

EDITORIAL
Creighton University Press
2500 California Plaza
Omaha, Nebraska 68178

MARKETING & DISTRIBUTION
Fordham University Press
University Box L
Bronx, New York 10458

Printed in the United States of America

I dedicate this book to my father and mother, Peter and Mary Clark, for instilling in me their love of knowledge, their courage to question, and their faith that with God's help all things are possible.

Contents

Preface

Medical and ethical decisions concerning whether or not to treat handi-capped neonates have confronted parents and health care professionals for decades.[1] In the past these decisions were less complicated and con-troversial since hospitals and physicians lacked the medical technology and expertise to sustain the lives of these handicapped neonates. Years ago, medical decisions about treatment were made in the privacy of the delivery room or the nursery. Such medical decisions were typically viewed as private matters between physicians and parents and were not matters for public policy debate. This scenario, however, has changed dramatically with advances in neonatal medicine and technology during the past twenty-five years.

New medical technologies, surgical procedures, and pharmaceutical advancements have made neonatology a technologically complex medi-cal subspecialty. Techniques and procedures considered a medical im-possibility just a few years ago have become a medical reality today. "The development of technologies as complex as extracorporeal mem-brane oxygenation, use of inhaled nitric oxide, and as simple as the ad-ministration of exogenous surfactant have resulted in the survival of many infants who would have succumbed to their illnesses only a few years ago."[2] Unfortunately, this technological progress often takes place without the benefit of reflective analysis. Consequently, both medically and ethically, neonatology has entered into uncharted waters with no clearly defined moral goals in sight.

Even with dramatic technological advances, diagnostic and prognos-tic certainty for many neonatal conditions remains elusive. Dr. John Ar-ras writes:

> Diagnoses are rarely 100 per cent certain and in spite of
> the traditional jargon, very few diagnoses are ever "ruled
> out." Prognosis is rarely certain at the time that a diag-
> nosis is entertained because all treatments vary in their
> efficacy from patient to patient and from time to time.

Furthermore, the risks of treatment are not always pre-
dictable.[3]

As a result, neonates with serious congenital anomalies, such as spina
bifida, anencephaly, intraventricular hemorrhage, etc., are often treated
aggressively. This treatment prolongs the lives of many neonates when in
the past they would have been allowed to die. Such life-prolonging
treatment decisions have far-reaching ramifications. Not only do medical
decisions to treat handicapped neonates create ethical problems for the
neonate but they also create emotional, social, and financial problems
well beyond the resources of families and society. At present, many in
society believe that all handicapped neonates must be treated. Such a
view raises a serious question. Does society have an ethical obligation to
meet the financial needs of these neonates and their families now and in
the future? Many ethicists believe that treatment decisions for handicapped neonates should no longer be considered private matters made in
the privacy of the delivery room. These decisions are complex and have
far-reaching medical, ethical, and financial ramifications for the neonate,
the family, and society at large.

It is relatively easy to observe a direct correlation between technological advances in neonatology and corresponding ethical dilemmas. As
neonatal technology continues to advance, crucial ethical issues likewise
have multiplied and diverse moral and policy arguments have prolifer-
ated.[4] There is little question that technology has provided new means to
save life. However, in recent years, questions are being raised about the
ethical nature of the means adopted and the quality of life being saved.

To address these questions, bioethicists have proposed a variety of
ethical criteria, that is, rules, standards, and guidelines concerning treatment decisions for handicapped neonates. These criteria have developed
from their ethical methodologies. A major problem for decision-makers
is that there is little or no consensus on which criterion or set of criteria is
ethically and medically more beneficial and appropriate. As a result of
this continuing debate, many handicapped neonates are suffering the
consequences. Some neonates are alive, but their lives are so completely
submerged in pain and suffering that their entire lives will be essentially
mere struggles for survival. In contrast, others are being allowed to die
when their deaths could be prevented. Parents and health care professionals search for a normative ethical criterion that will address the numerous treatment categories of handicapped neonates from an objective
standpoint. At the same time, this criterion ought to incorporate individual differences and personal value judgments. However, at the present
time there is no consensus and handicapped neonates are suffering as a
result.

One bioethicist who has struggled with these neonatal issues is Richard A. McCormick, S.J., described by some of his colleagues as the Dean of Roman Catholic moral theologians in the United States today.[5] McCormick proposes a patient-centered, quality-of-life approach to treatment decisions for handicapped neonates that appears to meet the needs of decision-makers. The primary focus of this book will be to articulate, analyze, and evaluate the three constitutive elements of McCormick's ethical methodology as they each relate to treatment decisions for handicapped neonates. McCormick's ethical methodology consists of three sets of claims: anthropological, epistemological, and criteriological. The analysis and critical evaluation of McCormick's ethical methodology will also consider alternative ethical positions that critique the positions he advances. This analysis will be accomplished by examining the writings of McCormick to show the foundational structure of his moral theology and how his ethical method can be useful in neonatal decision-making. The scope of this book will be an analysis of the writings of Richard A. McCormick and how his foundational moral theology serves as a basis for his ethical methodology, which can be applied to treatment decisions for handicapped newborns in an illustrative fashion.

Chapter One will examine Richard A. McCormick, S.J., as a moral theologian and his impact on bioethics in the United States. It will also place McCormick's ethical methodology within its proper context. In addition, this chapter will give a brief survey of neonatology from a United States perspective and examine the general ethical approaches used today in neonatal decision-making.

Chapter Two will consider McCormick's theological anthropology, which is rooted in the Christian story of Creation-Fall-Redemption. This forms the foundation upon which he grounds his notions of personhood, relationality, and human life as a relative good.

Chapter Three will treat McCormick's moral epistemology. He appears to have a dual moral epistemology; that is, it appears he has made a significant shift in his moral epistemology, at least at the level of synderesis. The first moral epistemology, which is prior to 1983, follows the school of John Finnis, J. Finance, G. de Broglie, and G. Grisez. Human persons seek the goods and values that define human flourishing by natural inclinations. The second epistemology, which begins after 1983, emphasizes prediscursive and discursive reasoning informed by the Christian story. Prediscursive reasoning discovers the basic human values, and discursive reason analyzes them, while the Christian story serves as a "corrective vision" to the cultural biases that may affect human reasoning.

Chapter Four will consider McCormick's moral criteriology. His moral criteria for treatment decisions for handicapped neonates are based on a patient-centered, quality-of-life approach. This approach is rooted in a normative understanding of what ought to be in the "best interests" of the handicapped neonate. This chapter will focus on McCormick's moral criteria for bioethical decision-making as it relates to never competent patients, since handicapped neonates may be grouped into this particular category. There appear to be dual criteria for McCormick's quality-of-life standard. The first criterion centers on the potential for human relationships associated with the handicapped neonate's medical condition. The second criterion is based on the traditional understanding of the benefit/burden calculus.

Chapter Five will apply McCormick's ethical methodology to five diagnostic treatment categories of handicapped neonates, established by this author, to determine if McCormick's normative method offers a practical and beneficial approach that can be used by appropriate decision-makers. The five treatment categories of handicapped neonates include: (1) The handicapped neonate whose potential for human relationships is completely nonexistent. An example is the anencephalic infant. (2) The handicapped neonate who has the potential for human relationships but whose potential is utterly submerged in the mere struggle for survival. An example is a neonate with a Grade IV massive intraventricular hemorrhage and hydrocephalus. (3) The handicapped neonate who has the potential for human relationships but the underlying medical condition will result in imminent death. An example is a neonate with hypoplastic left heart syndrome. (4) The handicapped neonate who has the potential for human relationships but after medical treatment has been initiated, it becomes apparent that the treatment is medically futile. An example is a neonate suffering from full-length large and small bowel necrotizing enterocolitis with perforation. (5) The handicapped neonate who has the potential for human relationships and has a correctable or treatable medical condition. An example is a neonate with Down syndrome and esophageal atresia with tracheoesophageal fistula. In this chapter, justification will be offered to explain why McCormick believes parents, in consultation with health care professionals, are the proper decision-makers. Throughout this chapter, criticisms of each methodological element will be addressed and applied, where applicable, to each treatment category.

Chapter Six offers a summary conclusion and overall evaluation of McCormick's ethical methodology as applied to treatment decisions for handicapped neonates. Two areas will be examined and critically analyzed. First, is McCormick's ethical methodology practical, beneficial, and appropriate for Christian parents and health care professionals in making treatment decisions for handicapped neonates? Second, can McCormick's ethical methodology be recommended to all decision-makers, both Christian and non-Christian, as a public policy option for the treatment of handicapped neonates? This chapter will also discuss future considerations where further explanation and clarification are necessary, and will offer this author's assessment of McCormick's ethical methodology and a recommendation on whether it can be recommended as a public policy option for the treatment of handicapped neonates.

There are two primary reasons for focusing this book on McCormick's ethical methodology. First, as one who has had enormous influence in the field of moral theology in the United States, McCormick has written extensively in the field of bioethics, and has formulated many useful guidelines, standards, and moral conclusions. In recent years, McCormick has applied these guidelines and standards to the issue of treatment decisions for handicapped neonates. Given the vast complexity involved, it is not surprising that his ethical methodology has met with considerable criticism. This criticism has been directed at McCormick's failure to articulate his theoretical foundations clearly and develop them systematically and coherently. While there may be inconsistencies and ambiguities with McCormick's ethical method, there are also many positive elements in it that may serve as appropriate and beneficial criteria that can be applied to treatment decisions for handicapped neonates. This book will attempt to construct a systematic analysis of McCormick's ethical methodology to determine if he advances Roman Catholic moral theology, especially in the area of bioethics.

Second, with rapid advances in neonatal medicine and technology, there is a serious need to examine whether McCormick's ethical methodology can assist parents, health care professionals, and other decision-makers in making these difficult neonatal treatment decisions. Decision-makers are searching for a public policy option that is both practical and beneficial in making treatment decisions for handicapped neonates. This book will seek to determine whether McCormick's ethical methodology can be applied in a consistent and helpful way to each of the five diagnostic treatment categories of handicapped neonates. The challenge for decision-makers is to determine how to apply this ethical criterion consistently to the wide diversity of neonatal defects. McCormick argues that he can address quality-of-life issues in a consistent way and can assist parents and health care professionals in practical, moral decision-making. This critical analysis of McCormick's ethical methodology, as applied to treatment decisions for handicapped neonates, will determine if his ethical methodology is appropriate and whether it can be recommended as a public policy option for all decision-makers. The importance of this critical examination can serve not only an academic, theoretical purpose—the advancement of moral theology—but it can also serve a clinical, practical purpose—giving assistance to parents and health care professionals in making well-discerned and sensitive moral decisions that affect the lives of handicapped neonates.

NOTES

[1]A neonate is a child from birth to one month of age. *The Merck Manual*, ed. Robert Berkow, M.D. (Rahway, NJ: Merck Research Laboratories, 1992), 1918. "Handicapped" refers to a deviation from standard functioning that is determined by medical standards. These defects would include congenital malformations, low birth-weight, genetic anomalies, asphyxia, etc.

[2]Richard L. Bucciarelli, "Neonatology in the United States: Scope and Organization," *Neonatology: Pathophysiology and Management of the Newborn*, eds. Gordon B. Avery, Mary Ann Fletcher, Mhairi G. Macdonald (Philadelphia: J. B. Lippincott Company, 1994), 12; and Leif Nelin, M.D. and George Hoffman, M.D., :The Use of Inhaled Nitric Oxide In A Wide Variety of Clinical Problems," *Pediatric Clinics of North America* 45 (June 1998): 531-548.

[3]John D. Arras *et al.*, "The Effect of New Pediatric Capabilities and the Problem of Uncertainty," *Hastings Center Report* 17 (December 1987): 10.

[4]Kathleen Nolan, "Imperiled Newborns," *Hastings Center Report* 17 (December 1987): 5.

[5]See Lisa Sowle Cahill, "Teleology, Utilitarianism, and Christian Ethics," *Theological Studies* 42 (1981): 601; Timothy J. Toohey, review of *Health and Medicine in the Catholic Tradition: Tradition in Transition*, by Richard A. McCormick, S.J., in *Journal of Pastoral Care* 39 (Spring 1985): 278; and Edward Collins Vacek, S.J., review of *The Critical Calling: Reflections on Moral Dilemmas Since Vatican II*, by Richard A. McCormick, S.J., in *Journal of Religious Ethics* 20 (Spring 1992): 209.

TO TREAT OR NOT TO TREAT

1

Introduction

This chapter will examine Richard A. McCormick, S.J., as a moral theologian; the ethical methodologies used in bioethics today; neonatology from a United States perspective; and general ethical approaches to treatment decisions for handicapped neonates.

RICHARD A. MCCORMICK, S.J.—MORAL THEOLOGIAN

The development of McCormick's ethical methodology can be situated by examining the background of this distinguished moral theologian. Richard A. McCormick was born on October 3, 1922, in Toledo, Ohio. He entered the Society of Jesus at the age of eighteen. His father, an eminent physician and past president of the American Medical Association, gave McCormick a distinct perspective on the medical profession. McCormick received his B.A. in 1945 from Loyola University Chicago, and an M.A. in 1950 from the same institution. He completed theological studies at the Jesuit theologate at West Baden, Indiana, and was ordained a priest in 1953. In 1957, McCormick received his S.T.D. (Doctorate in Sacred Theology) from the Pontifical Gregorian University in Rome, with a thesis on the removal of a probably dead fetus to save the mother's life. McCormick began his career as a moral theologian that same year, returning as a professor to the Jesuit theologate in West Baden, Indiana. After seventeen years in seminary education, McCormick was named the Rose F. Kennedy Professor at the Kennedy Institute, Georgetown University, in Washington, DC.

In 1986, McCormick accepted a teaching and research position as the John A. O'Brien Professor of Christian Ethics at the University of Notre Dame. He remained at Notre Dame University until his health began to fail in 1999. He then moved to Colombiere Center, the Detroit Province Infirmary, until his death on February 12, 2000. For many years, he

served on numerous local, state, national, and international ethics boards[1]
and has written extensively in the field of bioethics.[2]

McCormick has often emphasized the idea that "one's teaching and
writing reflect inescapably the historical context in which one lived."[3]
His training in a theology that was deeply rooted in the classicist mentality had a major influence on him as a moral theologian and has informed
his bioethical positions.[4] Wedded to neo-scholasticism,[5] the moral manuals were the textbooks that shaped the scope, method, and content of
moral theology up through 1965.[6] Following Vatican II, the Catholic
Church acknowledged a shift in worldviews from a classicist, legalistic
mentality to a modern, more historically conscious worldview. Actually
the "plausibility structures" of the classicist view had been in the process
of breaking down since the 1800s.[7] After the Council, Catholic moral
theology began to detach itself from neoscholasticsm and opened up
dialogue with a variety of philosophical partners. These theological,
philosophical and cultural shifts allowed McCormick to reexamine many
traditional formulations in a new light.[8] As a moral theologian, McCormick viewed himself fitting in somewhere between the classicist and the
historical consciousness mentality. McCormick writes: "Trained in the
classicist mentality, I have become conscious of both its strengths and its
weaknesses—and the need to correct or modify the latter."[9]

In an article entitled "Self-Assessment and Self-Indictment,"
McCormick sets forth three distinct stages in his methodological development: prior to Vatican II, Vatican II, and the debates about the encyclical *Humanae Vitae*.[10] This book will add a fourth, that is, the debates
about the "Curran Affair," which has had a profound impact on McCormick's more recent writings.[11] Prior to Vatican II, the Church viewed
itself as the guardian of God's law. The Church both determined and interpreted God's law and claimed the right and the duty to safeguard it
without question. The magisterium was viewed by many as being highly
or overly authoritarian and paternalistic; public dissent was almost unknown. Many held a very legalistic and juridical understanding of the
Christian life. The methodology of manualist moral theology tended to
be casuistic, unecumenical, unbiblical, "domestic" in its concerns, centrally controlled, natural law-oriented, and sin-centered. McCormick believed that he "escaped such pervasive influences first not at all, then
only gradually and more or less."[12]

Vatican II reversed many of the forces predominant prior to the
Council. Broader themes of Christian aspiration and living that were
biblically inspired began to replace the earlier emphasis on natural law,
casuistry, and a one-sided sin-centeredness. The authoritative teaching of
the magisterium, the self-understanding of the Church, the understanding
of moral norms, the relation of reason and morality, the place of the lay

voice in the formation of moral conviction in the Church, and the significance of non-Catholic witness and conviction all began to be questioned and debated. During this period, the Roman moral theologian Josef Fuchs, S.J., became a role model for McCormick.[13] McCormick writes:

> I needed someone of Fuchs' stature and undoubted loyalty to show me the possibility of change without unacceptable abandonment of essentials of "the Catholic idea." Without my explicitly averting to it, what was really changing were basic notions of ecclesiology and eventually moral methodology.[14]

During this period within moral theology there was a movement away from an act-centered, physicalist approach in judging the rightness and wrongness of human conduct to a person-centered approach.
For McCormick,

> Vatican II proposed as the criterion not "the intention of nature inscribed in the organs and their functions" but "the person integrally and adequately considered." Furthermore, to discover what is promotive or destructive of the person is not a deductive procedure.[15]

This basic change in worldview would restructure moral theology and would have a significant impact on how ethical decisions were discerned.

Following Vatican II, the papal encyclical *Humanae Vitae* was one of the most significant events of the twentieth century for the Roman Catholic Church. *Humanae Vitae* allowed theologians to wrestle with the meaning of "religious submission of mind and will."[16] This pivotal encyclical moved McCormick to reexamine two essential aspects of moral theology: the notion of the moral magisterium and the understanding of moral norms. McCormick came to understand that the proper response to authoritative teaching is not precisely obedience, but rather a docile personal attempt to assimilate the teaching. *Humanae Vitae* also initiated a much broader discussion among theologians that focused on the method of founding moral norms.

As a result, McCormick entered the proportionalism debate, a major turning point in the development of his ethical methodology. Despite the importance of the notion of the moral magisterium and the understanding of moral norms, McCormick believed that one problem overshadows them all: the relation of religious (Christian) belief to concrete areas of human behavior. McCormick believed his greatest failing as a moral theologian had been his inability to explore and make more clear and persuasive Vatican II's famous statement: "Faith throws a new light on everything, manifests God's design for man's total vocation, and thus directs the mind to solutions that are fully human."[17] But, he never gave up hope of rectifying this failing.

The fourth stage of development in McCormick's ethical methodology results from his involvement with the "Curran Affair." McCormick viewed the dismissal of Charles E. Curran from the theology faculty of the Catholic University of America as a great injustice. For McCormick, it violated the fundamental principles of academic freedom and institutional autonomy. The central issue in the "Curran Affair" concerns the right to public dissent from authoritative, noninfallible proposed teachings of the Church. McCormick writes: "Dissent is not an end product; it is a way of getting at things, a part of the human process of growth and understanding."[18] For McCormick, dialogue, debate, and dissent are necessary in the Church to ensure that moral teachings are free from error. Theologians must be willing to reexamine past formulations.[19] When the Congregation for the Doctrine of the Faith demanded that Curran be removed from his teaching position as a moral theologian, there were serious implications that followed from this approach for all theologians and Catholic universities.[20] The "Curran Affair" moved McCormick to become noticeably more vocal and pronounced in his criticism of the magisterium and bolder in his reexamination of tradition. McCormick saw the "restorationists" in the magisterium trying to claim the center as their own, making the true centrists in moral theology appear to be on the extreme left.[21] He also saw the goal of the "restorationists" to be the preservation of the pyramidal structure of the Church. McCormick viewed the "Curran Affair" as an important reminder that "when criticism is squelched and power enlists theology for its purposes, the entire Church suffers because theology has been politicized, i.e., corrupted."[22]

Prior to the "Curran Affair," McCormick had been more reactive than proactive in his approach to moral theology.[23] As a result of the "Curran Affair," McCormick realized that the very foundation of academic freedom and institutional autonomy were at stake, not to mention the role of moral theologians in the Church today. McCormick observed that "it takes little imagination to see how the climate of fear may lead theologians to 'stop exploring and challenging questions of the day,' or to hedge his or her bets."[24] The result would be devastating for the Church and for society. Fearing retrenchment by the magisterium, McCormick became less cautious in his criticism and adopted a more proactive approach to tradition while trying to move it forward.[25]

One result of these four stages in McCormick's development is the possibility of categorizing McCormick's writings into three distinct periods. First, from 1957-1967 he was still operating within the classicist mentality. His ethical methodology was dependent on the deductive method of the manuals and he used a revised form of casuistry. Second, from 1968-1983 he was writing "Notes on Moral Theology" for *Theological Studies* and was preoccupied with the distinctiveness of Christian ethics debate and the proportionalism debate. At this stage, a major paradigm shift occurred in McCormick's ethical methodology. His personalist orientation rooted in a "revised notion" of natural law compelled McCormick to move toward a teleological methodology. Finally, from 1983-2000, McCormick decided to turn his attention to bioethics and to approach bioethics from a theological viewpoint. His ethical methodology entailed the use of prediscursive and discursive reasoning in conjunction with the Christian story. The importance of this categorization of McCormick's writings will become more clear when McCormick's ethical methodology is analyzed in the following chapters.

These four stages of McCormick's methodological development show a clear maturation or evolution in McCormick as a theologian and bioethicist. He began his career as a moral theologian trained in the juridical, physicalist approach of the classicist worldview rooted in neo-scholasticism. Later he was drawn by Vatican II into a less juridical, more personalist approach of the historically-conscious worldview rooted in a "revised notion" of natural law. McCormick developed, along with other moral theologians, the idea of proportionalism, and became the leading proponent in the United States, which, along with the influence of the "Curran Affair," led to his more proactive revision of the moral tradition.[26] This book will argue that McCormick always remained firmly within the moral tradition of the Roman Catholic Church. However, in many of his writings, McCormick interprets this tradition to be in the process of transition.

As a bioethicist, McCormick's respect for, and openness to, science and technology and his emphasis on human experience allowed him to explore how medical technology has challenged Catholic moral theology to rethink some of its positions on issues regarding human life. Despite the complexity and diversity of advances in medical technology, McCormick saw a common denominator: more control means more responsibility, or at least a different kind of responsibility. This new sense of responsibility poses new ethical questions. How are we to exercise this responsibility? In what direction? With what criteria and controls? In light of what hopes and aspirations? And with what definition of the human? For McCormick, these are the questions at the heart of bioethics. In other words, the task of bioethics is not to apply mechanically old and presumably invariable injunctions to new facts, but rather to discover in changing times the very meaning of our value-commitments.[27] McCormick urged the Catholic Church to move beyond the positions of the past without forgetting the best of the tradition. This transition has not been an easy task, nor has it been without its pitfalls. McCormick argues:

> A transition involves both a "coming from" and a "going toward." The former dimension refers to the past that is historical but neither dead nor to be sloughed off like a decaying shell. This past is alive, with its own enduring visions, motives, and values that must continue to animate the "going toward" in ever-changing circumstances.[28]

Advancements in medicine and technology continue to challenge the Church tradition on various levels. Bioethical problems have two key characteristics: they are ever-changing and extremely complex. It is impossible for one individual to master and draw firm ethical conclusions valid for all times and cultures. Bioethical problems demand a convergence of competencies to discover what is truly humanly promotive or destructive.[29]

McCormick was well aware of the bioethical problems facing moral theology today. He was especially concerned about how science and technology can lull ethicists into a false sense of trust. Concerning this problem, McCormick writes:

> Our culture is one where: technology, especially medical, is highly esteemed; moral judgments tend to collapse into pragmatic cost-benefit calculations; youth, health, pleasure, and comfort are highly valued and tend to be sought and preserved at disproportionate cost; and maladaptations, such as senility, retardation, age, or defectiveness, are treated destructively rather than by adapting the environment to their needs. These factors suggest that the general cultural mentality is one that identifies the quickest, most effective way as the good way. Morality often translates into efficiency.[30]

McCormick understood that moral theology must be open to the challenges of medicine and technology and must always be ready to assist in confronting these ethical dilemmas in a realistic and ethical manner. For him, this does not mean that bioethicists must abandon the tradition of the Catholic Church, nor does it mean that such ethical dilemmas be resolved solely by tradition, power, fiat, prestige, political trade-off, or by economics. The value of human life continues to be challenged by new circumstances. Changing circumstances demand that imagination and creativity be employed to devise new formulations and understandings of this value in light of these new circumstances.[31] To accomplish this task, the bioethicist must remain in dialogue with health care professionals so that together a consensus may be reached to handle these difficult and complex ethical dilemmas. Even with enormous strides in the development of medical technology, no moral consensus exists on how to handle these ethical problems. In particular, there is little consensus on the required ethical methodology to address such ethical problems.

In recent years, a major area of ethical concern for bioethicists has focused on the subspeciality of neonatology. The impetus for McCormick's entry into the ethical problems facing neonatology, and in particular treatment decisions for neonates, was the now famous "Johns Hopkins Case."[32] McCormick was also influenced by an article written by Drs. Raymond S. Duff and A. G. M. Campbell in the *New England Journal of Medicine* that reported on 299 deaths in the special-care nursery of the Yale-New Haven Hospital between 1970 and 1972.[33] For McCormick, both situations were endemic to a culture and society that places higher value on some children over others to the point that some handicapped neonates may not even warrant treatment. McCormick began to question the criteria these physicians used to justify these decisions. He also inquired about the role parents played in the decision-making process. After involvement in a few neonatal ethical cases, McCormick soon came to the awareness that consensus on criteria regarding treatment decisions was lacking. He expressed concern that parents were often regarded and treated as third-party onlookers and not as co-patients in these tragic cases. In response to this situation, McCormick observed that "high technology came at parents in a rush. There is no indication that parents' wishes were consulted, their counsel sought, their consent obtained, their suffering assuaged. Things just happened to them, one after another."[34] From all of this it became evident that a serious need exists for an ethical methodology to address both the substantive and the procedural questions that are part of treatment decisions for handicapped neonates. In response, McCormick proposed a patient-centered, quality-of-life approach to treatment decisions for handicapped neonates.

McCormick's quality-of-life approach has been developed directly from his ethical methodology. However, this is but one specific ethical methodology among many. "Since its emergence some thirty years ago, bioethics in the United States has employed several methodologies. Principlism—the reliance on moral principles to address issues and resolve case quandaries—has come to dominate."[35] Over the past three decades, while recognizing the intellectual power and cogency of principlism, other ethical methodologies have emerged that suggest alternative treatments that either replace principlism entirely (though retain a role for principles as well as insights from principlism) or complement it, filling it out and providing correctives for its ills.[36] This next section will examine the various bioethical methodologies operative in the United States today.

BIOETHICAL METHODOLOGIES[37]

Before examining the ethical methodology of Richard A. McCormick, it is necessary to place his ethical methodology within its proper context. To accomplish this, one must first define ethical methodology. Second, one must examine the general types of ethical methodologies used in contemporary bioethics. Finally, McCormick's own ethical methodology must be located within the diverse field of bioethical methodologies.

Many ethicists begin their search for moral meaning and truth with the lived experiences that determine the value and worth of human persons. Once these foundational experiences are established, these ethicists then move to a process of reflection upon them to determine if these values are judged to be true and worthy of human well-being. In order to understand and judge human experience in the world, it is necessary to discover a method that will assist in determining the kinds of people we ought to be and the types of actions we ought to perform. For example, ethicist Trutz Rendtorff writes:

> If we define ethics as a theory of how we are to live, we are led to analyze the ethical question, and to describe and emphasize its basic elements. Now that these basic elements involved in living an ethical life have been described, we must look at the various elements of the ethical question in a methodical fashion so that they can be carefully considered. This will strengthen the role of ethics in orienting the discussion of how human life is to be lived. An ethical methodology of this sort is highly desirable, because the complexity of ethical experience demands a high degree of clarity, and clarity must extend to all the varied aspects that constitute ethical problems.[38]

A theory of ethics grows out of the human experience of reality. Through an ethical methodology, one can understand with precision the process in which the basic structure of an operative theory of ethics is explored and analyzed in its details.[39] An ethical methodology provides a strategy

which will be of assistance in living a good life in the midst of conflicting values.

Bioethical methodologies are a relatively new phenomenon. According to most assessments, bioethics began in the late 1960s or early
1970s. Many scholars believe that bioethics first began with the establishment of the Seattle Artificial Kidney Selection Committee in 1962.[40]
The growth of bioethics into a scholarly discipline did not begin until a
decade later when the Hastings Center and the Kennedy Institute were
established. Soon after, a few individuals were appointed to medical faculties, a literature in scholarly and professional journals emerged, and
conferences were convened.[41] Ethicists with both philosophical and
theological backgrounds were called to consult with health care professionals and families on various ethical dilemmas in the medical profession.

For the first decade of bioethics' existence, bioethicists tended to
stress principles; but as medicine advanced and technology became more
complex, many bioethicists began to see principlism as too fragile, too
constraining a structure to sustain the large issues that bioethics must
consider.[42] As a result, "new currents" began to emerge that either replaced principlism or complemented it. In addition to principlism, it is
possible to identify six major methodologies operative in the field of
bioethics today. These include: phenomenology, hermeneutics, narrative,
virtue-based, medical casuistry, and natural law. However, no single
methodology can adequately encompass the full dimensions of human
experience.[43] Each methodology offers a different path toward a common
ground as each aims to unpack the dense layers of human experience in
an effort to achieve shared insight and to promote informed action.[44] A
brief analysis of each of these seven ethical methodologies will be helpful in understanding how they impact contemporary bioethics.

PRINCIPLISM

As bioethicists began to consult with physicians and families about ethical dilemmas, a central question became: how were these ethical dilemmas to be analyzed so that all those involved could understand the terminology used? Albert Jonsen, a first-generation bioethicist, has suggested
that it was necessary to create a common language; this language has
become known as principlism. Jonsen writes:

> The philosophical ethics of that era had very little to say
> about the substantial content of moral decision and ac-
> tion. Theological ethics used terms that were incompre-

hensible to many who were not believers or were believers of another sort. We had to find an idiom that, at one and the same time, expressed substantive content and was comprehensible to many listeners. Although there were no consultations among us, no convocations to debate the issue, and no conspiracy to create an *ism*, almost all of us drifted away from the philosophical and theological languages of our intellectual tutelage. Like strangers in a strange land, we had to devise new forms of communication among ourselves, with our scientific and medical colleagues, and with the public.[45]

In 1974, the U.S. Congress passed the National Research Act which established the National Commission for the Protection of Human Subjects of Biomedical and Behavioral Research. The law mandated the following:

The Commission shall (1) conduct a comprehensive investigation and study to identify the basic ethical principles which should underlie the conduct of biomedical and behavioral research involving human subjects, (2) develop guidelines which should be followed in such research to assure that it is conducted in accord with such principles . . . [46]

The result of this commission was the issuance of the *Belmont Report*. Promulgated in 1978, this report settled on three basic principles: respect for persons, beneficence, and justice. The *Belmont Report* "became the classic principlist statement, not only for the ethics of human experimentation, but for bioethical reflection in general."[47] Ethicists James Childress and Thomas Beauchamp reevaluated these three principles and added a fourth principle called nonmaleficence, which was to be separated from beneficence. These basic ethical principles provided

scholars in this new field something that their own disciplinary traditions had not given them: a clear framework for a normative ethics that had to be practical and productive. They provided a focus for the broader, vaguer, and less applicable general reflections of philosophers and theologians of the era.[48]

As a result, a common language was established that most could comprehend. Following the *Belmont Report*, bioethics became principlist.[49]

As applied normative ethics, principlism is the application of general principles and rules to particular biomedical situations to determine the appropriate moral action by the agent. The four core principles (respect for persons, beneficence, nonmaleficence, and justice) are intended to provide a framework of moral theory for the identification, analysis, and resolution of moral problems in biomedicine. Deliberation and justification occur in applying the framework to cases.[50]

As bioethicsts became more involved in the complex dimensions of the medical profession, many realized that, despite the value of principlism, the approach had serious limitations. There existed a serious need to understand the full dimensions of the complexity and depth of human experiences that surrounded many ethical dilemmas in medicine. Principlism provided only one part of the puzzle. A major criticism leveled against principlism is that it is viewed as a "top-down" methodology that tries to impose abstract ethical principles on many diverse situations.[51] The result can be a tendency for principlism to obscure the full facts of a situation and to ignore the levels of complexity involved in each particular situation.

PHENOMENOLOGICAL METHODOLOGY

The phenomenological method examines situations from both objective and subjective dimensions. This approach places more emphasis on the subjective dimension since each situation is understood to be composed of a complex set of relationships. The focus is on the participants in the situation and how they experience and understand the situation. According to bioethicist Richard Zaner, the phenomenological method considers each situation as "context-specific" and works with and on behalf of persons. Therefore, the phenomenological method requires a strict focus on situational definitions. In clinical situations, moral issues are presented for deliberation, decision, and resolution solely within the "contexts" of their actual occurance. There is a need to penetrate and interpret each situation and relationship carefully, attentively, and completely. Every situational constituent, including any associated moral issue, is viewed solely within an ongoing relationship between the patient and the physician. In the phenomenological method, clinical ethics addresses the patient-physician relationship, always aware that all experience is in need of interpretation.[52]

HERMENEUTICAL METHODOLOGY

The hermeneutical method, according to philosopher Drew Leder, is an open-ended approach to a variety of interpretative perspectives. It rejects a "top-down" methodology that would impose uniform abstract principles on diverse situations. Within each medical situation there are a number of voices, each with its own narrative text that is open to multiple interpretations. The hermeneutical method approaches a case with a sense of respect for its "otherness" and allows a case to speak its own truth(s). The basic dynamic of bioethics is understood as an ongoing circle of experience-reflection-experience.[53] The hermeneutical approach is more open to the many influences that shape a text and thus to the many interpretative strategies that can be brought to bear upon it. Bioethicists operating within the hermeneutical approach believe that every text is susceptible to an infinite variety of readings. This is not to say that each text is equally significant or useful. It is important not to foreclose the possibility of multiple interpretations which overlap, supplement, clash, and converse with one another in ways that lead one to a deeper understanding of phenomena.

In the past, the bioethicist was viewed as the "answer person," showing what course of action was required by moral reasoning. A hermeneutically reframed notion of rationality requires new and productive roles for the bioethicist. The bioethicist becomes the articulator of the perspectives of the case participants and listens to the voice of each participant, allowing these voices to emerge more fully. The bioethicist is then better able to act as a facilitator of dialogue between the various parties, fostering mutual understanding and respect. The bioethicist recalls contexts and perspectives which often are systematically obscured and assists participants within the drama to tell and retell and to interpret and reinterpret their stories in order to achieve a consensus and mutual understanding in the face of the present ethical dilemma.[54]

NARRATIVE METHODOLOGY

The narrative method is similar to the phenomenological and hermeneutical methods. While this approach focuses on human experience, it also considers the richness of an individual's human story to reveal a fuller account of a particular situation. The narrative form can be described as "knowing-in-telling."[55] As cultures define their values through myth, individuals achieve identity and intimacy by telling and following stories. The narratival dimension moves beyond the realm of facts and searches for deeper and fuller meaning in human experience. This is accomplished by the awareness that each individual's story falls within a variety of contexts: the personal, religious, psychological, and historical. The bioethicist encounters this narratival dimension in every medical situation.

Rita Charon, a second-generation bioethicist, argues there are four fundamental stages to a narrative. These include: recognition, formulation, interpretation, and validation. These various stages assist the bioethicist in examining and interpreting the wider dimensions that surround an ethical dilemma. Autonomy, justice, beneficence, and nonmaleficence continue to guide ethical action and decisions within health care. Importantly, narrative competencies have the power to particularize health care decisions. The narrative method can increase involvement of both patients and providers in clarifying ethical choices as well as adopting timely longitudinal steps toward ethical recognition that will obviate quandary ethics.[56] The recognition of the narrative components in the actions of all bioethicists potentially can remove sources of bias, can assure a conceptual understanding of the personal contributions to ethical decision-making, and can favor a practice that respects the singular aspects of each clinical situation without raising relativistic or unduly situational fears.[57]

VIRTUE-BASED METHODOLOGY

The virtue-based method not only shifts the field of ethical analysis away from rules, principles, and rights; it moves beyond contextual questions that are the central focus of the phenomenological, hermeneutical, and narrative approaches. The virtue-based approach focuses on the character of the participants and is a personalist ethic, centering on the doctor-patient relationship.[58] Robert Veatch contends that this is not a relationship among "strangers"; rather, it is a relationship that depends on trust and confidence, if not friendship.[59] Ethicist James Drane views the character of the doctor as part of the therapeutic relationship and sees a structure to the doctor-patient relationship based on the patient's trust that the physician will do what is necessary to help the patient heal. The physician's primary task is not to cure illness but to care for patients, and such care depends on the character of the physician. The focus of attention in a virtue-based approach is on the inner realities of the persons involved, with particular attention to motives, dispositions, intentions, and attitudes. The character of a person is formed by the actions chosen and the values committed to over time. Character describes the person created by an individual's acts and omissions. A virtue-based approach focuses on the inner being of a person and the moral qualities brought to a situation rather than upon extrinsic principles. The refocusing of attention in mainstream biomedical ethics on "character" and "virtue" affords new dimensions to biomedical ethics not generally present within principlism. Ethicists working from a virtue-based methodology do not come to medicine with general principles justified in other contexts, that are to be applied now to "medical quandaries" or problem-points. Rather, medicine itself is seen as an exemplification of virtuous practices. The integration of the inner being of the doctor into a biomedical ethic of acts and rules will enhance medical ethics as a form of applied philosophy without diminishing any of the power of a mainstream principle's approach.[60]

MEDICAL CASUISTRY METHODOLOGY

Medical casuistry is the direct analysis of particular cases in clinical medicine. It deals directly with practical issues within clinical medicine and focuses on particular cases. The casuistic approach has its origins in the classical discipline of rhetoric. Two rhetorical techniques used by casuists include topics and the comparison of paradigm and analogy.[61] Particular cases are described by their circumstances and topics. Casuistical analysis then seeks to place each particular case into a context of similar cases. The technique of lining up cases, rather than viewing them in isolation, is the essence of casuistical analysis. The task of the medical casuist is to refer difficult cases arising in marginal and ambiguous situations to simpler, more nearly paradigmatic examples. Further, the casuist considers how far the simpler examples offer guidance in resolving the conflicts and ambiguities that awaken our moral perplexity. Paradigmatic cases provide the casuist a common basis for comparison and contrast. It is evident that the roots of medical casuistry are practical rather than theoretical and are based on the particular insights accumulated in the course of concrete practical experience. The medical information obtained in this approach is quite beneficial, but many ethicists question its intuitionist tendencies.[62]

NATURAL LAW METHODOLOGY

The final methodology to be considered is natural law, the cornerstone of the Roman Catholic tradition of ethics. Natural law in the Catholic tradition is based on the premise of "reason informed by faith." Natural law ethical theory is founded upon "an Aristotelian-Thomistic teleological model of moral agency and moral law."[63] Aquinas situates the natural law in his treatise on law in the *Summa Theologica* Ia-IIae, qq. 90-97.[64] The natural law is set within the theological context of the *exitus et reditus* (coming from God and returning to God) schema. The root of morality for Aquinas is in *ratio naturalis* (natural reason) which all human beings share. Aquinas believed that the will in every human person is drawn to the good. He viewed the natural law as a deliberative ethic which arrives at the good not through obedience to specific laws but by the deliberation of "right reason" (*recta ratio*). Every human person by nature possesses natural inclinations which guide toward self-realization and self-actualization. Reflecting on the Thomistic understanding of natural law, Frederick Copleston has written that

> Possessing the light of human reason, every human person can reflect on these fundamental inclinations of his nature and promulgate to himself the natural moral law, which is the totality of the universal precepts or dictates of right reason concerning the good which is to be pursued and the evil which is to be shunned. By the light of his own reason, therefore, man can arrive at some knowledge of the natural law. And since this law is a participation in or reflection of the eternal law in so far as the former concerns human beings and their free acts, man is not left in ignorance of the eternal law which is the ultimate rule of conduct.[65]

The fundamental principle of the natural law, which is regulative of all other precepts, is that "good is to be done and pursued, and evil is to be avoided."[66] Human nature is inclined toward certain intelligible goods. Aquinas refers to the precepts that govern our pursuit of these goods as the first precepts of the natural law.[67] The primary precepts are grounded in human nature and are self-evident, that is *per se nota*— known in themselves. However, the primary precepts themselves do not comprise a complete moral code. Practical reason reflecting on human nature as manifested in experience can discover less general and more particular precepts that Aquinas refers to as the secondary precepts. The secondary precepts are more detailed and are prudential conclusions following closely from the first principles. Aquinas maintained that the primary precepts of the natural law are unalterable. The primary precepts are the same for all persons and hold always and everywhere. However, with respect to the proper conclusions of practical reason, there is not the same truth and rectitude for all, nor are they equally known by all.[68] The secondary precepts can change for special reasons in some particular cases or in the event of some special causes preventing the observance of such precepts.

Of all the methodologies examined, natural law is perhaps the most ancient and historically persistent in Western ethics. However, natural law remains a very ambiguous term. Charles E. Curran points out that the word "nature" had over twenty different meanings in Christian thinking before Thomas Aquinas. Curran contends that the word "law" is also ambiguous, since it tends to have a very legalistic meaning for people today, whereas for Aquinas "law" was an ordering of reason. Curran writes:

> Natural law ethics has often been described as a legalis-
> tic ethic, that is, an ethic based on norms and laws; but in
> reality for Thomas natural law is a deliberative ethic
> which arrives at a decision not primarily by the applica-
> tion of laws, but by the deliberation of reason. Many
> thinkers in the course of history have employed the term
> natural law, but frequently have defined natural law in
> different ways. Thinkers employing different natural law
> approaches have arrived at different conclusions on par-
> ticular moral topics. Natural law in the history of thought
> does not refer to a monolithic theory, but tends to be a
> more generic term which includes a number of different
> approaches to moral problems. There is no such thing as
> *the* natural law as a monolithic philosophical system
> with an agreed upon body of ethical content from the
> beginning of time.[69]

While Roman Catholic moral theology is not committed to one par-
ticular natural law approach to moral problems, there are basic Catholic principles concerning moral objectivity that are held in official Catholic teaching and by Catholic scholars committed to the natural law tradition. Philip S. Keane, S.S., believes there are four such principles:

> First, there exists an objective moral order in which
> some actions are right and other actions are wrong; the
> moral order is not fleeting or capricious; it is not some-
> thing we can make up at will, granted, of course, that
> throughout history we continually gain insights into the
> exact nature of the moral order. Second, not only does
> the objective moral order exist but the human person (by
> reason even without the aid of faith) is able to know this
> order and understand that he or she ought to do what is

objectively morally good and avoid doing what is objectively morally evil. Third, once the human person and community come to objective moral knowledge, that knowledge is universalizable. Fourth, human persons do not always actualize their fundamental ability to know the objective moral order. Sometimes, either with or without fault or culpability, the human person will fail to be free enough to act on his or her knowledge. This failure, while it cannot be ignored, and while it may render the person less guilty or not guilty of sin, does not change the objective moral order.[70]

There does not appear to be any basic disagreement among Catholic natural law theologians regarding these basic principles. The questions among contemporary natural law theologians center on how to determine moral objectivity. Keane writes:

The basic question of moral objectivity is not whether external structures always yield the same moral object. The question is how much about the person and his or her action must be taken into account in order to grasp adequately the moral object of the act.[71]

The contemporary natural law ethicist believes a more complete analysis of the human person and his or her actions is necessary before one can give an adequate account of moral objectivity.

Catholic natural law theory has traditionally upheld two values of great importance for moral theology: (1) the existence of a source of ethical wisdom and knowledge that the Christian shares with all humankind, and (2) the fact that morality cannot be merely the subjective whim of an individual or a group of individuals.[72] Since bioethics encompasses matters of physiological well-being, moral choice, and justice, Roman Catholic moral theology claims that it is clear that natural law is indispensable to the framing and resolution of bioethical issues. Despite theoretical problems and disagreements, "nature" remains a useful standard for health. Modern technology urgently requires the investigation of the moral relevance of the contrast between nature and art.[73] Contemporary Catholic natural law, as it impacts on bioethics, is more person-centered in its approach in contrast to act-centered. This personalistic criterion is based on the essential dimensions of the human person. According to Louis Janssens, an action is moral if it is beneficial to the person integrally and adequately considered (i.e., as a unique, embodied spirit) and in the person's relations (i.e., to others, to social structures, to the material world, and to God).[74] The values upheld by the Catholic natural law theory and its personalistic criterion have helped create insights and perspectives that inform one's reasoning in the area of biomedicine.

All seven ethical methodologies reflect attempts by bioethicists to surface and better understand the complexity and density of human moral experience. Some of these methodological approaches focus more upon human relationships and human experiences. Others afford greater attention to the interpretation of human experience as well as the inner realities of individuals involved in these situations. Further, many of these approaches consider the direct analysis of particular cases in clinical medicine. McCormick is quite critical of many of these ethical methodologies. He contends that there is a "pervasive dissatisfaction with the status quo of bioethical reflection in the United States. A sense of malaise is unmistakably present and hovers over the subject like a dark cloud."[75] McCormick proposes that his ethical methodology, which is reasonable, objective, and rooted in the Catholic tradition, can counteract this malaise.

McCormick is firmly positioned in the natural law methodology of the Roman Catholic tradition. His understanding of natural law methodology has developed over the years from the more classicist view of natural law to the more revisionist view of natural law that is based in a historical conscious worldview.[76] Despite this revisionist view of the natural law it is clear that McCormick remains true to a very basic commitment that underlies the Roman Catholic tradition of moral teaching: moral values and obligations are grounded in a moral order known by human reason reflecting on experience. McCormick's commitment to an objective and reasonable morality is grounded in the thought of Aquinas, who in turn drew on Aristotle as well as on Christian sources. McCormick understands that humans and their abilities are limited, but it is at least in principle possible for them not only to become aware of those goods or values which enhance human life but also to consider these goods or values from viewpoints of persons and groups different in culture, religion, or historical era.[77]

McCormick's revisionist notion of Catholic natural law has been greatly influenced by the events of Vatican II. Lisa Sowle Cahill believes there have been four important shifts in the Catholic understanding of natural law that have shaken what appeared to be a prior unanimity of this tradition. Cahill writes:

> First, a shift *from a "classicist" to a historically conscious worldview*. Second, the theological ferment after Vatican II has brought a greater awareness that the teaching office of the Catholic Church *interprets natural*

law; it does not simply transmit revelation. Third, the Second Vatican Council represents an ecumenical movement toward dialogue with Protestant theology and ethics, and hence the enhanced Catholic *appreciation for scripture*. Fourth, a more integral appreciation of the importance of the *sociality and interdependence of human persons* characterizes recent Catholic thought.[78]

McCormick believed these shifts have enhanced the traditional natural law premise of "reason informed by faith." Reason is shaped by faith, and this shaping takes the form of perspectives, themes, insights associated with the Christian story. Reasoning about the Christian story reveals the deeper dimensions of the universally human.[79] As a result of this "compenetration" of faith and reason, McCormick shifted attention away from the principles and prescriptive norms that have occupied the focus of the Thomistic moral tradition, to a more experiential, commonsense basis of natural law thinking. This shift, not surprisingly, caused McCormick to be openly criticized by the "traditionalist" segment of the Catholic Church.[80] According to Lisa Sowle Cahill, it is possible to locate three main initiatives of McCormick's work in regard to the revision of natural law:

> First, to develop the traditional natural law method into a more experience-based and flexible form. Second, to unite Christian commitment with the natural law method, which in the past tended not to stress any special duties of discipleship. Third, to field issues of "dissent" in the Church, making dissent a partner in the constructive development of Catholic ethics.[81]

Cahill believes "it is fair to say that virtually all of McCormick's moral principles and conclusions come down to a matter of 'reasonableness'; but he increasingly uses Christian themes to flesh out and motivate."[82] Reason can discover and know the basic human goods. However, the Christian story nourishes the overall perspectives of the person and serves as a "corrective vision" to the secularism of the culture. For McCormick,

> The Christian story tells us the ultimate meaning of ourselves and the world. In doing so, it tells us the kind of person we ought to be, the goods we ought to pursue, the dangers we ought to avoid, the kind of world we ought

to seek. It provides a backdrop or framework that ought
to shape our individual decisions.[83]

Yet, for McCormick, the Christian perspective does not yield specific
moral rules for individual decision-making. Epistemologically these insights are not specific to Christians since they can be and are shared by
all people of good will.[84]

McCormick argues that because his ethical methodology is reasonable and objective, it can be applied to any situation. However, he is also
aware that because natural law is based on human experience, moral reasoning reflecting on experience always does so within a historical context. Applying an ethical methodology to a culture as diverse as that of
the United States and to the technologically complex field of neonatology presents serious challenges. There exists a plurality of views in our
culture even on matters as fundamental as saving the life of a neonate.
Confronted by this pluralism and the medical complexity of present day
neonatology, McCormick began to address these challenges by becoming
more knowledgeable in the specialization of neonatology. In this process
he learned quickly the importance of consultation with medical authorities and the need to be in dialogue with parents. McCormick once observed that:

> It remains true that if I, as a moral theologian, am going
> to reflect on the moral problem of terribly disabled neo-
> nates, I ought to learn all I can from neonatal intensive-
> care units, from nurses, from experienced physicians,
> from parents.[85]

McCormick has done this in various ways, and as a result he has gained
invaluable knowledge and experience. Following McCormick's example,
this next section will examine the specialization of neonatology from a
United States perspective.

NEONATOLOGY: A UNITED STATES PERSPECTIVE

Neonatology means knowledge of the human newborn. As a specialization, it has its roots in obstetrics, pediatrics, and physiology.[86] Prior to the
mid-1950s, medical care for handicapped neonates was primitive and
generally fell under the jurisdiction of pediatricians. Medical decisions
about the treatment of handicapped neonates were practically "non-
decisions" due to the lack of technology and medical information in this
area. During this time period, infant mortality was high. Ethical ques-

tions concerning treatment decisions were practically nonexistent since most handicapped infants were expected to die and were allowed to die. Before 1950, survival of the fittest along with a medical policy of gentleness with minimal intervention described the general approach to treatment decisions for handicapped neonates.

The specialization of neonatology became prominent during the late 1950s and the early 1960s. In 1960, the term "neonatology" was coined by Dr. Alex Schaeffer as interest continued to expand in the "neonate."[87] In 1975, neonatal-prenatal medicine became a board-certified subspeciality of pediatrics. Neonatal intensive care grew rapidly, bringing the technology of respirators, careful monitoring, computed tomography, ultrasonography, and aggressive intervention to the handicapped neonate. Unfortunately, little contemplative analysis accompanied this growth of medical technology. New ground was being broken, the lives of neonates were being saved, and new financial constraints on health care dollars led to the creation of large regional centers for neonatal intensive care.[88] Since the early 1960s, the United States has been at the forefront of neonatal medical advancements and in the creation of Neonatal Intensive Care Units (NICU). Describing neonatal medicine in the United States, various authors have collected the following data:

> In the United States approximately 4.0 million live births occur each year in about 5000 hospitals. Approximately 6-8% or 370,000 newborns will require special care of some variety, ranging from a few hours for observation to many weeks or months in the Neonatal Intensive Care Units. The percentage of infants born weighing less than 5.5 pounds rose 8% from 7% across the country in 1998, and remained steady at 9% in the cities. In an affluent middle-class community hospital approximately 3-4% of babies will require some special care or attention; in an inner-city, urban, lower socioeconomic setting as many as 15-20% of the babies will require special care. The overall infant mortality rate in the United States is 4.7 deaths per 1000 live births as of 2000. But specific ethnic and racial groups show no signs of improvement and in some cases their rates are, in fact increasing. African American, Native American, Alaskan Native and Puerto Rican infant death rates are above the national average. Infant mortality rates are 2-1/2 times higher for African Americans than for white Americans. The Native American rates are 1-1/2 times higher. Portions of several U.S. urban areas have infant mortality rates similar

to those of underdeveloped countries. Infant mortality
can be further divided into neonatal mortality (i.e., death
before 29 days of age) and post-neonatal mortality (i.e.,
death between 29 days and one year of age). One-half of
all neonatal deaths can be attributed to four leading
causes: low birthweight, acute perinatal asphyxia, congenital anomalies, and perinatal infections. There are approximately 792 hospitals providing 7,500 neonatal intensive care beds in the United States and close to 3,688
pediatricians subspecially trained in neonatology. The
number of neonatologists has doubled since 1985. It is
estimated that neonatal care costs about $8 billion per
year in the United States. Neonatal intensive care remains one of the highest single hospital costs—more
than 25% of the country's entire maternal-newborn
budget.[89]

As neonatal medical technology advanced, and as the lives of many
handicapped neonates were saved, the ethical dilemmas multiplied and
became more complex. Advances in neonatal technology raise numerous
problems: the meaning and definition of death, the duty to prolong life,
medical priorities, euthanasia, etc. However, the common denominator in
all these advancements is that more control means greater responsibility,
or at least a different kind of responsibility.[90] A central ethical question
confronting neonatologists and bioethicists today is how to set limits on
the use of this new technology.

In the United States, virtually all infants with any chance of survival
are treated aggressively in the delivery room. Later, these neonates are
stabilized in the intensive care nursery until further information is made
available to provide a more definite prognosis. This is the "wait until
certainty" approach. As more data is generated about diagnosis and
prognosis, recommendations are then made to withdraw current treatment or withhold future treatment when death or a terribly impaired life
seems inevitable. This approach to the uncertainty of neonatal care can
be contrasted with the "vitalist" approach of aggressive intervention for
all infants at all times, or the "statistical" approach which seeks to minimize the number of infants who die slow deaths or who live with profound disabilities, thus sacrificing some potentially healthy survivors by
not treating infants based on minimum weight or gestational age criteria.[91] Undoubtedly, there is a wide spectrum of treatment decisions for
handicapped neonates. A major concern of many ethicists is that with an
enormous bias to save life during the medical crisis in the nursery there

is limited provision of aftercare and support for families with handicapped or disabled children.[92]

The majority of these ethical dilemmas regarding treatment decisions for handicapped neonates are made daily in the privacy of the NICU by parents, health care providers, or a combination of the two. It is only when a conflict exists between the "best interests" of the neonate and the parental authority that treatment decisions become matters of public concern. Since 1980, decision-making powers of parents and health care providers have been challenged and placed under legal scrutiny. The threats of medical malpractice, civil or criminal liability, and failure on the part of physicians to be aware of judicial trends have caused additional problems.[93] However, not all the blame should be placed at the door of physicians. The federal government has played a major role and has caused and contributed to the confusion, uncertainty, and indecision in many treatment decisions for handicapped neonates.

Advancements in neonatal medical technology and the resulting ethical dilemmas have increased public awareness that some handicapped neonates have had medical treatments inappropriately withheld or withdrawn, leading to death in many cases. An early incident that raised public awareness to inappropriate use of treatment with handicapped neonates was the 1963 "Johns Hopkins case." This neonate was diagnosed with Down syndrome with an added complication of an intestinal blockage called duodenal atresia. After consultation with physicians on the case, the parents decided not to treat the duodenal atresia and eleven days later the infant died.[94] The publication of several articles in medical journals in the early 1970s about the practice of withholding and withdrawing medical treatment from handicapped neonates in neonatal intensive care units also raised public awareness of the issue.[95] While there was no significant public response to these events, other than a sense of agreement that parents in consultation with physicians ought to make these treatment decisions and ought to have the right to determine the outcome for handicapped neonates, there was a sense of guarded concern. Bioethicists, however, raised serious questions about the criteria used to make these clinical decisions. Thus, the ethical debate about the proper criteria for treatment decisions began. It was not until April of 1982 and the "Baby Doe" case in Bloomington, Indiana, that there began public outcry in the United States about withholding treatment from handicapped neonates.[96] The result of this case was the publication of two sets of federal regulations during the Reagan administration: the "Baby Doe" regulations of 1983 and the subsequent child abuse regulations established in 1985.

The "Baby Doe" regulations were written with the assumption that physicians and parents could not be trusted to give needed care to handicapped infants. These regulations mandated that every infant, unless permanently unconscious, irretrievably dying, or salvageable only with treatment that would be "virtually futile and inhumane," should be given life-sustaining treatment, no matter how small, young, or disabled the infant might be.[97] These regulations claimed to draw their authority from Section 504 of the Rehabilitation Act of 1973.[98] Hospitals were required to post notices that required health care professionals who observed that treatment was being withheld or withdrawn from a defective or handicapped infant to call a twenty-four-hour toll free "handicapped infant hotline" in Washington, DC. The government responded to these reports by dispatching a "Baby Doe squad" to investigate immediately the alleged discrimination against the neonate.[99] These regulations, mandating signs and creating "Baby Doe squads," were declared invalid by a federal judge on procedural grounds in April of 1983.[100] The regulations, now revised, were reintroduced on July 5, 1983, by the Department of Health and Human Services. In addition to signs and hotlines, the regulations advocated a process of decisional review called Infant Care Review Committees in order to encourage "informal, enlightened and fair decision making."[101] After considerable opposition, these regulations were again struck down. The basis of the regulations, the discrimination statute known as Section 504, was subsequently declared by the United States Supreme Court as inappropriate as the foundation of regulations concerning nontreatment of handicapped newborns.[102]

Additional efforts toward regulation were made by the U.S. President's Commission for the Study of Ethical Problems in Medicine and Biomedical and Behavioral Research (1983),[103] the American Academy of Pediatrics (1984),[104] and numerous writers on ethics in pediatric medicine. Concerned parties proposed the formation of an ethics review committee.[105] In 1984, the Federal Child Abuse Law was amended,[106] which added to each state's child protection agency the concern for withholding of medically indicated treatments from neonates. Currently in effect, these regulations do not mandate unnecessary or inappropriate treatments but allow physicians to use reasonable judgment in decision-making. Further, parents are allowed a role in the process even though the term "parent" is not part of the law or regulations. These federal regulations urge but do not mandate the formation of Infant Care Review Committees to facilitate decisional review and to assist in conflict resolution.[107] In 1992 the Americans with Disabilities Act (A.D.A.) went into effect, which protects a wide range of disabilities from discrimination. Whether the A.D.A. applies to handicapped neonates is not clear. However, in February 1994 a federal court specifically cited this act in mandating treatment for a 16-month old anencephalic infant named Baby K, who had been brought to a hospital emergency room in Virginia in respiratory distress. Time will tell whether handicapped neonates fall under the protection of the A.D.A.[108] Interest in the regulation of treatment decisions for handicapped neonates appears to be an American phenomenon. Other technologically advanced nations have not initiated such regulations.[109]

Despite these proposed federal regulations and medical guidelines that have gone a long way toward clarifying treatment issues, there is still no consensus on a specific criterion concerning treatment decisions for handicapped neonates. There is general agreement within the medical, legal, and ethical professions that there are some handicapped neonates whose lives need not be sustained. Consensus ends, however, when an attempt is made to determine which specific neonates should receive or should not receive treatment. Some argue that life should be preserved at all costs. For others, life may be ended, even by active means, when it has become too burdensome. Others hold opinions that are ambiguous and fall somewhere in between. The ethical perspectives concerning treatment decisions for handicapped neonates are equally diverse. Often this results in unnecessary suffering for some neonates and death for others. The diversity of ethical perspectives, not to mention legal and medical perspectives, has brought to the forefront the urgent need of parents and health care professionals for an ethical criterion to assist them in making these difficult and complex treatment decisions.[110] One caution must be stated clearly from the beginning. There do not exist ethical criteria that will bring about moral certitude in treatment decisions for handicapped neonates. Diagnosis and prognosis are almost always very speculative so value judgments are an important part of the entire decision-making process. However, despite this caution, various bioethicists have proposed ethical approaches to treatment decisions for handicapped neonates. The next section will survey these various ethical approaches.

GENERAL ETHICAL APPROACHES
TO TREATMENT DECISIONS FOR HANDICAPPED NEONATES

This section will present a summary of the various ethical approaches used by bioethicists in making treatment decisions for handicapped neonates. This survey is not intended to be exhaustive, but rather to present in a thoughtful and thought-provoking way the views that are representative of certain ways of thinking about treatment decisions for handicapped neonates.

Ethical criteria for treatment decisions concerning handicapped neonates must address both substantive and procedural issues. Substantive issues include consideration of appropriate standards for making treatment decisions and present various options. These options can be placed into four categories. First, treat every newborn as aggressively as possible. Second, base selective treatment in the balance between direct benefits and burden of care. Third, consider the personal and financial costs to the family and to society. Fourth, focus selective treatment on the "best interests" of the neonate, so that treatments should be limited only if suffering or a radically diminished quality of life would make existence a net burden to the infant. Procedural issues focus on (1) how decisions ought be made and (2) who the appropriate decision-makers are in the case. Potential decision-makers include parents, health care professionals, ethics or infant care review committees, and the courts.[111] The substantive and procedural issues are inseparable, and together they form the basis of ethical criteria concerning treatment decisions for handicapped neonates.

Much of the debate about various approaches centers on the notion of "objectivity." Objective data on which to base the decision must be considered to determine how and whether value judgments play an integral part in determining ethical criteria. Paul Ramsey, who was a leading Protestant ethicist, proposed a "medical indications policy." Medically indicated criteria suppose that the judgment is not only objective (not determined by personal value judgments) but is determined by scientific evidence alone.[112] Ramsey's categorical imperative is "never abandon care." For him, all nondying neonates must be treated, if they can be so benefited by the treatment. The patient's best interests, medically speaking, are to be the focus of any treatment decision for these patients. Every neonate's life, whether handicapped or not, is viewed to be of equal and independent value. The physician has the primary responsibility for determining if the neonate is dying and whether or not treatment offers the potential for medical benefit. Regrettably, Ramsey is less clear about the role of parents in decision-making even though he does speak of parental consent.[113]

Warren T. Reich, John R. Connery, S.J., and Leonard J. Weber each adopt "the ordinary/extraordinary means" approach. These ethicists reject the quality-of-life formulation. The ordinary/extraordinary means approach is a patient-centered, burden-to-benefit calculus and insists that each human life is inherently good regardless of condition. In this sanctity-of-life ethic,

> each individual life is inherently good regardless of condition and all lives are of equal value. There is no justification for discrimination based on quality or condition of life and no justification for killing, unless a person has

forfeited his right to life by certain actions which are themselves a destruction of or a threat to life itself.[114]

Reich, Connery, and Weber argue that, since parents have the primary responsibility in raising their children, they must be recognized as having primary responsibility for making treatment decision for their handicapped neonates.[115]

Michael Tooley and Peter Singer present an approach called "termination of selected nonpersons." This view is based on the functional definition of personhood. Tooley and Singer equate personhood with the mental capacity to become a moral agent. Ultimately, their position results in a benefit/burden calculus weighed on the side of the parents and other moral agents affected by the infant nonperson's life prolongation or death.[116] Mary Anne Warren's approach is similar to that of Tooley and Singer's. Infants are considered to be human beings in the genetic sense, but Warren questions if they are humans or persons in the moral sense.[117] Warren holds that neonates are nonpersons and should be allowed to continue living because they are wanted by their parents or since others are willing to pay for their care. For Warren, when an unwanted or handicapped neonate is born into a society that cannot afford and/or is not willing to take care of it, then its destruction is permissible. This action is not murder because only persons have a full right to life.[118]

H. Tristram Englehardt's position is based on the "child's best interests." Selective nontreatment is justifiable only when death appears to be in the best interests of a nondying infant. Such a decision is guided by the expected lifestyle and the cost in parental and societal pain and money for its attainment. Englehardt writes:

> When this perspective is adopted, there is a moral framework for withholding treatment or intentionally killing in cases where, in the parent's judgment, the child's existence after treatment will primarily be characterized by severe pain and deprivation. Even though the cost of the proposed treatment is not high—thus not making the treatment "extraordinary"—the treatment may still be withheld when it is judged to be in the child's best interests.[119]

David Smith's position is similar to Englehardt's as he argues selective nontreatment by parents is sometimes necessary for the sake of the child's best interests. However, Smith believes this argument is more problematic and less inclusive than Engelhardt seems to suggest. Smith understands the best interests test as a test that errs in favor of prolonging life. He acknowledges that there can be rare instances in which non-treatment would be in the best interests of the child, but in general, the best interests test amounts to a prohibition of active or passive infanticide on most newborns.[120]

Robert Veatch uses the "reasonable person standard," which is drawn from legal parlance. He maintains that a guardian has the right to refuse even lifesaving treatments for a handicapped neonate if the treatment is "unreasonable because of its uselessness or the burden it generates."[121] This is a patient-centered perspective that is based on the reasonableness of the treatment. A parent may morally refuse treatment for a handicapped neonate if it would seem "within the realm of reason to reasonable people."[122]

Next there is the quality-of-life approach. There are a number of approaches that form a spectrum moving from a more conservative quality-of-life position to a more radical quality-of-life position. Albert Jonsen and Michael Garland present a minimalist quality-of-life approach. The responsibilities of parents, the duty of physicians, and the interests of the state are conditioned by the medico-moral principle, "do no harm, without expecting compensating benefit for the patient." Life-preserving intervention is understood as doing harm to an infant who cannot survive infancy, or will live in intractable pain, or who cannot participate even minimally in human experience.[123] Joseph Fletcher can be generally situated within the quality-of-life approach, though his position is further down on the spectrum than that of Jonsen and Garland's. Fletcher argues that ethical analysis of nontreatment decisions begins with an inquiry into the "nature" of the life of the infant to be prolonged or terminated. Parents and physicians must determine if the proposed treatment will promote human well-being and reduce suffering for all individuals involved. It must be asked if such treatment will simply prolong the life of the infant who will end up in an institutional "warehouse" for the mentally and/or physically handicapped. The continued existence of a handicapped neonate is evaluated not only by the quality of its projected future but also by the quality of its projected impact on the lives of those affected by it. A number of practical elements are included in this evaluation.[124] Once a decision is made that the neonate's projected quality of life is insufficient to prolong life through medical treatment, Fletcher suggests that the means chosen to terminate the neonate do not really matter.[125]

Earl Shelp also advocates a quality-of-life approach founded on a property-based theory of personhood. For Shelp, to be a person in the full sense as a member of the moral community one must possess the qualities of "minimal independence."[126] Since neonates do not posses these qualities, for Shelp they are considered persons only in the social sense.

In his view, persons in the strict moral sense, that is, parents, siblings, or anyone the neonate might affect, have priority over neonates. Therefore, if the burdens imposed on others are disproportionate or unreasonable, then parents may make a moral decision to forego or withdraw medical treatments. Shelp even allows for infanticide in certain cases.[127] Parents are the primary treatment decision-makers, because they stand in a "quasi-fiduciary role" to their children.[128] Shelp's quality-of-life approach is a form of socially-weighed calculus.[129]

Finally, Richard A. McCormick also advocates a patient-centered, quality-of-life approach based on the potential for human relationships associated with the infant's medical condition. His approach also considers the traditional understanding of the burden/benefit calculus. McCormick's way of proceeding may be viewed as a reformulation of the distinction between ordinary/extraordinary means of life support. In this case, treatment decisions are morally optional when they are too burdensome for the patient even though treatment may extend the length of life. For McCormick, quality-of-life judgments are an extension of a sanctity-of-life ethic.[130] He argues that quality-of-life treatment decisions ought to be made by parents in consultation with the appropriate health care professionals.

This brief survey of the ethical approaches reveals both the broad diversity of ethical approaches to treatment decisions for handicapped neonates and the significant lack of consensus within the general categories of these approaches. Therefore, it is not surprising that many parents and health care professionals are often left in a state of ambiguity and confusion when attempting to make treatment decisions for handicapped neonates.

Today, parents and health care professionals are drawing lines between neonates who will be treated and those who will not be. If these lines are being drawn, then there must be an ethical methodology that these appropriate decision-makers can use. McCormick believes that his ethical methodology is both practical and beneficial for all decision-makers in making treatment decisions for handicapped neonates. To determine if this is true, the three distinct elements of McCormick's ethical methodology (theological anthropology, moral epistemology, and moral criteriology) will be critically analyzed and examined in the following chapters. Once his ethical methodology has been examined, it will be applied to the five diagnostic treatment categories of handicapped neonates to determine if it is appropriate and can be recommended to all decisions-makers, both Christian and non-Christian, as a public policy option on the treatment of handicapped neonates.

NOTES

[1]McCormick has served on the ethics committees of the American Hospital Association, Catholic Health Association, American Fertility Society, and the National Hospice Association. In addition, he has served on the Ethics Advisory Board of the Department of Health, Education, and Welfare, and on the President's Commission on Bioethics.

[2]Charles E. Curran, "Introduction: Why This Book?" in *Moral Theology: Challenges for the Future*, ed. Charles E. Curran (New York: Paulist Press, 1990), 6.

[3]Richard A. McCormick, S.J., *Corrective Vision: Exploration in Moral Theology* (Kansas City: Sheed & Ward, 1994), 40.

[4]For McCormick, the classicist mentality "conceives culture normatively and abstractly and represents a certain disengagement from the forces shaping the contemporary world. It seeks and easily finds certainties and views departure from them as unfaithfulness, pluralism as bordering on anarchy." Ibid.

[5] "Neo-scholasticism is a term used for the revival, from 1860 to 1960, of the philosophical tradition of the medieval and baroque universities. After the rise of the Enlightenment, Catholic theology found difficulty in using the empiricist and idealist philosophies to express orthodox theological concepts. By 1850 some were suggesting that a return to the 'Scholastic' tradition of the older Catholic universities might be the best solution. This received papal approbation in Leo XIII's encyclical *Aeterni Patris* (1879), which held up the 'Christian philosophy' of Thomas Aquinas as the best model for *philosophia perennis* for all Catholic education but urged that it be freed of obsolescent elements and that it assimilate the best of modern thought....By the time of the Council the weaknesses of neo-scholasticism were recognized by Catholic theologians: its lack of historical perspective and the eclectic confusion of Thomism with the alien doctrines of Francisco de Suárez, Duns Scotus, René Descartes, G. W. Leibniz, Immanuel Kant, and idealism; its failure to deal adequately with the findings of modern science and to recognize human historicity and subjectivity; and its teaching methods that tended to conceptualism, while neglecting to ground principles and definitions in experience." *The Harper-Collins Encyclopedia of Catholicism*, ed. Richard P. McBrien (San Francisco, CA: Harper-Collins Publishers, 1995), 911.

[6]In the manual tradition the objective norm of morality was viewed almost exclusively in terms of law, both in the Church and in civil society. Law included the eternal law, divine positive law, natural law, and human law. Conscience was the subjective norm of morality and con-

science had to conform itself to the various laws comprising the objective norm of morality. An extrinsic and voluntaristic mindset supported such a legal model. For the voluntarist the source of obligation comes not from the moral reality itself, but from the will of the legislator: something is good because it is commanded. This approach claims to be Thomistic. However, critics claim that it deviates dramatically from positions of Thomas Aquinas who had insisted on an intrinsic and rational approach to morality. For Aquinas, something is commanded because it is good. For a more detailed analysis of the manual tradition, see Charles E. Curran, "Introduction: Why This Book?" in *Moral Theology: Challenges for the Future*, 2.

[7]For McCormick, "It has become commonplace to say that the Council reinserted the Church into history, the wider context of Christianity and the world. It is also commonplace to interpret this as meaning the abandonment of a classicist consciousness for a renewed historical consciousness. To me 'historical consciousness' means taking our culture seriously as soil for the 'signs of the times,' as framer of our self-awareness. That means a fresh look at how Christian perspectives ought to be read in the modern world so that our practices are the best possible mediation of gospel values in the contemporary world . . ." Some emphases which cluster about the new historical consciousness in moral theology are the following: "a more dynamic, less aprioristic notion of natural law; collegiality by the teaching office of the Church in the discovery of moral truth; respect for the religious liberty of others in implementing our convictions in the public forum; a fresh look at our pastoral policies and practices where certain irregularities are involved (e.g., the divorced and remarried); a new awareness of the conflict model of decision-making, and of the sinfulness of the world in which we must pattern our lives and grow in Christlikeness; a more positive and pastoral pedagogy in the communication of moral values." Richard A. McCormick, S.J., *The Critical Calling: Reflections on Moral Dilemmas Since Vatican II* (Washington, DC: Georgetown University Press, 1989), 9, 22.

[8]It should be noted that Vatican II ratified an allowance for Catholics to engage in modern historical emphasis. Many theologians such as Bernard Häring, Pierre Teilhard De Chardin, S.J., and other Catholic modernists, were doing this already. The question is: was Vatican II the leader or was it following the lead that others had established? Paulinus Odozor believes that McCormick began to subscribe to a form of personalist morals well before the Council. This author would agree with Odozor that McCormick was one of the many Catholic theologians engaging in modern historical emphasis prior to the Council. For a more detailed analysis on McCormick and historical emphasis, see Paulinus Ikechukwu

Odozor, *Richard A. McCormick and the Renewal of Moral Theology*
(Notre Dame, IN: University of Notre Dame Press, 1995), 89. To under-
stand how McCormick subscribed to a form of personalist morals, see
Richard A. McCormick, S.J., "The Primacy of Charity," *Perspectives*
(August-September 1959): 18-27.

[9]McCormick, *Corrective Vision*, 41.

[10]*Humanae Vitae* is the 1968 encyclical of Pope Paul VI that reaf-
firmed the condemnation of artificial contraception for Roman Catholics.

[11]McCormick's article "Self-Assessment and Self-Indictment" was
published in 1987 prior to Rome's final judgment on Charles Curran. It
is my assessment that McCormick has entered a distinctive fourth stage
since 1987 even though he has never stated it explicitly in any of his
writings.

[12]McCormick, *Corrective Vision*, 42.

[13]Fuchs continued to serve not only as a role model for McCormick
until McCormick's death; McCormick often referred to Fuchs as "my
mentor in Rome." This relationship began when McCormick was doing
his doctoral studies at the Pontifical Gregorian University in Rome where
Fuchs has served as a faculty member. Richard A. McCormick, S.J.,
"Reproductive Technologies," Lecture-Ob/Gyn Grand Rounds, May 17,
1995, Loyola University Medical Center, Maywood, Illinois.

[14]McCormick, *Corrective Vision*, 43.

[15]McCormick, *The Critical Calling*, 339-340.

[16]"In matters of faith and morals, the bishops speak in the name of
Christ and the faithful are to accept their teaching and adhere to it with a
religious assent of the soul. This religious submission of will and of mind
must be shown in a special way to the authentic teaching authority of the
Roman Pontiff, even when he is not speaking *ex cathedra*." "Dogmatic
Constitution on the Church," *The Documents of Vatican II*, ed. Walter M.
Abbott, S.J., (Piscataway, NJ: New Century Publishers, 1966), no. 25,
48. McCormick writes: "The problem prior to *Humanae Vitae* was
whether the positive doubts surrounding traditional teaching had en-
countered a true teaching statement....The problem after *Humanae Vitae*
is the extent to which this document, obviously a teaching statement, has
truly resolved the doubts." McCormick objected to the encyclical's main
thesis that it is intrinsically evil to engage in artificial contraception. For
a more detailed analysis of McCormick's position on *Humanae Vitae*,
see McCormick *Notes on Moral Theology: 1965 through 1980*, (Washington, DC: University Press of America, 1981), 215-231.

[17] "Pastoral Constitution on the Church in the Modern World," *The
Documents of Vatican II*, no. 11, 209.

[18]McCormick, *The Critical Calling*, 120.

[19]For McCormick, "We know that at any given time our formulations—being the product of limited persons, with limited insight, and with imperfect philosophical and linguistic tools—are only more or less adequate to the substance of our convictions. It is the task of theology constantly to question and challenge these formulations in an effort to reduce their inadequacy." Ibid., 17.

[20]As McCormick puts it, "The first is that, to be regarded as a Catholic theologian, one may not dissent from *any* authoritatively proposed teaching. The second is that 'authentic theological instruction' means presenting Church teaching, and never disagreeing with it, even with respect and reverence. Third, and correlatively, sound theological education means accepting, uncritically if necessary, official Catholic teaching." Ibid., 119. Emphasis in the original.

[21]The term "restorationist" means the radical Catholic right. The goal of these "restorationists" is to restore the pyramidal structure of the Church and, as a result, the heavily obediential character given to the teaching-learning process of the Church.

[22]McCormick, *The Critical Calling*, 126.

[23]Curran also believes this to be true. Curran writes: "In his attempt, as a moral theologian in the Catholic Church, to make this tradition a living reality, our author has been more reactive than proactive. He has responded to the work of others in the 'Notes' and thereby has pushed forward his own understanding and agenda. This is one very important way of dealing with a tradition and keeping it alive. Others will adopt more innovative and even more radical approaches in their dealing with the tradition and trying to move it forward. The genre of the 'Notes' makes its most expert practitioner an incrementalist and reformer by definition." Curran, "Introduction: Why This Book?" in *Moral Theology: Challenges for the Future*, 9.

[24]McCormick, *Corrective Vision*, 15.

[25]This can be seen in McCormick's response to *Veritatis Splendor*. See McCormick, "*Veritatis Splendor* and Moral Theology," *America* 169 (October 30, 1993): 8-11; and Idem, "Some Early Reactions to *Veritatis Splendor*," *Theological Studies* 55 (September 1994): 481-506.

[26]McCormick refers to some of the best known names in moral theology as proportionalists: Josef Fuchs, S.J., Bruno Schüller, S.J., Franz Bockle, Louis Janssens, Bernard Häring, Franz Scholz, Franz Furger, Walter Kerber, S.J., Charles Curran, Lisa Cahill, Philip Keane, Joseph Selling, Edward Vacek, S.J., David Hollenbach, S.J., Maurice de Wachter, Margaret Farley, James Walter, Rudolf Ginters, Helmut Weber, Klaus Demmer, Garth Hallett, S.J. The leading published opponents of this methodological move are Germain Grisez, John Finnis, Joseph

Boyle, William May, and the late John R. Connery, S.J. Common to all so-called proportionalists is the insistence that causing certain disvalues (ontic, nonmoral, physical, premoral evils) in our conduct does not *ipso facto* make the action morally wrong as certain traditional formulations supposed. The action becomes morally wrong when, all things considered, there is no proportionate reason. McCormick, *Corrective Vision*, 8-9.

[27]Richard A. McCormick, S.J., "The New Medicine and Morality," *Theology Digest* 21 (1973): 308.

[28]Richard A. McCormick, S.J., *Health and Medicine in the Catholic Tradition: Tradition in Transition* (New York: Crossroad, 1987), 160.

[29]Richard A. McCormick, S.J., "'*Gaudium et Spes*' and the Bioethical Signs of the Times," in "*Questions of Special Urgency*": *The Church in the Modern World Two Decades After Vatican II*, ed. Judith A. Dwyer (Washington, DC: Georgetown University Press, 1986), 94.

[30]McCormick, *How Brave a New World?: Dilemmas in Bioethics* (Washington, DC: Georgetown University Press, 1981), 84.

[31]Richard A. McCormick, S.J., "A Proposal for 'Quality of Life' Criteria for Sustaining Life," *Hospital Progress* 56 (September 1975): 76.

[32]For a more detailed analysis of the Johns Hopkins Case, see James M. Gustafson, "Mongolism, Parental Desires and the Right To Life," *Perspectives in Biology and Medicine* XVI (1973): 529-559.

[33]Of these, forty-three (14%) were associated with discontinuance of treatment for children with multiple serious anomalies, trisomy, cardiopulmonary crippling, meningomyelocele and other central nervous system defects. After careful consideration of each of these forty-three infants, parents, and physicians in a group decision concluded that the prognosis for "meaningful life" was extremely poor or hopeless, and therefore rejected further treatment. Duff and Campbell state: "The awful finality of these decisions, combined with a potential for error in prognosis, made the choice agonizing for families and health professionals. Nevertheless, the issue has to be faced, for not to decide is an arbitrary and potentially devastating decision of default." Richard A. McCormick, S.J., "To Save or Let Die," *How Brave a New World? Dilemmas in Bioethics*, 340. See also Raymond S. Duff, M. D. & A. G. M. Campbell, M. D., "Moral and Ethical Dilemmas in The Special-Care Nursery," *The New England Journal of Medicine* 289 (October 25, 1973): 889-894.

[34]Richard A. McCormick, S.J., "Best Interests of the Baby," *Second Opinion* 2 (1986): 18.

[35]Edwin R. DuBose, Ronald P. Hamel and Laurence J. O'Connell, "Introduction" in *A Matter of Principles?: Ferment in U. S. Bioethics*,

eds. Edwin R. DuBose, Ronald P. Hamel and Laurence J. O'Connell (Valley Forge, PA: Trinity Press International, 1994), 1.

[36]Ibid., 9.

[37]There are a number of terms to describe this specific field of study—bioethics, medical ethics, biomedical ethics, health care ethics, etc. This book will use the term "bioethics" because in light of its origin, this term incorporates the global sense of bioethics as an ethics of the life sciences and health care. Warren T. Reich argues that this means "bioethics goes beyond ethical issues in medicine to include ethical issues in public health, population concerns, genetics, environmental health, reproductive practices and technologies, animal health and welfare, and the like. This broader scope, with which both Van Rensselaer Potter and Andre Hellegers (originators of the term) agreed, was the original intent of the Hastings Center, which from the start was interested in 'ethics and the life sciences.' Since 1972 the *Encyclopedia of Bioethics* advocated an approach to bioethics that is global in both scope and range of ethical sources. Noting that the word 'bioethics' is a composite derived from two Greek words—*bios* (life; hence life sciences) and *ethike* (ethics), it established a broad scope for the field in the following definition, which became standard in many parts of the world: 'the systematic study of human conduct in the area of the life sciences and health care, insofar as this conduct is examined in the light of moral values and principles.'" Warren Thomas Reich, "The Word 'Bioethics': The Struggle Over Its Earliest Meaning," *Kennedy Institute of Ethics Journal* 5 (March 1995): 29. See also Warren Thomas Reich, "The Word 'Bioethics': Its Birth and the Legacies of Those Who Shaped Its Meaning," *Kennedy Institute of Ethics Journal* 4 (December 1994): 319-335.

[38]Trutz Rendtorff, *Ethics: Basic Elements and Methodology in an Ethical Theology* (Philadelphia: Fortress Press, 1986), 86.

[39]Ibid.

[40]For a more detailed analysis of the Seattle Artificial Kidney Selection Committee, see Gergory E. Pence, *Classic Cases in Medical Ethics* 3rd Ed., (New York: McGraw-Hill, 2000), 323-326.

[41]Albert R. Jonsen, forward to *A Matter of Principles?*, ix..

[42]Ibid.

[43]It should be noted that Hauerwas, MacIntyre and others would remind us that what goes by the name "human experience" is always reported via the lens of a particular culture. Thus, human experience is never raw, but theory-laden and assumption-laden. See Stanley Hauerwas, *Vision and Virtue* (Notre Dame, IN: Fides Publishers, 1974); Idem, *Character and the Christian Life: A Study in Theological Ethics* (San

Antonio, TX: Trinity University Press, 1975); and Alasdair MacIntyre, *After Virtue* (Notre Dame, IN: University of Notre Dame Press, 1984).

[44]DuBose, Hamel, and O'Connell, "Introduction" to *A Matter of Principles?*, 16.

[45]Ibid., xii.

[46]Ibid., xiv.

[47]Ibid., xv.

[48]Ibid., xvi.

[49]According to Jonsen, bioethics became principalist, then, for several reasons. He writes: "First, the first bioethicists found in the style of normative ethics current at that time, the style of theory and principle, a *via media* between the arid land of metaethics and the lush but generally inaccessible visions of theological ethics. Second, the *Belmont Report* was a foundational document that met the need of public-policy makers for a clear and simple statement of the ethical basis for regulation of research. Third, the new audience of doctors and medical students had to be led through dilemmas and paradoxes by ideas and language that clarified rather than complexified the issues." Ibid.

[50]Thomas L. Beauchamp and James F. Childress, *Principles of Biomedical Ethics*, 3rd ed. (New York: Oxford University Press, 1989), 16.

[51]At best, these critics charge, principles serve as a checklist of considerations worth taking into account when addressing an issue. At worst, they "obscure and confuse moral reasoning by their failure to be guidelines and by their eclectic and unsystematic use of moral theory . . ." Other critics are troubled by the paramount status principlism accords to the "value complex of individualism," with its emphasis on autonomy, self-determination, and individual rights. See DuBose, Hamel and O'Connell, "Introduction," in *A Matter of Principles?*, 2.

[52]For a more complete analysis of the phenomenological method, see Richard M. Zaner, "Experience and Moral Life: A Phenomenological Approach to Bioethics," in *A Matter of Principles?: Ferment in U.S. Bioethics*, 211-239. See also Idem, *The Context of Self: A Phenomenological Inquiry Using Medicine as a Clue* (Athens, Ohio: Ohio University Press, 1981); Idem, *Ethics and the Clinical Encounter* (Englewood Cliffs, NJ: Prentice Hall, 1988); and Mary Rawlinson, "Medicine's Discourse and the Practice of Medicine," in *The Humanity of the Ill: Phenomenological Perspectives*, ed. V. Kestenbaum (Knoxville, TN: University of Tennessee Press, 1982), 69-85.

[53]DuBose, Hamel, and O'Connell, "Introduction," in *A Matter of Principles?*, 10.

[54] For a more complete analysis of the hermeneutical method, see Drew Leder, "Toward a Hermeneutical Bioethics," in *A Matter of Prin-*

ciples?: Ferment in U.S. Bioethics, 240-259. See also David C. Thomasma, "Clinical Ethics As Medical Hermeneutics," *Theoretical Medicine* 15 (June 1994): 93-112; Stephen L. Daniel, "Hermeneutical Clinical Ethics: A Commentary," *Theoretical Medicine* 15 (June 1994): 133-140; and M. Wayne Cooper, "Is Medicine Hermeneutics All the Way Down?" *Theoretical Medicine* 15 (June 1994): 149-180.

[55]DuBose, Hamel, and O'Connell, "Introduction" in *A Matter of Principles?*, 11.

[56]Quandary ethics focuses on moral dilemmas and problems, which then have to be resolved. One common criticism of principlism is that it fosters a conception of bioethics as quandary ethics. For a more detailed analysis of quandary ethics, see Ibid., 92-93.

[57]For a more complete analysis of the narrative method, see Rita Charon, "Narrative Contributions to Medical Ethics," in *A Matter of Principles?: Ferment in U.S. Bioethics*, 260-283. See also Kathryn M. Hunter, "Narrative," in *Encyclopedia of Bioethics* , rev. ed., vol 4, ed. Warren T. Reich (New York: Simon & Schuster & Macmillan, 1995), 1789-1793; Barbara Smith, "Narrative Versions, Narrative Theories," in *On Narrative*, ed. W. J. T. Mitchell (Chicago, IL: University of Chicago Press, 1983), 99-117; and Patricia Benner, "The Role of Experience, Narrative, and Community in Skilled Ethical Comportment," *Advances in Nursing Science* 14 (1991): 1-21.

[58]A personalist ethic in response to another person is an ethic of responsibility, or a relational ethic that seems obviously appropriate to medicine, where everything starts and finishes with a doctor-patient relationship and where most of the doctor-patient contacts have nothing to do with quandaries or dilemmas or conflict of rights. For a more detailed analysis, see James F. Drane, "Character and the Moral Life: A Virtue Approach to Biomedical Ethics," in *A Matter of Principles?: Ferment in U.S. Bioethics*, 286. See also, James F. Keenan, "Virtue Ethics," in *Christian Ethics*, ed. Bernard Hoose (Collegeville, MN: Liturgical Press, 1998), 84-94; and Douglas Birsch, "Virtue Ethics," in *Ethical Insights* (Mountain View, CA: Mayfield Publishing, 1999): 81-93.

[59]See Robert Veatch, "Against Virtue: A Deontological Critique of Virtue Theory and Medical Ethics," in *Virtue and Medicine: Explorations in the Character of Medicine*, ed. Earl E. Shelp (Dordrecht, Netherlands: D. Reidel, 1985), 175-200.

[60]For a more complete analysis of the virtue-based method, see James F. Drane, *Becoming a Good Doctor: The Place of Virtue and Character in Medical Ethics* (Kansas City, MO: Sheed & Ward, 1988); Idem, *Religion and Ethics* (New York: Paulist Press, 1976); Stanley Hauerwas, "Virtue and Character," in *Encyclopedia of Bioethics*, rev.

ed., vol. 5, 2525-2531; and Idem, *Vision and Virtue* (Notre Dame, IN: Fides Press, 1974).

[61]Albert R. Jonsen, "Casuistry," in *Encyclopedia of Bioethics*, rev. ed., vol. 1, 344-350.

[62]For a more complete analysis of the medical casuistry method, see Stephen Toulmin, "Casuistry and Clinical Ethics," in *A Matter of Principles?: Ferment in U.S. Bioethics*, 310-318; See also Albert R. Jonsen, "Casuistry," in *Encyclopedia of Bioethics*, rev. ed., vol. 1, 344-350; and Albert R. Jonsen and Stephen Toulmin, *The Abuse of Casuistry* (Berkeley, CA: University of California Press, 1988).

[63]Lisa Sowle Cahill, "Teleology, Utilitarianism, and Christian Ethics," 601.

[64]Aquinas maintains that for something to be called law, it must be (1) reasonable, in the sense of directing action; (2) ordained to the common good; (3) legislated by the proper authority; and (4) duly promulgated (*Summa Theologica* Ia-IIae, 90). The eternal law, whereby the world is ruled by divine providence, satisfies these criteria in an exemplary way (*Summa Theologica* Ia-IIae, 91, 1). Natural law, however, is principally that part of divine reason accessible to the human intelligence. It is not to be confused with the order of the physical or biological world. Law is predicated only by a kind of similitude with the order found in nonrational entities (*Summa Theologica* Ia-IIae, 91, 2, 3). Russell Hittinger, "Natural Law," in *Encyclopedia of Bioethics*, rev. ed., vol. 4, 1806; see also Richard Gula, *Reason Informed by Faith: Foundations of Catholic Morality* (New York: Paulist Press, 1989), 220-249.

[65]F. C. Copleston, *Aquinas* (New York: Penguin Books, 1955), 221.

[66]Thomas Aquinas, *Summa Theologica* Ia-IIae, 94, 2 (Westminster, MD: Christian Classics, 1948), 1,009.

[67]The first precepts of the natural law are: self-preservation (common to all substances), procreation and care of offspring (common with other animals), knowing the truth about God, and living in society (common to rational creatures alone). For a more detailed analysis of the first precepts, see Ibid.,1009-1010.

[68]For a more detailed analysis, see Aquinas, *Summa Theologica* Ia-IIae, 94, 4, 1,010-1,011.

[69]Charles E. Curran, "Natural Law In Moral Theology," in *Readings in Moral Theology No. 7: Natural Law and Theology*, eds. Charles E. Curran and Richard A. McCormick, S.J. (New York: Paulist Press, 1991), 253-254. Emphasis in the original.

[70]For a more complete analysis of these four basic Catholic principles, see Philip S. Keane, S.S., "The Objective Moral Order: Reflections On Recent Research," *Theological Studies* 43 (1982): 260-262.

[71]Ibid., 265.

[72]Curran argues that in the last few years Catholic thinkers have been developing and employing different philosophical approaches to understanding morality. One could suggest that such approaches are modifications of natural law theory because they retain the two important values mentioned above. Others prefer to abandon the term natural law entirely since the concept is very ambiguous. There is no monolithic philosophical system called natural law, and the term has been somewhat discredited because of the tendency among some to understand "natural" in terms of the physical structure of human acts. Curran sees three alternative approaches which have been advanced in recent years—personalism, a relational and communitarian approach, and a transcendental methodology. See Charles E. Curran, *Contemporary Problems in Moral Theology* (Notre Dame, IN: Fides Publishers, Inc., 1970), 138-139.

[73]Hittinger, "Natural Law," 1811.

[74]Louis Janssens, "Artificial Insemination: Ethical Considerations," *Louvain Studies* 8 (Spring 1980): 13.

[75]For a more detailed analysis of McCormick's criticism of these ethical methodologies, especially principlism, see McCormick, "Beyond Principlism is Not Enough: A Theologian Reflects on the Real Challenge For U.S. Biomedical Ethics," in *A Matter of Principles?: Ferment in U.S. Bioethics*, 344-361.

[76]For McCormick, the classicist mentality "conceives culture normatively and represents a certain disengagement from the forces shaping the contemporary world. It seeks and easily finds certainties and views departure from them as unfaithfulness, pluralism as bordering on anarchy." McCormick, *Corrective Vision*, 40. McCormick understands historical consciousness as "taking our culture seriously as soil for the 'signs of the times,' as framer of our self-awareness. This means taking a fresh look at how Christian perspectives ought to be read in the modern world so that our practices are the best possible mediation of gospel values in the contemporary world. Fresh look often leads to new emphases and modifications of more ancient formulations—formulations and emphases appropriate to one point in history but not necessarily to all." McCormick, *The Critical Calling*, 9.

[77]Lisa Sowle Cahill, "On Richard McCormick: Reason and Faith In Post-Vatican II Catholic Ethics," in *Theological Voices in Medical Ethics*, eds. Allen Verhey and Stephen E. Lammers (Grand Rapids, Michigan: William B. Eerdmans Publishing Company, 1993), 81-82.

[78]Ibid., 84. Emphasis in the original.

[79]McCormick, *The Critical Calling*, 204.

[80]The traditionalist segment of the Catholic Church believes that the reasonableness of extant specific norms is not to be challenged nor the norms substantially revised. Loyalty in faith to Jesus and his Church is measured by fidelity to the Catholic Church's authoritative moral interpretations. McCormick insists that the magisterium is not exempt from the ordinary process of inquiry in ethics. See Lisa Sowle Cahill, "On Richard McCormick," 84.

[81]Ibid.

[82]Ibid., 87.

[83]McCormick, *Health and Medicine in the Catholic Tradition*, 50.

[84]Ibid., 59.

[85]McCormick, "Public Policy on Abortion," *How Brave a New World?*, 201.

[86]For a more extensive historical review of neonatology as a specialization, see Gordon B. Avery, "Neonatology: Perspectives in the Mid-1990s," in *Neonatology: Pathophysiology and Management of the Newborn*, 4 th ed., eds. Gordon B. Avery, Mary Ann Fletcher & Mhairi G. Macdonald (Philadelphia: J.B. Lippincott Company, 1994), 3-7.

[87]Clement A. Smith, "Neonatal Medicine and Quality of Life: An Historical Perspective," in *Ethics of Newborn Intensive Care*, eds. Albert R. Jonsen & Michael Garland (Berkeley, CA: University of California Press, 1976), 32.

[88]Alan R. Fleischman, "Ethical Issues In Neonatology: A U.S. Perspective," *Annals New York Academy of Sciences* 530 (June 1988): 83.

[89]It should be noted that between 1985 and 1988, neonatal mortality declined more than five times as fast as post-neonatal mortality. In 1989 and 1990 provisional rates of 6.25 deaths per 1000 live births and 5.74 deaths per 1000 live births are thought to be a reflection on the marked improvement in death related to perinatal conditions that declined by 8.5% in 1989 and an additional 6.3% in 1990. Again minority neonatal mortality rates are considerably higher than Caucasian. From 1998 to 2000, the infant mortality rate in Caucasians was 3.9 per 1000 live births. For African Americans it was 9.5 per 1000 live births. For a more detailed analysis of neonatal medicine in the United States, see Reuters Medical News, "Rate of Prenatal Care in US Has Increased Over Last Decade," *Medscape Inc.*, February 21, 2001; Mike Mitka, "Neonatal Intensive Care: Costs vs Results," *Journal of the American Medical Association* 287 (June 26, 2002): 3200; Centers for Disease Control and Prevention, "National Linked Birth/Infant Death Data Set," (National Center for Health Statistics, 2002); Fleischman, 84; Emergency Cardiac Care Committee and Subcommittees, American Heart Association, "Neonatal Resuscitation," *Journal of the American Medical Association* 268 (Octo-

ber 28, 1992): 2276-2281; John D. Lantos & Kathryn L. Moseley, "Medical Aspects and Issues in the Care of Infants," in *Encyclopedia of Bioethics*, rev. ed., vol. 3, ed. Warren T. Reich (New York: Simon & Schuster & Macmillan, 1995), 1195; U.S. Congress, Office of Technology Assessment, "Neonatal Intensive Care for Low Birthweight Infants: Costs and Effectiveness," Office of Technology Assessment, Washington, DC, December, 1987; Richard L. Bucciarelli, "Neonatology in the United States: Scope and Organization," in *Neonatology: Pathophysiology and Management of the Newborn*, 12-31; Robert Wood Foundation, "Challenges in Health Care: Perspective 1991" (Princeton, NJ: RWJ Foundation, 1991); and J. Lemons, C. Bauer, W. Oh et al., "Very Low Birth Weight Outcomes of the National Institute of Child Health and Human Development Neonatal Research Network, January 1995 through December 1996," *Pediatrics* 107 (January 2001):e1.

[90]Richard A. McCormick, S.J., "The New Medicine and Morality," *Theology Digest* 21 (1973): 308.

[91]Fleischman, 85. The international perspective among pediatricians is both similar and different. In Sweden they use the "statistical prognostic" strategy. This approach seeks to minimize the number of infants whose deaths would come slowly as well as those whose lives would be characterized by profound disabilities. This approach uses statistical data, like birth weight, gestational age, and early diagnostic tests, to make selective nontreatment decisions. Pediatricians in Britain and Australia use the "individualized prognostic" strategy. They are willing to engage in time-limited trials to give various treatments a chance to work, even when the child being treated is likely to have ongoing disabilities. This strategy reflects an ethical perspective that realizes the inherent uncertainty in medicine, permits some role for parental discretion, and affirms the appropriateness of selective nontreatment decisions once the child's progress appears poor. In much of the world the differences in medical management that have just been described have no significance. The shortages of medicine, the obsolescence of medical equipment, the inadequacies of prenatal care, the limited number of pediatricians, and the ongoing problems of malnutrition and infectious disease contribute to the social context in which the lives of infants are frequently short and often characterized by disease and disability. For a more detailed analysis, see Robert F. Weir, "Ethical Issues," in *Encyclopedia of Bioethics*, rev. ed., vol. 3, 1209-1210.

[92]Gordon B. Avery, "The Morality of Drastic Intervention," in *Neonatology: Pathophysiology and Management of the Newborn*, 8.

[93]Many physicians are often uncertain regarding the legality of abating life-sustaining treatment for nonautonomous patients. Because most

physicians do not usually read the literature in bioethical ethics and health law, they are frequently unaware of the consensus that has developed in recent years regarding the ethics and legality of making decisions to withdraw or withhold treatment on the behalf of nonautonomous patients. In addition, physicians are often given very conservative legal advice by the attorney(s) working for their hospitals. Because the professional responsibility of hospital attorneys is to protect the hospital's legal and financial interests, they are frequently inclined to give advice on cases that is unduly conservative in terms of the patients' or physicians' interests. Especially in cases that involve decisions to abate life-sustaining treatment with nonautonomous patients, the legal advice to physicians is often to continue the medical status quo for an indefinite period of time to minimize even the possibility of the patients' surrogates becoming upset and initiating legal action against the physician and hospital. The combination of these factors results in considerable uncertainty on the part of many physicians regarding the ethical standards for decisions to abate life-sustaining treatment for nonautonomous patients and the legal liability involved in such decisions. In particular, physicians are often troubled by the prospect of civil or even criminal liability for failure to provide the full panoply of life-sustaining treatments. The 1983 California case of *Barber v. Superior Court* (an appellate court decision to drop murder charges against two physicians) still rings an alarm for physicians, at least in part because it was incorrectly portrayed in the media. Yet all states to have considered the question of liability have adopted the view of the *Barber* court that a physician who acts "in good faith" and within established professional standards of care cannot incur civil or criminal liability. See Robert F. Weir & Larry Gostin, M.D., "Decisions to Abate Life-Sustaining Treatment from Nonautonomous Patients," *Journal of the American Medical Association* 264 (October 10, 1990): 1846.

[94] There is some confusion about the date of this case. Some state it occurred in 1963 but others set the date in 1971. The confusion may be caused by the fact that a film about this case was widely circulated in 1972. Richard Sparks states: "In late 1963, at the Johns Hopkins Medical Center in Baltimore, an infant boy was born who lived for only fifteen days. The circumstances surrounding his brief life and the fact that he was the subject of a widely circulated 1972 film *Who Shall Survive?* have made the 'Johns Hopkins Baby' one of a handful of well-known, ethically troubling cases regarding decisions not to treat handicapped or so-called 'defective' newborns." See Richard Sparks, *To Treat or Not to Treat?: Bioethics and the Handicapped Newborn* (New York: Paulist Press, 1988), 2. For a detailed description of the Johns Hopkins case, see

Robert Weir, *Selective Nontreatment of Handicapped Newborns* (New York: Oxford University Press, 1984), 50-51.

[95]R.S. Duff & A.G.M. Campbell, "Moral and Ethical Dilemmas in the Special Care Nursery," 889-894; J. Lorber, "Results of Treatment of Myelomeningocele," *Developmental Medical Child Neurology* 13 (1971): 279-303; and A. Shaw, G. Randolph, & B. Manard, "Ethical Issues in Pediatric Surgery: A Nationwide Survey of Pediatricians and Pediatric Surgeons," *Pediatric* 59 (1977): 588-599.

[96] "Baby Doe was afflicted with Down syndrome, a chromosomal abnormality resulting in mental retardation and a propensity for cardiac and other congenital malformations. The infant had such a congenital defect, a tracheo-esophageal fistula (an abnormal passage connecting the trachea and esophagus), which if not surgically corrected results in death. The parents, after consultation and with the concurrence of their attending physician, refused to consent to surgery, primarily on the grounds that a child with Down syndrome could not attain a 'minimally acceptable quality of life.' That conclusion was, and continues to be, strongly disputed. A trial court, (Indiana Supreme Court) however, ruled that the parents had the right to refuse surgery for their child (In *re Infant Doe*, 1982)." Anne M. Dellinger and Patricia C. Kuszler, "Public-Policy and Legal Issues," in *Encyclopedia of Bioethics*, rev. ed., vol. 3, 1215.

[97]Weir, "Ethical Issues," 1208. For a more complete analysis, see Department of Health and Human Services, "Nondiscrimination on the Basis of Handicap," *Federal_Register* 48 (1983), 9630-9632; Department of Health and Human Services, "Nondiscrimination on the Basis of Handicap Relating to Health Care of Infants: Proposed Rules," *Federal Register* 48 (1983), 30846-30852; and Fleischman, "Ethical Issues in Neonatology," 86.

[98]Section 504 is the basic civil rights statute for handicapped individuals. Section 504 states: "No otherwise qualified handicapped individual . . . shall, solely by reason of his handicap, be excluded from the participation in, be denied the benefits of, or be subject to discrimination under any program or activity receiving federal financial assistance . . ." Weir, *Selective Nontreatment of Handicapped Newborns*, 127.

[99]Fleischman, "Ethical Issues in Neonatology," 86.

[100]On March 18, 1983, the American Academy of Pediatrics announced its lawsuit against the Department of Health and Human Services, and on April 14, 1983, Judge Gerhard A. Gesell in *American Academy of Pediatrics v. Heckler* invalidated the rule on procedural grounds. See Kenneth Kipnis & Gailynn M. Williamson, "Nontreatment Decisions for Severely Compromised Newborns," *Ethics* 95 (October 1984): 93.

[101]Fleischman, "Ethical Issues in Neonatology," 86.

[102]Ibid.

[103]In the volume entitled *Deciding to Forego Life-Sustaining Treatment*, the U.S. President's Commission recommended: "When the benefits of therapy are unclear an ethics committee or similar body might be designated to review the decision making process . . . cases included in this category should certainly encompass those in which a decision to forego life-sustaining therapy has been proposed because of a physical or mental handicap." President's Commission for the Study of Ethical Problems in Medicine and Biomedical and Behavioral Research, *Deciding to Forego Life-Sustaining Treatment*, U.S. Government Printing Office, Washington, DC (1983), 227.

[104]The bioethics Committee of the American Academy of Pediatrics developed a set of guidelines for the establishment and operation of Infant Bioethics Review Committees. These committees would facilitate review of any cases where there was the consideration of foregoing life-sustaining treatment. The hope was that conflict situations could be resolved within these committees. See American Academy of Pediatrics, "Joint Policy Statement: Principles of Treatment of Disabled Infants," *Pediatrics* 73 (1984): 559-560; and American Academy of Pediatrics "Guidelines For Infant Bioethics Review Committees," *Pediatrics* 74 (1984): 306-310.

[105]Given the complexity of some pediatric cases and the life-and-death nature of selective nontreatment decisions, the common recommendation was to have an ethics committee consult on the case and give advice to the physicians in the case. The ethical perspective at the heart of this recommendation was straightforward: in truly difficult cases, the most prudent procedure for decision-making is the achievement of consensus by a multidisciplinary committee that is knowledgeable, emotionally stable, and consistent from case to case. For a more detailed analysis, see Weir, "Ethical Issues," in *Encyclopedia of Bioethics*, rev. ed., vol. 3, 1208.

[106]A new definition of withholding of medically indicated treatment is added to Section 3 of the Act to mean the failure to respond to an infant's life-threatening conditions by providing treatment (including appropriate nutrition, hydration and medication) which in the treating physician's reasonable medical judgment will be most likely to be effective in ameliorating or correcting all such conditions. Exceptions to the requirement to provide treatment may be made only in cases which: (1) the infant is irreversibly comatose; or (2) the provision of such treatment would merely prolong dying or not be effective in ameliorating or correcting all of the infant's life-threatening conditions or otherwise be futile in terms of the survival of the infant; or (3) the provision of such

treatment would be virtually futile in terms of the survival of the infant and the treatment itself under such circumstances would be inhumane. For a more detailed analysis of the Federal Child Abuse Law, see Fleischman, "Ethical Issues in Neonatology," 87; Department of Health and Human Services, "Child Abuse and Neglect: Prevention and Treatment," reprinted from *The Federal Register* 50 (April 15, 1985), No. 72: Rules and Regulations, part 1340, 14887-14892.

[107]Concerns were raised about the Infant Care Review Committees. First, many fear that parental authority for decision-making for infants will be circumvented and supplanted by such committee structure. Second, there is a fear that the ethics committees will be too narrowly focused on the law and that ethical analysis will be less part of the committee's deliberations than concern for the law and institutional liability. See Fleischman, "Ethical Issues in Neonatology," 87.

[108]For a more detailed analysis of the "Baby K case," see Mark A. Bonano, "The Case of Baby K," *Trends in Health Care, Law, and Ethics* 9 (Winter 1994): 1-48. It should be noted that federal regulations require hospitals to treat all patients needing care who arrive at an emergency room. The particular interest with this case is that the A.D.A. was cited in this case. Baby K had been on a respirator since birth. When the case was heard, her physicians wanted to disconnect it and let her die; but her mother insisted on continued care, for religious reasons. At its heart, Baby K's case was about whether or not physicians may, without incurring charges of discrimination against the handicapped, overrule parents' decisions about continuing treatment which seems to be medically futile and pointlessly expensive. See Lawrence Schneiderman and Sharyn Manning, "The Baby K Case: A Search for the Elusive Standard of Medical Care," *Cambridge Quarterly of Healthcare Ethics* 6 (1997): 9-18 and Gregory Pence, ed. *Classic Cases In Medical Ethics*, 3rd ed. (New York: McGraw-Hill, 2000), 219-220.

[109]See Weir, "Ethical Issues," in *Encyclopedia of Bioethics*, rev. ed., vol. 3, 1208.

[110]For an extensive survey of the legal and medical perspectives regarding treatment decisions for handicapped neonates, see Weir, *Selective Nontreatment of Handicapped Newborns*, 59-142.

[111]Aaron L. Mackler, "Neonatal Intensive Care," *Scope Notes* 11 (Washington, DC: Kennedy Institute of Ethics, 1993): 1-2.

[112]Richard A. McCormick, S.J., *Notes on Moral Theology 1981 through 1984* (Lanham, MD: University Press of America, 1984), 35.

[113]Paul Ramsey, *Ethics at the Edges of Life: Medical and Legal Intersections* (New Haven: Yale University Press, 1978); Idem, *The Pa-*

tient as Person: Explorations in Medical Ethics (New Haven: Yale University Press, 1970).

[114]Leonard J. Weber, *Who Shall Live?: The Dilemma of Severely Handicapped Children and its Meaning for Other Moral Questions* (New York: Paulist Press, 1976), 82-83.

[115]Reich and Weber affirm that there is a binding obligation to accept all "ordinary" means to sustain or prolong life, while there is no strict obligation to use "extraordinary" means. Extraordinary is any means that (1) does not hold out a reasonable hope of medical benefit or which (2) also has the effect of causing or perpetuating an excessive hardship for the patient (and for one's principal caretakers). Connery rejects the movement by Gerald Kelly, S.J., to incorporate medical benefit into the very definition of what constitutes a means as "ordinary" or "extraordinary." According to Connery, benefit and burden "deal with different issues" and ought to remain distinct. Connery has merely reinstated the older language of obligatory/optional for that of ordinary/extraordinary, relegating the latter to one half of the equation, namely "burden" viewed from the patient's perspective. Richard Sparks argues that Connery's preference for the older language is ultimately more a matter of semantics than of actual differences in content. See Richard Sparks, *To Treat or Not to Treat?*, 102-103. See also Leonard J. Weber, *Who Shall Live?*, 82-87; Warren T. Reich, "On the Birth of a Severely Handicapped Infant," *The Hastings Center Report* 3 (September 1973): 10-11; Warren T. Reich & David E. Ost, "Infants: Ethical Perspectives on the Care of Infants," *Encyclopedia of Bioethics*, vol. 2, ed. Warren T. Reich (New York: The Free Press, 1978), 727-729; and John R. Connery, S.J., "Prolongation of Life: The Duty and Its Limits," *Linacre Quarterly* 47 (May 1980): 151-165.

[116]Michael Tooley, "Abortion and Infanticide," *Philosophy and Public Affairs* 2 (Fall 1972): 3, Idem, "A Defense of Abortion and Infanticide," in *The Problem of Abortion*, ed. Joel Feinberg (Belmont, CA: Wadsworth Publishing Company, 1973), 51-91; Idem, "Decisions to Terminate Life and the Concept of Person," in *Ethical Issues Relating To Life and Death*, ed. John Ladd (New York: Oxford University Press, 1979), 62-93; Peter Singer, *Practical Ethics* (New York: Cambridge University Press, 1979); Idem, "Unsanctifying Human Life," in *Ethical Issues Relating to Life and Death*, ed. John Ladd (New York: Oxford University Press, 1979), 41-61; Idem, "Life: The Value of Life," *Encyclopedia of Bioethics* ed. Warren T. Reich, 822-829; and Sparks. *To Treat or Not to Treat?*, 236-242.

[117]For Warren, there are five traits necessary for personhood: consciousness, reasoning ability, self-motivated activity, the capacity to

communicate, and the presence of self-awareness. See Weir, *Selective Nontreatment of Handicapped Newborns*, 156.

[118]Mary Anne Warren, "On the Moral and Legal Status of Abortion," *The Monist* 57 (January 1973): 43-61; and Idem, "Do Potential People Have Moral Rights?" *Canadian Journal of Philosophy* 7 (June 1977): 275.

[119]H. Tristram Engelhardt, Jr., "Ethical Issues in Aiding the Death of Young Children," *Beneficent Euthanasia*, ed. Marvin Kohl (Buffalo, NY: Prometheus Books, 1975); Idem, "Bioethics and the Process of Embodiment," *Perspectives in Biology and Medicine* 18 (Summer 1975): 486-500; Idem, "Euthanasia and Children: The Inquiry of Continued Existence," *Journal of Pediatrics* 83 (July 1973): 170-171; Idem, "Medicine and the Concept of Person," *Ethical Issues in Death and Dying*, eds. Tom Beauchamp & Seymour Perlin (Englewood Cliffs, NJ: Prentice-Hall, 1978); Sparks, *To Treat or Not To Treat?*, 242-250; and Weir, *Selective Nontreatment of Handicapped Newborns*, 174.

[120]David H. Smith, "On Letting Some Babies Die," *Hastings Center Studies* 2 (May 1974): 37-46; Idem, "Death, Ethics and Social Control," in *Medical Wisdom and Ethics in the Treatment of Severely Defective Newborns and Young Children*, ed. David J. Roy (Montreal: Eden Press, 1978), 74; Idem, "Our Religious Traditions and the Treatment of Infants," in *Which Babies Shall Live? Humanistic Dimensions of the Care of Imperiled Newborns*, eds. Thomas H. Murray & Arthur L. Caplan (Clifton, NJ: Humana Press, 1985), 59-70; Weir, *Selective Nontreatment of Handicapped Newborns*, 175-176; and Weber, *Who Shall Live?*, 61-63.

[121]Robert M. Veatch, "Shall We Let Handicapped Children Die?" *Newsday*, 8 August 1982, 1, 8-9.

[122]A reasonable person would find a refusal unreasonable (and thus treatment morally required) if the treatment is useful in treating a patient's condition (though not necessarily life-saving) and at the same time does not give rise to any significant patient-centered objections based on physical or mental burden; familial, social, or economic concern; or religious belief. See Robert Veatch, *Death, Dying and the Biological Revolution* (New Haven, CT: Yale University Press, 1976), 112; and Paul Ramsey, *Ethics at the Edges of Life*, 163-171.

[123]A. R. Jonsen *et al.*, "Critical Issues in Newborn Intensive Care: A Conference Report and Policy Proposal," *Pediatrics* 55 (1975): 756-768; and A. R. Jonsen & Michael J. Garland, *Ethics of Newborn Intensive Care*.

[124]Fletcher writes: "First, the extent to which the parents are counseled; second, the parents' attitude toward defects; third, the size or pro-

portion of the risk in terms of a projected distribution of chances; fourth, the severity of the risk; fifth, the economic resources of the family; sixth, the welfare of other children involved, as well as the parents' physical and emotional capacity to cope." Joseph Fletcher, "Moral Aspects of Decision-Making," in *Report of the Sixty-Fifth Ross Conference on Pediatric Research: Ethical Dilemmas in Current Obstetric and Newborn Care*, ed. Thomas D. Moore (Columbus, OH: Ross Laboratories, 1976), 70. See also Weir, *Selective Nontreatment of Handicapped Newborns*, 169.

[125]Joseph Fletcher, "Four Indicators of Humanhood—The Enquiry Matures," *Hastings Center Report* 4 (December 1974): 6-7; Idem, "Medicine and the Nature of Man," in *The Teaching of Medical Ethics*, eds. Robert M. Veatch, Willard Gaylin & Councilman Morgan (New York: Institute of Society, Ethics, and the Life Sciences, 1973), 52-57; Idem, "Ethics and Euthanasia," *American Journal of Nursing* 73 (April 1973): 670-675; Idem, "Infanticide and the Ethics of Loving Care," in *Infanticide and the Value of Life*, ed. Marvin Kohl (Buffalo, NY: Prometheus Books, 1978), 15-20; and Weir, *Selective Nontreatment of Handicapped Newborns*, 168-169.

[126]The qualities of "minimal independence" would include a capability to relate, communicate, ambulate, and perform tasks of basic hygiene, feeding, and dressing. Clearly there are technologies available today that can supplement or compensate for one's deficiencies in any of these areas. If competent medical opinion is that a particular newborn is physically and/or mentally impaired to the degree that these capabilities are not attainable even with technological assistance, then parents and society are not obliged to attempt the impossible. Either or both may elect to sustain this class of newborns, but there can be no moral obligation to do the impossible. This conclusion obviously rests on the belief that independence and these criteria for minimal independence are morally defensible ends upon which duties to attain them are grounded. For a more detailed analysis, see Earl E. Shelp, *Born To Die?: Deciding the Fate of Critically Ill Newborns* (New York: The Free Press, 1986), 48.

[127]Shelp writes: "In those instances today when the baby is born with a disease or defect such that it can be judged reasonably to foreclose (1) the attainment of capacities for minimal independence, (2) the attainment of capacities sufficient for personhood, (3) whose survival would impose a burden on the infant such as to render life a net disvalue, or (4) whose severely impaired survival would impose upon others an unreasonable, grave, disproportionate, or incommensurable burden, a decision that intends death for the newborn could be morally justified. When death for a newborn is a morally justifiable intention and outcome, it is as morally

licit to bring about this end by merciful means as it would be to stand aside while death occurs by so-called natural means." Ibid., 175.

[128]Parents are guided in their decision-making role about the reasonableness of treatments by the principles of autonomy, beneficence, and justice. Ibid., 70-76.

[129]Earl E. Shelp, *Born To Die?*; Idem, "Courage and Tragedy in Clinical Medicine," *Journal of Medicine and Philosophy* 8 (November 1983): 417-429; Idem, "To Benefit and Respect Persons: A Challenge for Beneficence in Health Care," in *Beneficence and Health Care*, ed. Earl E. Shelp (Dordrecht, Netherlands: D. Reidel Publishing Co., 1982), 200-217; and James J. Walter, "Termination of Medical Treatment: The Setting of Moral Limits from Infancy to Old Age," *Religious Studies Review* 16 (October 1990): 305-307.

[130]McCormick writes: "Quality-of-life assessments ought to be made within an overall reverence for life, as an extension of one's respect for the sanctity of life. However, there are times when preserving the life of one with no capacity for those aspects of life that we regard as *human* is a violation of the sanctity of life itself. Thus to separate the two approaches and call one *sanctity* of life, the other *quality* of life, is a false conceptual split . . ." Richard A. McCormick, S.J., "The Quality of Life, The Sanctity of Life," *How Brave a New World?*, 407. Emphasis in the original.

2

Theological Anthropology

In the most generic sense, anthropology may be considered as the human person's description and explanation of himself or herself. As an empirical science, anthropology is usually divided into cultural and physical: the study of human beings' social behavior, languages, world views, family life, and communal organizations as distinguished from the investigation into the evolution of human beings, the functional capacities of the human body, the development of races, etc.[1] Likewise, anthropological claims may also be considered as a subset of a full theological system.

Theological anthropology is "the critical reflection on the origin, purpose, and destiny of human life in the light of Christian belief."[2] It considers human persons precisely in terms of their relationship to God. As J. J. Mueller notes:

> Karl Rahner correctly reflected that whatever we say about God says something about us; and whatever we say about ourselves says something about God. God and humanity are correlative terms. If either God or humanity did not exist, theology would be meaningless. It is no wonder that theology begins in the human experience of God.[3]

Being in relation to God forms the basis for viewing the human person as centrally related to, totally dependent on, and responsible to God. The human person is dependent upon God for his or her origin, nature, condition, dignity, and destiny. To understand this relationship between God and the human person, theological anthropology draws upon a variety of disciplines. Robert Krieg writes:

> Theological anthropology employs a variety of methods (e.g., transcendental reflection, historical investigation, phenomenological inquiry) in its study of Scripture, the Jewish-Christian tradition, the findings of social sciences, contemporary life and thought (e.g., philosophy), and the Church's current experience (e.g., worship, communal life, and service).[4]

Theology's openness to, and dialogue with, the social sciences, history, and various forms of philosophy has had a significant bearing on theological anthropology.[5]

Influenced by these data, theology proceeds to reflect on the human person within the scope of revelation. The human person has been created by God, has been redeemed by God, and is destined for God. God is perceived as the metaphysical ground of the human person's receptivity through his or her finite resources oriented to the infinite. The acknowledgment of this tension and its implications for the person as both limited and transcendent is the foundation for the open-ended anthropology without which religion and revelation become totally extrinsic to the human. The final fulfillment of this tendency becomes explicit for the Christian in the mystery of the incarnate Word, the ultimate union of God and the human person who is the paradigm for all humankind. Christology becomes, therefore, the culmination of Christian theological anthropology.[6] For many contemporary theologians, theological anthropology, with its emphasis on the human person as a knowing subject, has become the core of theology's foundation.

For McCormick, theological anthropology concerns the human person in all his or her fullness as viewed within the context of the Christian mysteries. McCormick writes:

> The Christian tradition is, or better ought to be, an outlook on the human, a community of privileged access to the human. The Christian tradition is anchored in faith in the meaning and decisive significance of God's covenant with persons, especially as manifested in the saving incarnation of Jesus Christ and the revelation of His final coming, His eschatological kingdom, which is here aborning but will finally only be given. Faith in these events, love and loyalty to their central figure, yields a decisive way of viewing and intending the world, of interpreting its meaning, of hierarchizing its values of reacting to its apparent surds and conflicts.[7]

The Christian mysteries provide a framework for understanding the full dimensions of the human person. The person understands what is human because the Christian mysteries underline the truly human against cultural biases and distortions. Within these mysteries the very meaning, purpose, and value of the human person is grounded.

McCormick believes the basic structure of human life has been revealed in God's self-disclosure in Jesus. The acceptance of this disclosure by the human person transforms the person's values, attitudes, perspectives, and dispositions, which impact how he or she understands God, self, others, and the world.[8] These attitudes and values sharpen and intensify the human focus on what is good and definitive of human flourishing. McCormick writes:

> One who has accepted in faith God's stupendous deed in Christ, one who sees (and accepts) in the Christ God's self-disclosure and therefore who sees (and accepts) in the Christ-event the central fact of human history, will come to be (by God's healing grace) stamped by the dispositions associated with that event. Some are putting others' needs ahead of our own; seeking God's will in hard times; carrying one's cross in imitation of Christ; giving one's life for one's friends; turning the other cheek; seeing Christ in the neighbor; subordinating everything to the God-relationship; trusting in God's providential care. Such dispositions do not, of course, solve problems. They do, however, powerfully incline us to seek out and do morally *right* things.[9]

From within the context of the Christian mysteries, the human person can discover and communicate what it means to be fully human and how this impacts human existence. Thus for the Christian there is an inner dynamic of the faith experience. McCormick argues that, "the person of Jesus is testimony to the fact that no effort of man to know himself, find himself, be himself, is a viable possibility outside the God-relationship."[10] The person of Jesus constantly reminds the human person that what God did for humanity is an affirmation of the human and therefore must remain the measure of what the persons may reasonably decide to do to and for themselves.[11]

In essence, McCormick's theological anthropology is important because it is the foundation for his ethical methodology. The context in which McCormick views the human person has a direct influence on both his moral epistemology and his moral criteriology. The person viewed in terms of the Christian mysteries is not only modified as a decision-maker, but has been given a standard by which to judge particular situations. McCormick believes that informed moral judgments are always made within a context. For the Christian, that context consists in a complex interrelationship of anthropological and theological presuppositions. These presuppositions, which inform the person's moral thinking and judgment, are derived from and rooted in God's actions and purposes as they impact the inner dynamics of the person.

To understand the full dimensions of McCormick's doctrine of the human person one must examine and analyze his notion of God and God's providential wisdom, as well as the relations between divine and human agency. This will be the central focus of this chapter, because these positions profoundly affect the shape and direction of his understanding of the human person, and ultimately, how McCormick discerns moral decisions. After analyzing the human person in terms of the Christian mysteries, McCormick will infer various value judgments. From these value judgments McCormick will derive moral norms and human rights that form the basis for his positions on treatment decisions for handicapped neonates.

The remainder of this chapter will examine McCormick's theological anthropology from the perspective of salvation history described in terms of creation-fall-redemption. An effort will be made to specify the practical implications of McCormick's theological anthropology as it pertains to treatment decisions for handicapped neonates. Finally, this chapter will consider various criticisms of this part of McCormick's ethical methodology.

MCCORMICK'S THEOLOGICAL ANTHROPOLOGY

The center of McCormick's theological anthropology is the human person "integrally and adequately considered," which he views within the context of the Christian mysteries. By "theological anthropology" McCormick means

> a doctrine of the human person that views the human
> person in terms of the great Christian mysteries: crea-
> tion-fall-redemption. It is a doctrine that would yield an
> appropriate emphasis on vision, perspectives, and char-
> acter and the stories, metaphors, and images that gener-
> ate and nourish these elements.[12]

McCormick argues that Vatican II summarizes theological anthropology very cryptically. For the Council, "faith throws a new light on everything, manifests God's design for man's total vocation, and thus directs the mind to solutions which are fully human."[13] For McCormick the terms "God's design" and "total vocation" are shorthand for what he means by theological anthropology.

McCormick's view of the doctrine of the human person has developed through his writings. He began his career as a moral theologian trained in the manualist tradition that emphasized the juridical and physicalist approach of the classicist mentality. "This mentality conceives culture normatively and abstractly and represents a certain disengagement from the forces shaping the contemporary world."[14] The classicist image of the human person was one of the "agent as solitary decisionmaker."[15] In this view, moral norms were understood as generalizations about the significance or meaning of human conduct.[16] The criterion for rightness and wrongness was not the whole person, but isolated dimensions of the human person. This criterion McCormick refers to as "faculty finality" or "physicalism," which offers an analysis of faculties and finalities.[17] Vatican II reversed many of the predominant forces prior to the Council and thus McCormick began to favor a less juridical and more personalist approach. This approach gives priority to a historically-conscious worldview with a "revised" conception of the human person.[18] Vatican II broadened previous conceptions of the "human person" when it explicitly introduced the notion of the person "integrally and adequately considered." For example, *The Pastoral Constitution on the Church in the Modern World* asserts that "the moral aspect of any procedure . . . must be determined by objective standards which are based on the nature of the person and the person's acts."[19] The official Vatican Commentary on this wording notes two important points for consideration:

> (1) The expression formulates a general principle that applies to all human actions, not just to marriage and sexuality where the phrase occurs. (2) The choice of this expression means that "human activity must be judged insofar as it refers to the human person integrally and adequately considered."[20]

Vatican II proposed as the criterion for rightness and wrongness of human conduct not "the intention of nature inscribed in the organs and their functions" but "the human person integrally and adequately considered" (*personam humanam integre et adequate considerandam*).[21] This not only represents a significant shift in the criteria of moral conduct from a deductive to an inductive procedure; it also leads McCormick into the realm of theological anthropology.[22] Lisa Sowle Cahill observes that, "to base moral evaluation on the 'nature of the person' means increasingly to look beyond the individual, and certainly beyond physical functions and capacities, placing the person in relationship to others."[23] Vatican II's emphasis on the centrality of the human person has made moral theologians more aware of the need for a sound theological anthropology.

McCormick's understanding of the person "integrally and adequately considered" builds on the anthropology of Vatican II. It can also be inferred from McCormick's writings that he has adopted Louis Janssens' concept of a human person, which seeks to understand the human person in all his or her essential aspects.[24] Janssens suggests that to consider the person adequately all the essential aspects of the person must be considered. It is necessary to consider the person in himself or herself and in his or her relations to the world, to others, to social groups, and to God. Janssens considers eight aspects of the human person.[25] All human actions that promote the person adequately considered in this way are morally right; those that attack or undermine the person are morally wrong.[26] Since McCormick cites Janssens' eight essential aspects of the human person several times in his writings and in very favorable terms, it is fair to conclude that these essential aspects of the human person reflect McCormick's own anthropological views.[27]

McCormick believes that the Christian tradition provides the human person with two heuristic devices for understanding the full dimensions of the human person and the dynamic nature of life. The first device looks at the human person from the inside. McCormick writes:

> Salvation history is described in terms of creation-fall-redemption. This is not only temporal history but it is the shape of our own personal history. We bear the marks of this temporal history in ourselves, in our attitudes, habits and values. As Thomas Clarke has noted, our everyday lives in Christian perspective are simultaneously an act of continuing creation, a struggle with evil and a personal campaign for the victory and prospering of good.[28]

McCormick's notion of the great Christian mysteries throws light on the fact that the human person has been created by God, is redeemed by God, and is destined for God.[29] "God's Christ tells us what God thinks of us, and therefore we are—in spite of darkness, estrangement, sickness, and brokenness—basically loveable."[30] Created in the image and likeness of God, the human person is the central focus and crown of God's creation.[31]

The triad of creation-fall-redemption will be the vehicle for discovering and communicating how Christ gives new meaning to the world. It will be the vehicle for how the human person continues the process of redemption until the time when all humankind in the eschaton will be totally redeemed. There are various models and metaphors for viewing the human experience of creation-fall-redemption. There also exist secular variants of these models.[32] However, the advantage of the Christian models is that "they have an ultimacy of reference—what God does for us in creation, what we do to ourselves in sinfulness, what God does for us in redemption."[33] This device assists the human person in understanding the internal dimension of being, but human persons are more than internal beings. Human persons exist and act in the concrete world.

The second heuristic device is a view from the outside. McCormick uses Thomas Clarke's notion of "climates" to explain that the human situation is made up not only of the characteristics of personhood (interiority, subjectivity) but also of climates (symbols, institutions, structures, manner of living, lifestyles, etc.). McCormick argues:

> These "climates" refer not only to laws and structures of a formal kind, but to informal climates like accepted habits of speech, physical settings, the influence of tradition and customs, mind-sets, popular and public values, etc. Such climates have a profound influence on how we think, feel, behave. They seep through our pores and become the shapers of our decisions and even our lives. The danger we daily face: that the values and priorities of a secular, material and unbelieving world will seep through and strengthen our lack of freedom and truth and run our lives in a kind of silent slavery. The opposite is also true. Personal attitudes and freely chosen relationships affect the climates in which we live and decide.[34]

In order to counteract these exterior climates that may bias the human person, Christianity has given much attention to "climates of grace." Grace shapes our priorities, values, habits, attitudes, and eventually our decisions. McCormick observes that "when this climate gets into decisions and relationships, it will get into our world and have a transforming effect. Good people create good climates. And good climates support good people and their decisions."[35]

Emerging out of the triad of creation-fall-redemption comes the ultimate fact that Jesus Christ is God's total gift of self. For the Christian, this fact transforms the inner-person and gives the person a new context and basis for understanding God, self, others, and the world. Although humanity has not yet realized its full redemption, the love of Christ challenges humanity to move forward in the process of redemption to the time when all humanity will be totally redeemed, that is, when Christ comes to claim the redeemed world. For McCormick, the response of faith by the human person is a response of the whole person to God's stunning and aggressive love in Jesus.[36]

In order to analyze the full dimensions of how salvation history affects the human person, each element of the creation-fall-redemption triad will be examined and evaluated, because each of these elements play a foundational role in understanding McCormick's moral epistemology and moral criteriology. An examination and evaluation of McCormick's positions on Christology, the incarnation, and eschatology will also be undertaken. McCormick's views on these three doctrines play a major role in his theological anthropology even though they are not included explicitly in the creation-fall-redemption triad. In order to maintain the integrity of the triad, McCormick's views on these three doctrines will be treated separately at the end of this section.

DOCTRINE OF CREATION

The foundation of McCormick's theological anthropology is rooted in the doctrine of creation. The doctrine of creation is about the lasting relationship between God and all creation. God is the author and preserver of all life. God willed not only to create the world out of nothing and continually sustain it, but also to enter into a relationship with it. This relationship can never be overestimated. It is the basis for the fundamental Christian truth that human persons have their origin from God and are destined for God.

The Christian tradition is anchored in the belief that God relates to and covenants with God's people. This covenant is the basis for the human person's social and relational nature. God would love all creation and all creation would love God in return. The special sense of intimacy God has with humanity, and not with the rest of the created world, is the basis for understanding the human person as the crown and glory of God's creation. Each individual human person is graced with the gifts of reason and freedom, making each unique and existing in a special relationship with God. This relationship finds its fulfillment in the love one has for God and is manifest in the love human persons have for one another. It is primarily in others that human persons are able to recognize and love God. This love, which has as a standard the love of Jesus Christ, is the crowning achievement of human relationality. It is through social, relational, and interdependent persons that the work of creation is advanced and humankind moves toward its ultimate destiny. Each person is an integral part of God's action and plan. Through the responsible use of the goods of creation, human persons assist God in bringing creation to its fulfillment.

In order to understand the significance of the doctrine of creation for McCormick's theological anthropology, the various aspects of the doctrine will be examined—the *imago Dei*, the uniqueness and diversity of the human person, covenant as a metaphor for human sociality and relationality, and McCormick's view concerning humans as co-creators— and analyzed in depth. This will be done because each one plays an integral role in the doctrine of creation, but also because each aspect has a profound influence on McCormick's moral epistemology and moral criteriology.

Imago Dei. As the author and preserver of life, God created human life out of nothing and thus gave life its ultimate meaning.[37] McCormick writes:

> Just as God called the world out of chaos (nothing), just as He created a people (Israel) out of next to nothing and the new Israel out of insignificant beginnings, so He calls into being each one of us. Thus, Psalm 139: "Truly you have formed my innermost being; you knit me in my mother's womb." This is the thought-form that governs the biblical account of human life.[38]

The ultimate meaning God gave human life is that all human life is sacred, because all human persons are unique and equal in the eyes of God. Created in the image of God, the human person "is a member of God's family and the temple of the spirit."[39] Therefore, God confers on humanity a sense of dignity, which makes everyone equally valuable. Sustained and preserved by God, the human person is totally dependent on God for human existence. The human person is dependent on God because being a creature implies finitude. That is to say, it imposes limitations on our being and on our doing. Human persons can make choices, but their choices are limited by time, space, and matter.[40] As the preserver of life, and the ultimate destiny of the human person, God sustains humanity by God's self-gift of love. God created each human person out of love, which is the basis for the relationship of each person with God. Persons also fulfill their destiny by responding to God through others in a loving manner. Christians understand this God-relationship, that is, total self-gift, in and through Jesus Christ. God is self-gift and human persons are created in God's image and likeness.[41]

The *imago Dei* is an important aspect in understanding McCormick's doctrine of creation. The problem is that he never defines precisely what he means by it. McCormick writes that "we are images of God in our humanity."[42] However, he never explains what that image entails. One could infer from McCormick's writings that what he means by the *imago Dei* is the capacity of humans to be filled with the Spirit of God, which allows the person to reflect the qualities of God. If Jesus Christ, the exemplary human person, is God's total self-gift of love, and this gift is offered to all human persons, then human persons image God in their ability to love. When the human person responds to others in love, he or she is reflecting the qualities of kindness, generosity, and fidelity that characterize God.

In summary, the *imago Dei* is the foundation for McCormick's doctrine of creation. Created in the image of God, each human person has been created by God out of love. Each human person has an intrinsic dignity that is not subject to whims or calculations.[43] Finally, each human person has a destiny that can be fulfilled by responding to God through relating to others lovingly. For McCormick, the *imago Dei* is not a static concept given once-for-all. Rather, it is as dynamic as the human person is dynamic. The human person deepens in the *imago Dei* by responding to God, others, and the world lovingly.[44]

Uniqueness and diversity of the human person. McCormick argues that "uniqueness and diversity (sexual, racial, ethnic, cultural) are treasured aspects of the human condition. Theologically viewed, we are images of God in our humanity, in its enchanting, irreplaceable uniqueness and differences."[45] Created in the image and likeness of God, with the same origin, nature, and destiny, human persons share not only a basic uniqueness and equality but also a basic individual dignity. The Judaeo-Christian tradition has always viewed human persons as "in relationship to God." McCormick writes:

> This means that persons are the bearers of an "alien dignity," a dignity rooting in the value God puts in them.... The greatest affirmation of this alien dignity is, of course, God's Word—become flesh. As Christ is of God, and Christ is *the* man, so all persons are God's, his darlings, deriving their dignity from the value He is putting on them. This perspective stands as a profound critique of our tendency to assess persons functionally, to weaken our hold on the basic value that is human life. It leads to a particular care for the weakest, most voiceless, voteless, defenseless members of society: orphans, the poor, the aged, the mentally and physically sick, the unborn.[46]

There are certain common features of humanity that every human person shares. However, because each person is an individual, each person embodies these common features differently and to different degrees. No two people can be expected to respond to the same situation in the same way. Each person is the same but different because of the gifts of reason and free will bestowed upon them by God. What the human person thinks and how the human person responds form the basis of human individuality.

As rational beings, human persons have the ability to discover and analyze the basic values of life. Our dispositions, perspectives, and beliefs are the mark of our unique character. These dispositions and perspectives have their roots in the affections, feelings, and sensitivities of each person as well as our discursive reasoning. Human persons have also been given the gift of free will that allows them to make choices. McCormick places great emphasis on human freedom in regard to the uniqueness and individuality of the person. McCormick believes:

> Freedom is often presented as a quantity, something I possess at the age of reason and unpackage as I mature. Contrarily, freedom is much more accurately described as a task, something to be built and acquired. We do not have it; we must first earn it. It is the increasing ability to dispose of myself.[47]

McCormick argues that freedom is not just the freedom of choice to do a certain thing or not. Rather, the freedom to which McCormick refers is what Karl Rahner calls "basic or fundamental freedom." Concerning basic human freedom, McCormick writes:

> It is the more basic choice with respect to the whole meaning and direction of my life. It is "yes" or "no" to the whole moral order. It is the free determination of one's self with regard to the totality of existence, a fundamental choice between love and selfishness, between ourselves and God our Savior. It is the fundamental acceptance or rejection of the grace that is the person of Jesus into my life as invitation of the Father. It is our acceptance or rejection deep in our persons of God's enabling love.[48]

Basic freedom presupposes that the moral order "is properly and primarily constituted by the order of personal response," which involves the exercise of a basic choice between self and God and between love and selfishness.[49] Therefore, it refers to the relationship between the agent as a free person and his or her actions. Like freedom of choice, it is expressed through one's choice of particular goods. However, whereas freedom of choice concerns the psychological motivations or principles behind our choice of particular objects, fundamental freedom involves a basic orientation or a fundamental option on the part of the self-conscious subject to realize himself or herself either in openness to God and thus to other conscious subjects or through withdrawal from them.[50]

For McCormick, it is human intention, or the basic direction of human actions governed by one's knowledge and freedom that is the core of human individuality and uniqueness. Every human person shares the common features of humanity, but who we are as historical beings, will determine the different uses of these common features. By historical beings McCormick is referring to our being rooted in time and space and to our characteristic as changing beings whose self-definition and experience of self emerge from a consciousness in contact with a rapidly changing world.[51] As historical beings, each person matures through stages, each with specific challenges and possibilities. Furthermore, persons live in social groups that have their own cultural history and development.[52] This means that a person's racial, religious, ethnic, and sexual characteristics will play a role in determining one's distinctiveness or uniqueness.[53] The cultural, religious, and familial values a person holds will determine who that person is and the types of decisions that person will make. Created by God in our uniqueness and "diversity," all human persons should respect and value one another for who and what they are. Jesus Christ, the perfect human person, stands as a model for the uniqueness and "diversity" of the human person.[54] The self-giving of Christ is not only the basis for this individuality and "diversity," it is also the core of who we are as human persons—social and relational beings.

Covenant: Human Sociality and Relationality. The Christian tradition is anchored in faith, based on the belief that God relates to and covenants with a people. McCormick observes that "God covenanted with the Jewish *people*, with a group. It was within a group and through a group that the individual was responsible and responsive to God."[55] This loving, graced relationship or covenant between God and God's people is a metaphor to explain the human person's social and relational nature.[56] McCormick argues that "if a person's dignity is radically in his relationship to God, and if this is a relationship pursued and matured only through relationships to other persons, then this relationship to God is unavoidably social."[57] The Hebrew scriptures offer a number of stories about God's covenant with the Jewish people that attest to this fact. But this is even clearer in the New Testament with Paul's notion of "being in Christ" as a shared existence. Paul refers frequently to the human per-

son's new being which is being in a community.[58] To be a Christian is to
be a part of a believing community, an *ecclesia*. McCormick states: "Our
being in Christ is a shared being. We are vines of one branch and sheep
of the same shepherd."[59]

McCormick argues that this sense of community, which is at the core
of Christian consciousness, has two implications. He writes:

> First, it has meant that my freedom to realize my poten-
> tialities as a person is conditioned by the authenticity of
> the members of the community, and vice versa—that is,
> the community exists for the individual. Second, it
> means that we cannot exist in isolation, neither can we
> know as Christians in isolation, and it would be un-
> Christian to think we do or hope that we could. Our
> shared knowledge is concerned with God's wonderful
> saving events and their moral implications.[60]

Each individual has been given gifts and talents by God, but to reach
self-fulfillment as individuals and as a people it is necessary that these
gifts and talents be shared with and complemented by those of others.
This sense of radical sociality suggests that the well-being of persons is
interdependent. Further, the well-being of one person cannot be conceived of or realistically pursued independently of the good of others
since being a social creature is part of human being and becoming.[61]
McCormick argues:

> We exist in relationships, and are dead without them.
> This is not surprising for those who believe that man is
> created in the image and likeness of God. For the more
> we know of God, the more we know that He is *relation*,
> that His very being is "being-in-and-for-another."[62]

McCormick argues that to be a human person "means to have the capacity, actually or potentially, for significant human relationships. It is, I
believe, not a Christian discovery, but a typically Christian insistence
that the crowning achievement of human relationships is love."[63]

The ultimate meaning of the relational constitution of the human person is love. Human relationships are the very possibility of growth in the
love of God and neighbor. McCormick writes:

> As my ability to love God is His gift to me, so our ability
> to love each other is our gift to each other. The greatest
> human need is to be loved. For unloved, I remain un-

loving, withdrawn, self-encased. But when I am loved in
a full human way, selfhood, personal dignity, a feeling
of security, a sense of worth and dignity is conferred
upon me—the very things which enable me to respond
to others as persons, to love them. Thus it is clear that
because my greatest fulfillment is the other-centeredness
of love (and charity), my greatest human need is for that
which created the possibility; that is love from others,
their acceptance of me as a person. Similarly my greatest
gift to them is my self-donation to them because this is
also their greatest need.[64]

It is the ability to relate to others that allows the human person to love
God. This ability occurs within a group and through a group. McCormick
understands that to love our neighbor is in some real sense to love God.
He quotes 1 John 4: 20-21 to clarify this point. "If any man says, I love
God, and hates his brother, he is a liar. For he who loves not his brother,
whom he sees, how can he love God, whom he does not see?" The good
our love wants to do for God and to which God enables the human person, can be done only for the neighbor. This is a point Karl Rahner has
argued, and McCormick accepts his position. For Rahner and McCormick, the love of God and the love of neighbor are inseparable. It is the
love of neighbor that unites the human person with God.[65] McCormick
writes:

It is in others that God demands to be recognized and
loved. If this is true, it means that in Christian perspective, the meaning, substance, and consummation of life
are found in *human relationships*.[66]

In summary, in the covenantal relationship God has with us, God
gives God's love freely and waits for a response. McCormick argues that
"our radical acceptance of God is tied to love of the neighbor—a love
that secures rights, relieves suffering, promotes growth. God is speaking
to us in history and we are not free to be uninvolved."[67] Response to God
must be both individual and corporate and can occur only by relating to
others lovingly. As social beings, in loving relationship with God
through others, human persons are interdependent, and should never seek
self-fulfillment independently of the goods of others. This quality of relationality will define McCormick's understanding of the human person
and forms the basis of his theological anthropology.

Human Persons as Co-Creators. As part of the loving covenant God
has with us, God calls human persons to bring creation to its fulfillment,

its ultimate destiny, when "all will be all."[68] One can infer from McCormick's writings that his view of co-creatorship is based both in the anthropology of Vatican II and Janssens' first aspect of the human person's essential dimension where the person is a subject, normally called to consciousness, to act according to conscience, in freedom and in a responsible way.[69] Human persons are beings-in-the-world whose challenge is to transform not only humanity but the natural order.[70] According to the *Pastoral Constitution on the Church in the Modern World,* the Council teaches:

> Man, created in God's image, received a mandate to subject to himself the earth and all that it contains, and to govern the world with holiness and justice; a mandate to relate himself and the totality of things to Him who was to be acknowledged as the Lord and Creator of all. . . . They can justly consider that by their labor they are unfolding the Creator's work, consulting the advantages of their brother men, and contributing by their personal industry to the realization in history of the divine plan.[71]

Since the human person has been gifted with a creative intellect and free will, then God is to be viewed as an enabler of human abilities and potentialities. McCormick argues that this perspective is adopted by Thomas Aquinas in the *Summa Theologica* Ia-IIae, 91, 2: *Rationalis creatura . . . fit providentiae particeps, sibi ipsi et aliis providens* [creatures endowed with reason participate in providence by providing for themselves and others]. God committed the natural order to us as intelligent and creative persons. In this sense he is not only the creator of the natural order, but the enabler of our potentialities through our innovative interventions.[72] McCormick interprets Aquinas to mean that God has graced the human person with the means to bring creation to its fulfillment. When these means are used to help others and to serve God, then creation is advanced toward its ultimate destiny. Further, the human person also has the ability to misuse the goods of creation for self-serving motives. McCormick writes: "Thus our attitude toward the world must live in paradoxical tension, combining both appreciation and manipulation."[73] On the one hand, human persons are creatures and completely dependent on God for their existence. On the other hand, they are also responsible for playing a role in bringing creation to its fulfillment. An example of how the human person combines both an appreciation and a manipulation of creation would be gene therapy associated with adenosine deaminase (ADA) deficiency syndrome.[74] Gene therapy in this situation involves "the removal of bone marrow cells, then treatment of them with modified viruses in order to insert a new and normal gene, and finally replacement of the bone marrow cells back into the patient's body where the new gene would code properly for the deficient enzyme or protein."[75] Saving a person's life by this type of gene therapy is an example of how creation can be manipulated responsibly. The human person is to love and respect what God has created and at times manipulate it in order to bring creation to its ultimate destiny. Such a realization in history of God's divine plan is only to be accomplished by the responsible manipulation of creation for the good of God and humanity. However, the human person can also misuse the goods of creation for selfish motives. This is a direct effect of the Fall.

DOCTRINE OF THE FALL

The Christian tradition teaches that the first man and woman disobeyed God. As a result, the covenant with God was broken. Enfranchised with the gifts of reason and free will, the Fall took place and sin entered the world (Genesis 3:1-24). In the wake of the Fall, many Catholic theologians teach that the *imago Dei* was not entirely lost; rather, it was only badly damaged or weakened. This translates into the Catholic position that humanity, which is fallen, remains essentially good and with the grace of God can distinguish between what is morally right and should be done and what is morally wrong and should be avoided. Catholic theologians have historically based their theological anthropology predominantly in the doctrines of Creation and Incarnation.

McCormick's interpretation of the Fall follows a traditional Catholic understanding. Human beings have been gifted with reason and free will, and while the Fall and its effects have weakened both, reason and free will are not utterly destroyed. The life, death, and resurrection of Christ have transformed the human situation, but not totally. Sin exists in the world, and the human person, being imperfect, is still susceptible to its effects. McCormick writes:

> The tradition has viewed man as redeemed but still affected by the *reliquiae peccati* (remnants of sin). In the words of the scholastics, man is *totus conversus sed non totaliter* (a total convert but not totally). This means that notwithstanding the transforming gift of God's enabling grace, we remain vulnerable to self-love and self-deception (sin) and that these noxious influences affect our evaluative and judgmental processes ('*primi hominis culpa obtenebrate*'—'obscured by the fault of the first human being').[76]

In McCormick's writings he distinguishes original sin, individual-personal sin, and social sin. Original sin is the direct result of the Fall. The consequence of original sin is that the human person has been diminished, and his or her path to fulfillment has been blocked. Sin entered the world, and along with human creaturehood and finitude, ambiguity became part of the human condition.[77] As a result of the Fall, both human reason and freedom have become even more vulnerable. McCormick writes:

> Human beings are not disincarnated spirits with instantaneous understanding and freedom. Their knowledge comes slowly, painfully, processively. Their freedom is a gradual achievement. Their choices are limited by space, time, and matter. The good they achieve is often at the expense of the good left undone or the evil caused. In Bergson's words, "every choice is a sacrifice." Every commission involves an omission. Thus our choices are mixed, ambiguous. This intertwining of good and evil in our choices brings ambiguity into the world. The limitations of human beings become eventually the limitations of the world, and the limitations of the world return to us in the form of tragic conflict situations.[78]

Humanity has been redeemed, but because of the Fall, there is a need for daily redemption. Temptation is now part of life. McCormick argues:

> We know that the just are those who have turned to God and embraced His holy will in faith. Yet we also know that they are exposed to temptation. The pilgrim people just have not achieved the ultimate depths of free adherence to God. Their charity is, in this sense, incomplete.[79]

McCormick argues that there are two facts of human experience that make this obvious. He writes:

> First, is our lack of freedom. St. Paul stated: "For I do not do the good I want, but the evil I do not want is what I do" (Romans 7:10). As a result of the Fall there is a certain lack of freedom in our condition as human beings, an inconsistency in acting according to our basic option. Second, our human condition is accurately described as lack of truth. We lie to ourselves and to one

another. We turn away from the evil (and the good) in ourselves and in our actions. We prefer not to face it. It is uncomfortable, unflattering, unsettling. We are generous to a fault, especially our own.[80]

The human person lives this daily tension. On the one hand, the human person is confronted by the acceptance of God's enabling love into one's being. On the other hand, there exists the ratification of sin in the unfolding of one's life. Life is a struggle between charity, which is the center of all virtues, and self-love, which is the root of all sin.

McCormick understands individual-personal sin to be a change in one's basic orientation toward God. He believes: "Sin involves a conversion to the creature, but its principal element is aversion from God. That is, sins concerned with this or that object are signs of a deeper rebellion, even though this deeper rebellion is not real except in particular acts."[81] For McCormick, conversion is a reestablishing of the fundamental posture which is the acceptance and deepening of God's enabling love into the very being of the person.   Individual-personal sin for McCormick is an internal act, which contravenes the moral order in different ways. It is the heart that is sinful. McCormick uses scripture to clarify his position. He writes:

> In the parable of the prodigal Son (Luke 15: 11-31) sin is not only an action against God, but above all a withdrawal of a son from the supremacy and charity of the father. Similarly, St. John treats individual sins as manifesting the internal situation (*anomia*) of the sinner (1 John 3:4). Individual sins are consequences of this internal situation. In St. Paul, *hamartia* is sin personified, a kind of power in man. This power originates with the sin of Adam but is freely accepted by the sinner and becomes the font of various sins.[82]

For McCormick, individual-personal sins are the manifestation of the fundamental sin that occurred as a result of the Fall. McCormick further clarifies his position on individual-personal sin by making a distinction between mortal sin and venial sin. For McCormick, mortal sin is an act of fundamantal liberty by which a person disposes of self before God who is calling him or her through grace. It is therefore a fundamantal option, in which an individual turns in rejection from the charity of Christ whether Christ is thematically known or not.[83] Venial sin is not an act of fundamental or core liberty. It is rather a relatively superficial act involving only peripheral or slight freedom.[84]

Sin has more than an individual, personal manifestation. It also has a social manifestation. Social sin is the result of the power of sin in the world.[85] The human person must focus on both the interior and exterior components of sin in order to understand the reality of sin in the world. As social and relational beings, sin cannot be conceived of as only an isolated act of an individual since it also has societal, structural dimensions. For example, McCormick writes: "We began to see that the sins and selfishness of one generation became the inhibiting conditions of the next. The structures and institutions that oppress people, deprive them of their rights and alienate them are embodiments of our sinful condition."[86]

For McCormick, there is an inevitable relationship between individual-personal sin and social sin, because the love of God and neighbor are inseparable. Therefore, it follows that the love of neighbor must also be inseparable from justice to the neighbor. As social beings, individuals participate in society by helping to create social structures. Some of these social structures are the direct cause of various forms of oppression, injustice, and exploitation. Because human persons share in the creation of these structures and the maintaining of them, individuals also share in the responsibility for the sinfulness they cause. Examples of social sin would include: racial discrimination, economic systems that exploit the worker such as migrant farm workers, exclusion of women from certain positions, etc. There are many biblical images that attest to this: "the prince of this world," "the power of darkness," "the elements of this world," "principalities and powers." These phrases convey the idea that sinfulness can be embodied in our very institutions and ways of doing things, in the air we breathe.[87]

As a result of the Fall, the presence and influence of sin pervades all creation. However, sin does not destroy the basic goodness of all that God has created. For McCormick, there is always hope. That hope is Jesus Christ, the supreme liberator. In Jesus Christ the human person has been transformed. For McCormick, this transformation has far-reaching ramifications for all of creation.

DOCTRINE OF REDEMPTION

McCormick understands redemption to be God's saving activity through Jesus Christ in delivering humanity from sin and evil. As a pilgrim people who have been adversely affected by the Fall, humankind has been redeemed by the life, suffering, death, and resurrection of Jesus Christ. The human condition that is imbued by sin, suffering, and ambiguity is now opened to mercy, forgiveness, and redemption. McCormick writes:

> Jesus came to liberate us all by his graceful presence (life-death-resurrection) from the grips of sin and from its structural manifestations. This he did by offering to us the capacity to love after his example, and thus fulfill our potential as human beings. A lifetime work.[88]

For McCormick, the effect of being redeemed by Christ is that human persons have been totally transformed into "new creatures" in a community of the transformed.[89] In Jesus' life, death, and resurrection, sin and death have been overcome and have met their victor.[90] McCormick argues that "we are offered in and through Jesus Christ eternal life. Just as Jesus has overcome death (and now lives), so will we who cling to him, placing our faith and hope in him and taking him as our law and model."[91]

As redeemed, something profound has happened to the human person. The love of Christ, which is God's gift of charity, has been poured into the very being of the human person. McCormick argues that "it is our task—and one with eternal stakes—to protect, nourish, support, extend, and deepen that great gift."[92] For McCormick, it is the love of Christ that guides the "new creature" to the ultimate end. This end, however, is not always realized. Redeemed in Christ, the "new creature" is still threatened by the *reliquiae peccati* [remnants of sin]. Humans have a tendency to make idols and to pursue the basic goods of life as ends in themselves. McCormick writes:

> This is the radical theological meaning of secularization: the loss of the context which subordinates and relativizes these basic human goods and which prevents our divinizing them. The goods are so attractive that our constant temptation is to center our being on them as ultimate ends, to cling to them with our whole being.[93]

It is only with Jesus as the standard of human love that human persons are able to avoid this type of idolatry, because as "new creatures" we are free and powerful in Christ's grace.[94] Human persons have been redeemed, but they must also grow into the fullness of their redemption.[95]

What McCormick means specifically by becoming a "new creature" as the effect of redemption is not clear. It is only in McCormick's later writings that one finds this notion of "new creature." The reason for this is that between 1983 and 1999, McCormick wrote primarily in the area of bioethics from a theological perspective. As a result, he introduced certain theological notions that have not had the advantage of being fully developed over the years.[96]

One can infer from McCormick's writings since 1983 that it is Jesus' love that empowers the human person and makes him or her a "new creature." It empowers the human person to love God in and through one's neighbor. McCormick writes:

> . . . in Jesus, God confronts us to tell us who we are and what we may become, to enlarge our humanity, to create and deepen our capacity for the Godlife. He confronts us to mirror to us our true potential, and by mirroring to confer it. This conferring liberates us from those cultural, hereditary, and personal hang-ups and deformities that drain self-respect and stifle our growth.[97]

As "new creatures" McCormick believes the human person is liberated and empowered. Liberated from self-distrust to self-esteem, from anxiety to peace, from emptiness and alienation to joyful hope, and from the slavery of compromised secular value judgments to fearless Christian value judgments. Empowered, the human person can recognize and fulfill his or her true potential and help others realize the fullness of their potential.[98]

Jesus Christ, as the standard of love, shapes the basic priorities of the "new creature" and suggests the shape of Christian love for one another. The effects of redemption for McCormick include both individual redemption and social redemption. He argues that, if human beings allow the grace of Christ to transform them totally, then

> it will inevitably get into our habits, values, and attitudes and thus into our decisions small and large. It will shape our priorities. And when this climate gets into our decisions and relationships, it will get into the world and have a transforming affect [sic].[99]

Christ's love relativizes all human goods in a world that has a tendency to absolutize them. As McCormick writes:

> Christ's suffering and cross were both a symbolic contextualizing of human goods *and* the profoundest act of love. Therefore, those who strive to follow Him ("as I have loved you") are performing the profoundest act of love for the world by pursuing in interpersonal life the basic *goods within their context, as* subordinate. In this sense, both Christ's love for us as standard, and there-

fore our love for each other, constitutes a profound relativizing of basic human values.[100]

As "new creatures" in Christ, Christians are called to challenge any tendency to absolutize not only individual goods, but institutions, structures, and ideas. Human beings are called to an ongoing conversion until they reach the ultimate destiny of their combined journeys—the coming of the kingdom. The present can never be absolutized because it is always incomplete. It is only in the future, with the return of the glorified Christ to claim the redeemed world, that human beings as a pilgrim people redeemed in Christ will reach fulfillment.

Conversion is central in understanding what McCormick means by the effects of redemption. McCormick argues:

> Too often we have viewed forgiveness in its narrowest sense as a definitive act or declaration of non-imputation. In a larger and richer sense, it is the whole process of withdrawal from sin, of deepening antipathy to sin, of refashioning of the sinner. It is a many-sided process of liberation capable of infinite increase and perfection. One's deepening inner revulsion for and psychological opposition to sin is part of the process. Conversion is, we might say, a deepening of the fundamental option.[101]

The radical acceptance of God is tied to the love of neighbor—a love that secures rights, relieves suffering, and promotes growth.[102] This entails not only a personal conversion but the conversion and transformation of creation. McCormick writes further that conversion means

> not simply individual one-on-one action for those we generally avoid (the mentally ill, the starving, the sick, criminals, poor minorities, etc.); it means organizing the corporate power of the community in such a way that so-called "sinful structures" are changed. The structures which oppress people, alienate them, deprive them of rights, are embodiments of our sinful structure.[103]

As social and relational beings, human persons live in community and are responsible for one another. For example, as persons, Christians are called to bind every wound, shelter the sick, share possessions with the poor, educate the young, offer compassion to the bereaved, protect the innocent, and bring therapy to the mentally ill—but above all to work to change the structures that allow human deprivations to exist—and always with the intent to expand a person's capacity to love by loving that person in every concrete way possible. Human persons learn to love by being loved.[104] Conversion is an ongoing process, which challenges individual Christians to expand the capacities of love in their own lives and to expand the capacities of others to love by liberating them from all that prevents love from growing and flowering.

In conclusion, for McCormick, it appears that love is the basis of being a "new creature" in Christ. As a standard, Christ not only sensitizes humanity to the meaning of persons, but also to how the world should be viewed and intended. Human beings are called to an ongoing conversion and to transform not only self but also others and the world. This is a lifelong process that will find its completion only when the glorified Christ comes to claim the redeemed world.

CHRISTOLOGY, INCARNATION, AND ESCHATOLOGY

McCormick states that his own theological anthropology consists in viewing the human person in terms of the great Christian mysteries of creation-fall-redemption. We are created by God, redeemed by God, and called back into loving union with God. However, it is evident from his writings that the doctrines of Christology, the incarnation, and eschatology, also play significant roles in his theological anthropology. McCormick's positions on Christology, the incarnation, and eschatology are presented as inchoate theories. He refers to them throughout his writings; however, he fails to present them systematically. It appears that McCormick implicitly includes them within the triad without explicitly classing them as part of the great Christian mysteries.

Christology serves as a major element in McCormick's theological anthropology. By "Christology" McCormick means the critical theological reflection upon the Christian confession that Jesus is the Christ. Jesus Christ is God's self-disclosure as self-giving love. McCormick argues:

> If Jesus is God-become-man, God's self-gift and self-revelation, the second person of the Triune God, then knowing Him is knowing God. His actuality is at once insight-injunction for us, insight into who God is and who we are, injunction as to what we should become. "Lord," Philip said to him, "show us the Father and that will be enough for us." "Philip," Jesus replied, "after I have been with you all this time, you still do not know me? Whoever has seen me has seen the Father" (John

14: 8-9). Knowing Jesus' qualities, ideals, and injunctions is a direct insight into God's gracious governance of the world. More importantly, *knowing who He is* is knowing both the Godhead and ourselves in relationship with the Godhead, and therefore knowing some things about God's plan for us.[105]

McCormick's Christology, while not systematically detailed in his earlier writings, is the bond that unites the great mysteries. McCormick writes:

For the believer, Jesus Christ, the concrete enfleshment of God's love, becomes the meaning and *telos* of the world and of the self. God's self-disclosure in Jesus is at once the self-disclosure of ourselves and our world. "All things are made through him, and without him was not anything made that was made" (John 1:3). Nothing is intelligible without God's deed in Christ.[106]

He argues that the human person is illumined by the person, teaching, and achievement of Jesus Christ.[107] The experience of Jesus is regarded as normative for McCormick because Jesus is believed to have experienced what it is to be human in the fullest way and at the deepest level.[108] Jesus Christ provides the context by which the human person can view the relationships of God, self, others, and the world. Jesus' love is the paradigm and model of what our love must be for God and others. McCormick writes:

To be molded in Christ's image means a deepening or radicalizing of our love. We grow to love the Heavenly Father as Christ did. But love after the fashion of and in the manner of Christ's love is essentially different from other good works, from any other act we perform. In other words, one might say, we give something; in love we give ourselves. It is this growth in surrender to ourselves, this giving in Christ's image that the Spirit is attempting to operate in us. In this sense, all our actions are mediations or expressions of Christlike love.[109]

For the Christian, all things lack full meaning and intelligibility without reference to God's deed in Jesus Christ. The believer's response to this specific, momentous, and supreme event of God's love is a total and radical commitment of faith.

McCormick's position on Christology becomes more specific in his later writings. In an article entitled, "Moral Theology in the Year 2000," McCormick offers six assertions to serve as the foundation of theological ethics. These are rooted in the Christian fact that in Jesus something has been done to and for the human person. Jesus Christ is a prior action of God at once revelatory and response-engendering.[110] These six assertions form the core of McCormick's Christology which serves as the unifying bond of his theological anthropology. McCormick writes:

> First, God's self-disclosure in Jesus Christ as self-giving love allows of no further justification. It is the absolutely ultimate fact. The acceptance of this fact into one's life is an absolutely originating and grounding experience. Second, this belief in the God of Jesus Christ means that "Christ, perfect image of the Father, is already law and not only law-giver. He is already the categorical imperative and not just the font of ulterior and detailed imperatives." Third, this ultimate fact reveals a new basis or context for understanding the world. It gives it a new (Christocentric) meaning. Fourth, this "new fact and center of thinking" that is Jesus Christ finds its deepest meaning in the absoluteness and ultimacy of the God-relationship. Fifth, the God-relationship is already shaped by God's prior act in Jesus (self-giving). "To believe in Jesus Christ, Son of God, is identical with believing that God— the absolute, the meaning—is total gift of self." Therefore, the "active moment of faith takes place in the recognition that meaning is to give oneself, spend oneself, and live for others." Sixth, the empowered acceptance of this engendering deed (faith) totally transforms the human person. It creates new operative vitalities that constitute the very possibility and the heart of the Christian moral life.[111]

These assertions give credence to the fact that McCormick's Christology is the dominant force that brings together the various aspects of his theological anthropology. In and through Jesus the human person comes to know that the God-relationship is total self-gift. Charles E. Curran has written that a more functional Christology, one concerned with the saving work of Christ, has greater implications for moral theology than a one-sided ontological or metaphysical Christology. In a Christology from above, salvation is abstract, individual, and extrinsic, whereas in a Christology from below, salvation is concrete, communal, and intrinsic.[112] McCormick's Christology by this analysis would seem to fall into Curran's functional category, because as McCormick's theological anthropology will show, salvation is concrete, communal, and intrinsic.[113]

Fundamental to McCormick's theological anthropology is his view on the decisiveness of God's covenant with humanity manifested in the saving incarnation of Jesus Christ.[114] For McCormick, the incarnation "no matter what the depth of its mystery, was, as Vatican II repeatedly noted, an affirmation of the human and its goodness."[115] God so loved humankind that God was willing to enter the human situation completely. McCormick writes:

> The incarnation is necessarily affirmation about humanhood and is the Christian theological basis for asserting that "the glory of God is humanhood alive." After Jesus and because of what we know in Jesus, humans are indeed the measure of all things. To say less is to undermine the implicit affirmations of the incarnation.[116]

By the incarnation—the supreme epiphany of God's self and our potential selves—God's immanent presence, his love in the flesh, became visible in the person of Jesus Christ.[117] The "good" became identified with the divine person of Jesus Christ. Charity, which flows from our experience of God's own love in Christ, became the heart of the Christian moral life.[118]

One cannot understand the full dimensions of the mystery of the incarnation without an appreciation for the complexity of sin and an understanding of the ultimate destiny of humanity's combined journeys in the coming of the kingdom. The incarnation confirms the basic goodness inherent in human nature, fallen but redeemed. In reaffirming the goodness of creation, the incarnation reestablishes the covenant with God's people, and gives human life new significance. Humanity is open to God and longs to enter into relationship with God. The social and communitarian nature of the human person is further developed and brought to fruition by the incarnation. Jesus enters completely into the fullness of human fellowship. The love of God has been made visible in the world by the mystery of the Incarnation. As a result, the Word made flesh is the standard, the center of mind and heart, and charity is at the root of human behavior.[119] The Incarnation becomes not only the foundation of reasoning in ethics, but the source of the Church's moral magisterium.[120]

McCormick's notion of eschatology has its origin in the Christian mysteries. God is the creator, redeemer, and destiny of all creation. McCormick states clearly that

> we are pilgrim people, having here no lasting home. . . .
> The ultimate destiny of our combined journeys is the
> "coming of the kingdom," the return of the glorified
> Christ to claim the redeemed world.[121]

McCormick's notion of eschatology, along with his understanding of the doctrine of creation, serves as the basis for his view of humanity's co-creatorship. As relational creatures in a covenant with God, human persons are called to work together as co-creators to help bring about the kingdom of God. God acts through humanity by God's free gift of God's self in grace, and human persons cooperate with that grace to bring about the kingdom of God.

McCormick follows the Catholic theological tradition that teaches that the reign of God through Jesus Christ and the Spirit is already present in the mystery of the world. However, the fullness of this reign will come only at the end of time. There exists both a continuity and discontinuity between this world and the next. Human persons must strive to cooperate in bringing about the kingdom of God, but their efforts will always be imperfect, insufficient, inadequate, because the kingdom of God is a gracious gift to us.[122] Despite all human efforts, McCormick argues that "we are led to admit that the final validation and transformation of human effort is given by God with the ultimate coming of His kingdom."[123] The "already but not yet" is the central focus of McCormick's eschatology and is the basis for his prophetic view of eschatology.[124]

McCormick's prophetic perspective concerning eschatology is developed out of his views on the Church and on the doctrine of creation. His eschatology is in contrast to both the apocalyptic and the teleological views of eschatology as Harvard theologian Harvey Cox has dubbed them.[125] Prophetic eschatology offers a more balanced view of the continuity and discontinuity between this world and the next. Harvey Cox distinguishes prophetic eschatology from both the apocalyptic and the teleological by stating:

> Prophetic eschatology visualizes the future of this world
> not as an inferno that ushers in some other world but as
> the only world we have and the one which man is un-
> avoidably summoned to shape in accord with the human
> person's hopes and memories. Against the teleological
> view, it sees the *eschata* transforming the *arche*, rather
> than vice versa. It sees the future with its manifold pos-
> sibilities undoing the determinative grip of the past, of
> the beginning. In contrast to most forms of teleology,
> prophecy defines the human person as principally his-

torical rather than as natural. Without denying his kinship to the beasts it insists that his freedom to hope and remember, his capacity to take responsibility for the future, is not an accident but defines his very nature. But, most importantly, prophecy sees everything in the light of its possibilities for future use and celebration. Without rejecting the influence of historical continuities, it insists that our interest in history, if it is not merely antiquarian, arises from our orientation toward the future. We write and rewrite the past, we bring it to remembrance, because we have a mission in the future. The Israelite prophets called the past to memory not to divinize it but to remind people that the God of the covenant still expected things from them in the future.[126]

Cox's view of prophetic eschatology could serve as a framework for interpreting McCormick's eschatology. While McCormick has not addressed the eschatological issue in depth, it is possible to deduce his understanding of prophetic eschatology from his ecclesiology and his understanding of the human person "integrally and adequately considered."

McCormick states clearly that the Church is eschatological. First, as a pilgrim Church it is "a tentative and unfinished reality. It is *in via*. A fortiori its moral and ethical judgments are always *in via* and share the messy, unfinished and perfectible character of the Church itself."[127] This eschatological experience of the Church is evident in its understanding of the gospel message as never complete. God's revelation is perceived in the dynamic unfolding of history.[128] The Church moves forward into the future, but never forgets the past. Thus, there is a basic dynamism that involves both continuity and change. Second, McCormick's understanding of the doctrine of creation views the human person as a historical being who uses the past to advance the future. The human person has been graced by God with creative intellect and freedom in order to help transform creation. As co-creators with God, human persons have been enabled by God to use their abilities and potentials in a responsible manner that will help bring about the realization in history of the divine plan. McCormick's view of the Church and his understanding of the human person serve as the framework for his prophetic eschatology. His view of eschatology plays a distinctive role in both his moral epistemology and his reinterpretation of tradition, and has a profound influence on his criteria for moral decision-making.

In summary, the mystery of creation-fall-redemption is not only our history as a people; it is also our own personal history. Each human person is created in the image and likeness of God. As a result of the Fall, each human person is prone to sin, failure, and corruption. But with the eyes of faith, humankind has been redeemed by the love of Jesus Christ, which challenges each person to move forward in the process of redemption to the time when all humankind in the eschaton will be totally redeemed. For McCormick, "our lives are processes of enlightenment, liberation, reintegration, healing, reconciliation. These words are active and transitional. They suggest the past, acknowledge the ambiguous present, but point to the glorious future."[129] The bond that holds McCormick's theological anthropology together is the love of Christ—charity. While McCormick's position on Christology is not systematically spelled out, it plays a distinctive role in his theological anthropology. Jesus Christ, the perfect human being and concrete enfleshment of God's love, is the standard by which human persons must live, and his love is the ground of human behavior. With Jesus as the standard, it is now possible to draw some practical implications from McCormick's theological anthropology as it relates to treatment decisions for handicapped neonates.

PRACTICAL IMPLICATIONS OF MCCORMICK'S THEOLOGICAL ANTHROPOLOGY AS APPLIED TO TREATMENT DECISIONS FOR HANDICAPPED NEONATES

McCormick's positions on bioethical dilemmas develop their plausibility and force from his theological anthropology. Throughout his writings in bioethics, the very meaning, purpose, and value of a person is grounded in, and ultimately explained by, the Christian mysteries. Thus, his theological anthropology provides the framework that ought to shape a person's decisions on various bioethical dilemmas. McCormick writes:

> When decision-making is separated from this framework, it loses its perspective. It can easily become a merely rationalistic and sterile ethic subject to the distortions of self-interested perspectives and cultural drifts, a kind of contracted etiquette with no relation to the ultimate meaning of persons.[130]

Personal value judgments about bioethical dilemmas must have a standard by which they can be judged. For McCormick, that standard is Jesus Christ, who is the standard of love. If personal value judgments are separated from the Christian mysteries of creation-fall-redemption, they lose their meaning for the Christian and become controlled by the forces of science and technology.[131]

McCormick argues that in Western secularized society, value judgments have become technological as they have become separated from theological anthropology. Science and technology have become the standard because the Christian story that reveals the meaning of life is no longer regarded as functional. McCormick argues:

> Thus in our secularized society we have (1) the assertion of autonomy as the controlling value of the person; (2) the canonization of pluralism as instrumental to it. . . . It [autonomy] is surely a precious value. But it is the condition of moral behavior, not its exhaustive definition.[132]

For McCormick, technology cannot determine what it means to be truly human. To understand the human person comprehensively it is necessary to place the human person within the very matrix that is the only complete indicator of the truly human. The Christian mysteries will not give concrete answers or ready-made rules. But the Christian mysteries will "tell us who we are, where we come from, where we are going, who we ought to be becoming. It is only against such undertakings that our concrete deliberations can remain truly humane and promote our best interests."[133]

As human beings created by God, redeemed by God, and destined for God, the human person has been transformed. Although incomplete, this transformation must influence how the human person views bioethical issues. McCormick argues that for Christians faith can shed light on bioethics in three distinct but overlapping ways. He explains:

> 1. *Protective*: the human person perceives basic human values, but the perception is shaped by our whole way of looking at the world. Faith should and does sensitize us to the meaning of persons, to their inherent dignity regardless of functionality. In this sense it aids us in staying human by underlining the truly human against cultural pressures to distort it.

> 2. *Dispositive*: the Christian of profound faith will reflect in his or her dispositions the very shape of faith. That shape is the self-gift we call charity, love of God in others, charitable action. Although the non-Christian may choose the same action, which is shaped by charity, the act will be chosen and viewed by the Christian as a more intense personal assimilation of the shape of the Christ-event.

3. *Directive*: the biblical materials that occasion and ground faith yield themes or perspectives that shape consciousness.[134]

Having examined these three distinctive ways that faith sheds light on bioethics, it can be argued that McCormick applies the following value judgments, which are inferred from his theological anthropology, to treatment decisions for handicapped neonates.

HUMAN LIFE IS A BASIC BUT NOT ABSOLUTE GOOD

One of the basic notions of McCormick's theological anthropology is that human life is a precious gift with a purpose and destiny. Human beings are called to live life to its completion, knowing that self-fulfillment can only occur in the eschaton. McCormick argues: "The fact that we are pilgrims, that Christ has overcome death and lives, that we will also live with him, yields a general value judgment on the meaning and value of life as we now live it. It can be formulated as follows: life is a basic good but not an absolute one."[135] Therefore, human life is a relative good, because there are higher goods for which life can be sacrificed.[136] In this argument, McCormick draws upon Church teaching and Scripture as he writes:

> Life is basic because, as the Congregation for the Doctrine of the Faith worded it, it is the "necessary source and condition of every human activity and of all society." It is not absolute because there are higher goods for which life can be sacrificed (glory of God, salvation of souls, service of one's brethren, etc.). Thus, in John 15:13: "There is no greater love than this: to lay down one's life for one's friends." Therefore, laying down one's life for another cannot be contrary to the faith or story of meaning of humankind. It is, after Jesus' example, life's greatest fulfillment, even though it is the end of life as we now know it. Negatively, we could word this value judgment as follows: death is an evil, but not an absolute or unconditional one. [137]

Dying is a rhythm of nature, a natural part of life. However, for the Christian, it is not the absolute end. It is a transition, that is, the end of one stage—physical life—and the beginning of another—eternal life.[138] Christians have regularly refused to absolutize either life or death, because there is a higher spiritual good. For the Christian, the idolatry of physical life is unacceptable.

This value judgment has immediate implications for the care of handicapped neonates. McCormick argues: "It issues into a basic attitude or policy: not all means must be used to preserve life."[139] McCormick bases this argument on the words of Pope Pius XII in the Pontiff's 1957 address to the International Congress of Anesthesiologists. After noting that there exists an obligation to use only ordinary means to preserve life, Pius XII stated: "A more strict obligation would be too burdensome for most men and would render the attainment of the higher, more important good too difficult. Life, health, all temporal activities are in fact subordinated to spiritual ends."[140] McCormick interprets Pius XII as arguing that

> forcing (morally) one to take all means is tantamount to forcing attention and energies on a subordinate good in a way that prejudices a higher good, even eventually making it unrecognizable as a good. Excessive concern for the temporal is at some point neglect of the eternal. An obligation to use all means to preserve life would be a devaluation of human life, since it would remove life from the context or story that is the source of ultimate value.[141]

Human life is a basic good, but there may come a time when that life is no longer considered a precious gift. When a person no longer has the potential for human relationships—which are the very possibility for growth in love of God and neighbor—or these relationships would be so threatened, strained, or submerged that they would no longer function as the heart and meaning of the individual's life as they should, then one is no longer required to preserve that life by all human means.[142] To preserve a life in this situation would be to replace the "higher, more important good." "Physical life" would become the ultimate value. When that happens, the value of human life has been distorted.

The moral implication of this value judgment that human life is a basic but not absolute good can be applied to the handicapped neonate. If in the course of treatment there comes a time when such treatment is medically futile or may cause needless iatrogenic insults on the handicapped neonate, then one is not morally obliged to initiate or continue treatment. For McCormick, an example of a neonate in this situation would be one with severe necrotizing enterocolitis.[143] The Catholic tradition has sought a middle path between medico-moral optimism or vitalism (which preserves life with all means, at any cost, no matter what its condition) and medico-moral pessimism (which actively kills when life becomes onerous, dysfunctional, or boring).[144] McCormick seeks this same middle path since he understands treatment decisions to be more than mere technological judgments. For him, treatment decisions are also value judgments, and as such, they are rooted in the Christian mysteries of creation-fall-redemption.

HUMAN LIFE IS A VALUE TO BE PRESERVED ONLY INSOFAR AS IT CONTAINS SOME POTENTIALITY FOR HUMAN RELATIONSHIPS

For McCormick, to be human means to have a capacity, actually or potentially, for significant human relationships.[145] Human persons exist in relationship with God and others. For McCormick, "the crowning achievement of human relationships is love."[146] Therefore, significant human relationships are the very possibility of growth in love of God and neighbor. This emphasis on relationality, particularly that human relationship called "love," sums up briefly the meaning, substance, and consummation of life in the Judaeo-Christian perspective. For McCormick, the love of God is the "higher, more important good." In the Christian tradition it follows that

> life is a value to be preserved precisely as a condition for
> other values, and therefore insofar as these values remain
> at least minimally attainable or, as James Gustafson puts
> it, "as the *sine qua non* for other values." Since these
> other values cluster around and are rooted in human re-
> lationships, it seems to follow that life is a value to be
> preserved only insofar as it contains some potentiality
> for human relationships.[147]

McCormick reasons that, before any human experiences, responses, or achievements are possible, there must be human life. In this sense, human life is a condition for all other values and experiences. However, when a human life is devoid of the possibility of experiencing human love, that is, no experience or interrelation is possible, then that life has achieved its potential.[148] This is not to devalue the worth of the person.[149]

McCormick defines human personhood as a social state that requires a potential for human relationships.[150] He argues that "we exist in relationships and are dead without them."[151] If a human person is no longer able to love God, then that person has lost the potential for relationality and has achieved his or her potential. For McCormick, it is the ability to relate that grounds the human person's ability to love, and becomes the basis for determining personhood.[152]

In the case of handicapped neonates, when the potential for human relationships is simply nonexistent or the neonate would be utterly submerged in the mere struggle to survive, then for McCormick that life has achieved its potential.[153] In this situation, McCormick argues that it would be morally permissible to forgo or discontinue treatment. McCormick opines: "It is neither inhuman nor un-Christian to say that there comes a point where an individual's condition itself represents the negation of any truly human—that is, relational—potential. When that point is reached, is not the best treatment no treatment?"[154] On this subject he writes:

> Every human being, regardless of age or condition, is of incalculable worth. The point is not, therefore, whether this or that individual has value. Of course he has, or rather *is* a value. The only point is whether this undoubted value has any potential at all, in continuing human survival, for attaining a share, even if reduced, in the "higher more important good." This is not a question about the inherent value of the individual. It is a question about whether this worldly existence will offer such a valued individual any hope of sharing those values for which physical life is the fundamental condition.[155]

For McCormick, the potential for human relationships is based on his theological anthropology which emphasizes God's covenant with human persons. If the essential relationship of love (for others, God, and self) is the benchmark of a Christian life, then McCormick would conclude that a life lacking the basic capacity for such responsive love is a human life with no earthly potential, no personal future for the neonate, except death and whatever awaits thereafter.[156]

HUMAN LIFE AS SACRED

As the author and preserver of life, God created human life out of nothing and thus gave life its ultimate meaning. That ultimate meaning is that human life is sacred, because all persons are unique and equal in the eyes of God. McCormick writes: "Human life is sacred because of its origin and destiny, because of the value God places on it. Our grasp of this sacredness is marvelously deepened in Christ's costing love."[157] For McCormick, human life is sacred because it is created by God, redeemed by God, and destined for God. From this value judgment he draws out the moral obligation that human life must be treated with dignity and respect.

Human persons being unique and equal in the eyes of God are bearers of an "alien dignity," a dignity rooting in the value God puts in them. The greatest affirmation of this dignity is God's Word become flesh. This perspective stands as a profound critique of the human tendency to assess persons functionally, to weaken our hold on the basic value that is human life. The sacredness of human life and the dignity that is derived from it leads to a particular care for the most defenseless members of society.[158] McCormick argues that "sacredness of life demands reverential attitudes and practices."[159]

McCormick's view on the sacredness of life directly influences his positions on treatment decisions for handicapped neonates. There is a debate within bioethics concerning the "sanctity of life" vs. the "quality of life." Proponents of the sanctity of life position argue that focusing attention on the obligation to preserve life avoids degrees of discrimination in quality-of-life criteria. McCormick believes that these two approaches should not be set against each other.[160] As a result of this belief, McCormick draws a distinction between "every person is of equal value" and "every life is of equal value." He believes that every person is sacred, is of incalculable worth, and deserves to be treated with dignity and respect. However, he does not believe that every life is of equal value. According to McCormick:

> What the "equal value" language is attempting to say is legitimate: We must avoid *unjust* discrimination in the provision of health care and life supports. But not all discrimination (inequality of treatment) is unjust. *Unjust* discrimination is avoided if decision-making centers on the benefit to the patient, even if that benefit is described largely in terms of quality-of-life criteria.[161]

McCormick argues that "we must be concerned not just with keeping a patient alive by surgery or medication, but with a certain level of being alive, a certain acceptable mix of freedom, painlessness and ability to function."[162] Every human life is sacred in the eyes of God. However, when that human life is devoid of the potential for significant human relationships, it is a violation of the sacredness of human life to preserve it. An example McCormick gives would be the decision medically to treat an anencephalic infant as if it were to recover from its condition.

Once a decision has been made to forgo or discontinue treatment, because the neonate has no potential for significant human relationships, there is still a moral obligation to give comfort to that handicapped neonate. For McCormick, that comfort would consist in palliative care.[163] Since every human life is of incalculable worth, one can never abandon a neonate because a decision has been made not to treat. Every human life has value and should be treated with dignity and respect.

MEDICAL TREATMENT DECISIONS OUGHT TO INCORPORATE INDIVIDUAL AND SOCIAL FACTORS

God made a covenant with the Jewish people, that is, with a group. For McCormick, the implication of this is that it is only within a community and through a community that an individual is responsible and responsive to God. McCormick argues that this sense of community, which is sunk deep into the human consciousness, means two things. First, the community exists for the individual. Second, to be a Christian means one cannot exist in isolation, neither can one know as a Christian in isolation.[164] Therefore, for McCormick, to be a person is to be a social being. Since human beings are related, it is apparent that human persons need each other in order to reach self-fulfillment. Decisions made by one will affect others. There exists a clear relation between the individual and the community. There have been times when the individual and the community were viewed as two separable and competing values. The Judaeo-Christian tradition has resisted this view and recognizes that the individual and community are inseparable complementarities. McCormick argues:

> The individual and the community are related like only partially overlapping circles. At points there is identification of concerns and goods, at other points there is distinction. Thus, while the individual is an integral part of the community and must take it into account in defining his or her own prerogatives and rights, still the individual does not exist for the community in a way that totally subordinates him or her to it.[165]

This radical equality before God and the sense of being part of a community requires that the human person search for a delicate balance between the two.

Understanding human persons as radically equal and essentially social has far-reaching moral implications in regard to treatment decisions for handicapped neonates. Decisions about medical treatment will not only affect the individual neonate but will also have serious ramifications for the family and society as a whole. As radically equal, all neonates are entitled to medical treatment if such treatment will be beneficial for their condition. As essentially social, all neonates are members both of the community and of their particular families. Therefore, social factors such as cost, allocation of resources, better utilization of medical personnel; and familial factors, such as excessive psychological, emotional, and financial burdens, must be considered when determining treatment decisions for handicapped neonates. A delicate balance must be found between the right of every individual to medical treatment and social and familial factors.

McCormick includes not only the rights of the individual neonate in regard to treatment decisions but also includes familial and societal considerations.[166] He bases his inclusion of social factors on the Catholic theological tradition. As Pius XII taught: "normally, one is held to use only ordinary means—according to circumstances of persons, places, times, and culture—that is to say, means that do not involve any grave burden for oneself or *another*."[167] McCormick includes financial costs within this category of social factors. McCormick writes: "If the financial cost of life-preserving care was crushing, that is, if it would create grave hardships for oneself or one's family, it was considered extraordinary and non-obligatory."[168]

There exists a delicate balance between individual and community needs, and McCormick admits that these are in constant flux and tension. McCormick maintains that there are certain obligations which are part of the requirements for membership in society. Thus, individual membership in human communities goes hand in hand with obligations.[169] He argues: "Individuals ought to—indeed can—be rightly forced to make certain sacrifices for the common good (for example, conscription, proportionate taxation)."[170] Yet, for McCormick, the individual can never exist for the community in a way that totally subordinates the individual to the community. McCormick believes: "The common good of all persons cannot be unrelated to what is judged to be promotive or destructive to the individual—in other words, judged to be moral or immoral."[171] For McCormick, the balance between individual and social considerations entails making a value judgment, and the means for achieving this balance are to be found in the great Christian mysteries of creation-fall-redemption.

PAIN AND SUFFERING CAN HAVE REDEMPTIVE MEANING

McCormick follows the Catholic theological tradition and argues that pain and suffering have a special place in God's saving plan. Without glorifying suffering, the Catholic tradition has viewed suffering and even death within a larger perspective, that of the redemptive process. By suffering, Christians can participate in the paschal mystery. McCormick writes:

> Suffering is not mere pain and confusion, dying is not merely an end. These must be viewed, even if mysteriously, in terms of a larger process: as occasions for a growing self-opening after Christ's example, as various participations in the paschal mystery.[172]

For the Christian, pain and suffering must be seen as something more than that which is to be avoided. McCormick does not propose that suffering is to be caused, but rather believes that there are times when persons must at least endure it.[173]

Christians view life within the context of the Christian mysteries. McCormick writes: "Just as Christ suffered and died for us to enter his glory, so we who are 'in the Lord,' who are inserted into the redemptive mystery, must expect that our growth 'to deeper life' will share the characteristics of God's engendering deed in Christ."[174] For McCormick, grave illness is to be seen as an intensifying conformity to Christ. As the human body weakens and is devastated by disease and illness, the strength of Jesus Christ is shared by those who have been baptized into his death and resurrection. For McCormick, the Catholic conviction is that grave illness should be a time of grace, of the gradual shedding of the sinful self.[175] This conviction reinforces the view that human persons are completely dependent upon God's love. Christ manifested his supreme dignity by doing God's will—"Not my will but thine be done" (Luke 22:43). Christians are called to the same complete dependence on God's love as Christ showed on the Cross. This dependence on God manifests itself in human dependence on others. Therefore, suffering should lead not only to dependence on God but to dependence on others. When a human person is experiencing pain and suffering, that person needs the help and presence of others. Only through dependence on others and God can one truly become independent.[176]

McCormick's views on pain and suffering have a direct influence on his positions concerning treatment decisions for handicapped neonates. Some ethicists believe that it is morally right to dispatch or terminate infants' lives when they are in intractable pain,[177] or once a decision has been made that their quality of life is insufficient to prolong life through medical treatment.[178] McCormick has never defended infanticide. His position is quite clear: "there is no proportionate reason for directly dispatching a terminal or dying patient."[179] In situations of critical illness, death may only be brought about indirectly by acts of omission. Human life is sacred and the direct killing of an innocent life is a "virtually exceptionless norm."[180] McCormick's moral position on infanticide is grounded in his doctrine of creation and in the lordship of God over all creation. For example, McCormick writes: "If all persons are equally the creatures of the one God, then none of these creatures is authorized to play God toward any other. And if all persons are cherished by God, regardless of merit, we ought to cherish each other in the same spirit."[181] Thus, for McCormick, all human life is valued because of God's unconditional love. Therefore, no person has the right to take an innocent life simply because that person is experiencing pain and suffering. If every person is created by God, redeemed by God, and destined for God, then only God can decide when a person will attain his or her ultimate destiny.

SCIENCE AND TECHNOLOGY AS GOODS OF CREATION

Science and technology are goods of creation that make possible the otherwise impossible. Created in the image and likeness of God and graced with the gifts of free will and reason, the human person has been enabled by God to use these gifts in a creative way that will help transform self, others, and the world. Advances in science and technology are the result of God's gifts to humankind.[182] Consequently, these advancements must be used in a responsible manner that will advance the good of creation. As co-creators with God, the human person's "attitude toward the world must live in paradoxical tension, combining both appreciation and manipulation."[183]

In this technological age, human persons are confronted daily with the dilemma that because something can be done, does that mean it ought to be done? McCormick believes that the "power-plasticity model" of the human person, identified by Daniel Callahan, has shaped contemporary moral imagination and feelings. According to this model, human persons today view themselves corporately as *homo technologicus*, which means that if something can be done, it will be done. In society today, "the best solution to the dilemmas created by technology is more technology. We tend to eliminate the maladapted condition (defectives, retardates, and so on) rather than adjust the environment to it."[184] For McCormick, advancements in science and technology must be examined holistically. The responsible use of science and technology must consider the good of the whole person and the common good of society, not just a particular problem. McCormick argues that "moralism and excessive preoccupation with 'problems' and the rights and wrongs of omissions and commissions, too readily leads us to overlook the human quality of care and cure—that which we need no matter what our condition."[185] Responsibility in science and technology requires human persons to look not only at individual problems but at the future implications of such a technology in the light of what it means to be a human person "integrally and adequately considered." McCormick expresses concern with the danger that both the human and the morally good will be identified with what is technologically possible, with the result that technology creates its own morality.

Scientific and technological advancements play an integral role in deciding treatment decisions for handicapped neonates. Neonatal medical information and technology increase every day, and these advancements are often implemented almost immediately. Neonatal technology can now prolong the lives of many neonates, when in the past these neonates would have died. There is little doubt that technology has provided the means to save the lives of many neonates. However, McCormick frequently questions the ethical nature of the means adopted and the quality of the life being saved. He observes that technology "challenges us to grow beyond our past without forgetting it, to be informed by tradition without being enslaved by it, to move into the future while still clinging to the imperishable riches of the past."[186] While demonstrating great respect for medicine and technology, McCormick remains firmly grounded in the Catholic theological tradition and calls for the responsible use of the goods of creation. For him, just because something can be done does not necessarily mean it ought to be done. His thinking here is particularly applicable to treatment decisions for handicapped neonates. A need exists for an ethical criterion to assist decision-makers as they determine whether certain neonates should be aggressively treated. Such an ethical criterion must examine whether or not certain technologies are in the "best interests" of the person "integrally and adequately considered." According to McCormick, the great Christian mysteries provide the framework by which the Christian can judge what is truly human and in the "best interests" of the person against cultural attempts to distort it.

In conclusion, McCormick's view of the human person in terms of the creation-fall-redemption triad is the ground for the meaning, purpose, and value of the human person. The basic structure of human life has been revealed in God's self-disclosure in Jesus Christ. The acceptance of this self-disclosure by the human person in the form of values and attitudes has a profound impact on how the human person views, God, self, others, and the world. These values and attitudes keep the focus of the human person on what is good and definitive of human flourishing. McCormick's theological anthropology provides the framework for the various value judgments that influence his positions on treatment decisions for handicapped neonates. These value judgments form the basis for both the theological and anthropological presuppositions that will inform and shape the human person's moral thinking and judgment.

McCormick argues that the value judgments inferred from his theological anthropology are reasonable and firmly rooted in the Catholic theological tradition, an argument not shared by all his Catholic ethicist colleagues. Some critics argue that McCormick's interpretation and analysis of the Christian mysteries is lacking in clarity. Others criticize the vagueness and selective use of concepts within his anthropology. Still others argue that the practical implications of his theological anthropology have not been consistently applied to treatment decisions for handicapped neonates. To complete the analysis of McCormick's theological anthropology it will be necessary to articulate, analyze, and evaluate some of these criticisms.

CRITICISM

A variety of criticisms have been directed at McCormick's theological anthropology from a diverse group of critics. McCormick believes that such criticism by peers is a valuable tool that can lead to further clarification, reevaluation, and even the revision of one's positions. For example, McCormick has written that "I take seriously the suggestion that theologians should be ready, willing and able to admit mistakes—especially to each other. In that spirit it goes without saying that I would welcome criticism and correction."[187] Taking McCormick at his word, this section will evaluate four specific critiques directed at McCormick's theological anthropology.

First, McCormick's theological anthropology is shaped not only by the Christian mysteries of creation-fall-redemption, but also by the doctrines of Christology, the incarnation, and eschatology. These latter three doctrines are presented in McCormick's writings as inchoate theories. In his earlier writings, that is, prior to 1983, McCormick incorporated these three doctrines implicitly within the triad of creation-fall-redemption. It is not until after 1983 that these three doctrines appear more explicitly in an undeveloped form. One can speculate that the reason for this is that from 1983 onward McCormick writes primarily in the area of bioethics from a theological perspective. From this perspective it became necessary for him to articulate his positions on Christology, the incarnation, and eschatology. However, his positions on these three doctrines have never been articulated in a systematic manner.[188] This has resulted in a sense of ambiguity regarding McCormick's theological anthropology and its practical implications.

Presenting these three doctrines in a more developed fashion would clarify a number of important issues regarding McCormick's theological anthropology. For example, McCormick agrees with James Gustafson that Christology is the most critical doctrinal issue for any Catholic theology.[189] If McCormick is correct that it is in and through Jesus that human persons know the full dimensions of the God-relationship as total self-gift, and if God's self-disclosure in Jesus is at once a self-disclosure of humanity and the world, then it seems imperative that McCormick should have presented his position on the doctrine of Christology in a systematic manner. With this understood the human person can gain a deeper understanding of humanity and the God-relationship. In regard to the incarnation, McCormick states: "An ethics that takes the incarnation seriously, will be the very last to abandon moral reasoning and argument; for the incarnation, no matter what the depth of its mystery, was, as Vatican II repeatedly noted, an affirmation of the human and its goodness."[190] If the incarnation is an affirmation of the human and its goodness, and the "glory of God is humanhood alive," then to understand the human person "integrally and adequately considered," it would have been beneficial for McCormick to clarify his position on the incarnation by developing his view on the doctrine in more depth. Finally, McCormick's notion of co-creatorship has its origin in both his doctrine of creation and his doctrine on eschatology. His notion of co-creatorship has a significant influence on the formation of certain value judgments that influence treatment decisions for handicapped neonates. To understand the full significance of co-creatorship and how it influences these moral decisions, it would have been helpful for McCormick to clarify his position on eschatology and to state explicitly how it impacts co-creatorship.

Second, McCormick's theological anthropology affords great emphasis to the social and relational nature of the human person. For McCormick, the human person is essentially social, radically equal, and inherently relational. The origins of these positions are found in his understanding of the doctrine of creation. The human person, created in the image and likeness of God, is in a loving covenant with God. This relationship with God finds fulfillment through the love of one's neighbor. Unless a person can relate to and with others, that person can neither love nor develop his or her potential. The central theme of McCormick's doctrine of creation is the relational nature of God with humanity. Despite a significant amount of focus on relationality in his theological anthropology, McCormick never once mentions the theological concept of the Trinity. Rather, he emphasizes the significance of God as the Father, the centrality of Jesus Christ as the Son, and the guidance given to humanity by the Spirit. Yet he never mentions the notion of interrelations within the Trinity. McCormick does articulate the interdependence of human persons, the communitarian nature of human persons, and how the potential for human relationships is the basis for personhood. However, he fails to relate these concepts and communitarian themes directly to the Trinity. McCormick has a Trinitarian vision of the moral life, but he never clarifies it adequately.[191] This is an important issue because in McCormick's view on Christology he refers to the fact that, "knowing Jesus, the second person of the Triune God, is knowing God. Knowing who Jesus is is knowing both the Godhead and ourselves in relationship to the Godhead, and therefore knowing some rather basic things about God's plan for us."[192] Understanding the notion of "relation" in the Trinity can only deepen our knowledge of who God is and how human persons understand their relationship to and with God. That is important in any theological anthropology.

One explanation for McCormick's avoidance of the relational nature of the Trinity may be the complex and archaic language that has been used in the past to explain the theological nature of the Trinity. McCormick may have believed that such language would cause only confusion rather than clarity if he tried to relate it to the nature of the human person in regard to contemporary bioethical dilemmas. Theologian Kenneth R. Himes argues:

> Few Catholics today understand what the Greek-speaking theologians of Cappodocia meant by *hypostases* or even what Tertullian meant by *personae* when the formula three-in-one was used to describe the Trinity. The hallowed formulation simply does not communicate the substance of the tradition accurately to most believers.[193]

McCormick may have believed that the archaic language surrounding the Trinity would be misunderstood and thus render meaningless his communitarian notion of the human person. If true, then he could have benefitted from a more contemporary interpretation of the Trinity advanced by some present-day theologians. A number of contemporary theologians have expressed the notion "relation" in the Trinity in a more contemporarily relevant manner. Such clarity might strengthen significantly McCormick's position on the social and relational nature of the human person and give it an even stronger theological grounding as related to bioethical issues.[194]

Third, McCormick states explicitly that the human person is "essentially social," which he bases in the doctrine of creation.[195] For him, when deciding on treatment decisions for handicapped neonates, it is necessary to take into consideration the effects of these decisions on the family and society at large. He quotes Pope Pius XII[196] and Gerald Kelly, S.J.,[197] to show that the Catholic theological tradition has always included social factors in determining medical decisions. However, a number of ethicists suggest that McCormick offers a very narrow view of social factors as they influence treatment decisions for handicapped neonates. Richard Sparks and James McCartney, both Roman Catholic ethicists, criticize McCormick's view of these social factors.

The issue of including social and familial factors in determining treatment decisions for handicapped neonates will be examined and analyzed in a more complete manner in chapter four, which will deal with McCormick's moral criteriology. However, the social nature of the human person is the basis for including these factors, so it is pertinent to include this criticism under theological anthropology. Sparks believes that "the ultimate decision as to whether treatment is in a given patient's total best interest ought to incorporate not only medical or individualistic (i.e., experiential) burden factors, but also broader social factors, viewed from the patient's existentially-contexted vantage point."[198] Sparks argues that McCormick's interpretation of social factors is too narrow. He suggests that McCormick allows the patient's social nature to impact only to the extent that the person has physiologically-based potential to relate with others (determining one's minimal capacity to derive benefit from treatment). However, he rejects communality when it comes to the impact the patient's condition has on his or her family or society (burden in the fullest sense). Sparks further argues that it would be truer to the extraordinary/ordinary means tradition and fairer to the patient viewed as a social as well as personal being to allow familial and even societal burdens into the calculus concerning the handicapped neonates' best interests. Sparks states that "those who are broader interpreters of the quality of the patient's life echo the best of the extraordinary/ordinary means tradition in their insistence that the cost, psychic strain, and the degree of inconvenience born by others, a non-competent's social net-worth, ought rightly to be factored in as part of the patient's burden, holistically considered."[199]

In similar fashion, James McCartney criticizes the first guideline offered by McCormick and Paris in their joint *America* article[200] that specifies their criteria of the capacity for human relationships as a summary of the burden-benefit evaluation. That guideline states, "life-saving interventions ought not be omitted for institutional or managerial reasons."[201] McCartney writes:

> . . . since we are talking about the promotion of a positive good (the saving of the life of the child), there may be limitations and restrictions based not on the infant's

questionable ability to benefit from this treatment, but on
the sheer fact that it may cost too much, may involve
personnel who are more needed elsewhere, may utilize
resources that could more readily save many more lives,
may involve the family in genuinely excessive psychological, emotional, or financial burdens they are unable
to handle, or may involve the child's becoming a ward
of the state with the psychological trauma that entails.
While I agree that we ought to do all that we can to miti-
gate these factors, when they are irrevocably present I
hold that they would provide adequate justification for
the foregoing or discontinuance of treatment when they
are coupled with a fairly serious pathological anomaly.[202]

The major point of Sparks' and McCartney's criticism appears to be
that McCormick is not consistent in the application of some elements of
his theological anthropology. In a number of articles,[203] McCormick argues that social and familial factors ought to be considered in the burden-
benefit calculus. He argues that under specific guidelines, infants should
be allowed to participate in experimentation because as members of the
Christian community there is a sense of solidarity and Christian concern
for others. Sharing in sociality, infants are in some sense volunteer-able
to help the common good of society, provided that their individual well-
being is not thereby appreciably burdened.[204] McCormick further supports inclusion of social and familial factors in the burden-benefit calculus by appealing to the Catholic theological tradition's "extraordinary-
ordinary means" distinction. McCormick understands the tradition as
stating:

If the financial costs of life-preserving care was crushing—that is, if it would create grave hardships for oneself or one's family—it was considered extraordinary
and nonobligatory. Or again, the grave inconvenience of
living with a badly mutilated body was viewed, along
with other factors (such as pain in preanesthetic days,
uncertainty of success), as constituting the means extraordinary. Even now, contemporary moralist M. Zalba,
S.J., states that no one is obliged to preserve his life
when the cost is "a most oppressive convalescence"
(molestissima convalescentia).[205]

Sparks believes that, despite McCormick's statements on this topic, he has not applied social and familial factors in a consistent manner when dealing with handicapped neonates. Sparks argues that this may be due to the fact that McCormick is trying to address his critics who believe his quality-of-life criteria may lead to the slippery slope of selfish social utilitarianism.[206]

From the vantage point of McCormick's theological anthropology, it appears that Sparks' and McCartney's criticism of McCormick in this area may be accurate. McCormick affords significant attention to articulating the significance of the human person as essentially social and inherently relational. However, it also appears that McCormick does not apply the full dimensions of these concepts to treatment decisions for handicapped neonates. This issue of social and familial factors applied to treatment decisions is a complex issue that entails more than just the social and relational nature of the human person. There may be more to McCormick's position on these issues than just a failure to be consistent in the application of social and familial factors in a broad sense to treatment decisions for handicapped neonates. A final evaluation of this criticism will be deferred until chapter four when McCormick's moral criteriology is articulated, analyzed, and evaluated.

The final criticism directed at McCormick's theological anthropology concerns his view of redemption and the Pauline images he uses of being "in Christ" or "in the Lord." What does this mean at the level of concrete existence? Ethicist Kenneth Himes writes:

> McCormick's answer is quite sweeping: the experience of being in Christ "totally transforms the human person" creating "new operative vitalities." From here he proceeds to lay out an understanding of how charity, rooted in the experience of acceptance of Christ as Lord, forms the entirety of the moral life.[207]

Unfortunately, McCormick fails to articulate what he means precisely and concretely by "totally transformed," or by "new operative vitalities." Himes argues that "the statements read more like assertions that are not easily reconcilable with human experience. It appears that McCormick claims too much in his account of the experience of redemption."[208]

Himes believes that McCormick's abstractness in regard to redemption is because his account of redemption is insufficiently eschatological. "What is lacking is the element of the 'not yet' and the consequent role for processes of conversion and growth."[209] To address this deficiency, Himes argues that more attention must be given to the experience of grace given in Jesus as experienced by people in their everyday lives.

Himes' criticism is partially correct. McCormick's notion of salvation is quite concrete. Himes' criticism that it is "abstract" is due to the fact that McCormick's position on eschatology is presented in an undeveloped form. However, McCormick clearly states that human persons are transformed, redeemed, and divinized by the grace of Christ. He also states that even though the human person has been redeemed, because of the effects of the Fall, there is a need for daily redemption. Therefore, humans are called to grow in the fullness of their redemption. This is the basis for understanding the process of conversion and growth in the human person. Unfortunately, McCormick fails to articulate fully how the human person grows in the fullness of this daily redemption. Despite God's enabling grace, the human person remains vulnerable to sin. Sin endures but so does the redeeming love of Jesus Christ. The problem is that McCormick is ambiguous about what he means when he says the human person redeemed in Christ becomes a "new creature." How is the grace given in Jesus experienced by individuals in their everyday experiences? Stating that the human person becomes a "new creature" does little to explain how the ongoing process of conversion and redemption takes place. If Jesus is "God's incarnate self-gift" as McCormick states, and this is essential to understanding the human person, then Himes is correct in stating that attending to the implications of this fact in an experiential way requires more effort on McCormick's part. The relation of human nature and grace is essential to understanding McCormick's theological anthropology. To understand the human person "integrally and adequately" McCormick needed to be less ambiguous about how redemption is experienced in daily life.

In conclusion, if McCormick is serious when he states that theologians should be ready, willing and able to admit mistakes, especially to each other, then he should have examined these criticisms with an open mind. His theological anthropology is the foundation of his ethical methodology. McCormick's failure to address the criticisms directed at his theological anthropology has led to ambiguity concerning his moral epistemology and moral criteriology. This is not to say that he had to accept the above criticisms as correct. However, as he states, "unless a theologian is ready to examine criticisms and admit mistakes, differences degenerate into distance and ultimately disorder."[210] His failure to address these criticisms could lead to dire consequences in regard to treatment decisions for handicapped newborns.

CONCLUSION

McCormick's theological anthropology views the human person in terms of the Christian mysteries: creation-fall-redemption. These mysteries affect a person's instincts, attitudes, sensitivities, imagination and values, and ultimately, influence a person's perspectives, analyses, and judgments. McCormick argues:

> If God is present and self-communicative to us in his glorified Son—the exemplary human being—through his Spirit, and if this presence is mediated to us by a historical religious community, then surely this faith in that presence as formed by this community will have a powerful influence on one who tries to sort out the complexities of modern scientific problems.[211]

Faith in Jesus Christ, God's self-disclosure, grounds the Christian's attitudes and values toward life. Something profound has happened to the person of faith. The love of Christ has been poured into his or her being, and the result is a modification of the decision-maker.[212] For McCormick, "being-in-the-Lord" contains an inclination, an intention, a goodwill, a readiness to do what is right.[213] He argues that within the context of God's self-revelation in Jesus Christ, the Christian infers certain value judgments, from which he or she derives specific norms and moral obligations, which can be applied to treatment decisions for handicapped neonates. This process involves determining objectively what is supportive and promotive of others or conversely what undermines their well-being and even their human rights. How a person comes to know values/disvalues and moral obligations falls within the area of moral epistemology. It is necessary in the chapter that follows to examine how McCormick comes to informed moral judgments within the context of his theological anthropology.

NOTES

[1]T. M. McFadden, "Anthropology," *The New Catholic Encyclopedia*, vol. XVI (Washington, DC: The Catholic University of America Press, 1967), 12.

[2]Robert A. Krieg, "Theological Anthropology," in *The Encyclopedia of Catholicism*, ed. Richard P. McBrien (San Francisco: CA: Harper-Collins, 1995), 64.

[3] J. J. Mueller, S.J., *What Is Theology?* (Collegeville, MN: The Liturgical Press, 1988), 17.

[4] Krieg, "Theological Anthropology," in *The Encyclopedia of Catholicism*, 64.

[5] Without being exhaustive, the following are contributions of these disciplines as they have had a bearing on a contemporary theological anthropology: "First, man is a being-in-time in the sense that he experiences his own radical finitude; bounded by death, he perceives that he does not have a hold upon existence. He faces this realization with anxiety, and seeks to make sense of it in light of his orientation toward the fullness of being or eternity. Second, man is historical or social. His awareness of reality is not achieved in isolation from the cultural forces that variously shape his perspectives. Language, even though culturally conditioned and limited, is the necessary embodiment of truth. Third, freedom is an essential prerequisite for human fulfillment, without which cultural advance is an illusory veneer. Fourth, man is future oriented. As Marxists stress, the future is the dominant mode of time and a vision of an authentic although yet-to-be achieved model supplies the hope out of which a nonalienated society can be achieved." T. M. McFadden, "Anthropology," *New Catholic Encyclopedia*, vol. XVI, 12.

[6] Ibid.

[7] Richard A. McCormick, S.J., "Christianity and Morality," *Catholic Mind*, 75 (October 1977): 28.

[8] An example of some of the insights, perspectives, and value judgments that McCormick infers from the Christian mysteries as they relate to bioethics would be: life as a basic but not absolute value; the extension of this evaluation to nascent life; the potential for human relationships as an aspect of physical life to be valued; the radical sociality of the human person; the inseparability of the unitive and procreative goods; and the permanent, heterosexual marriage as normative. For a more detailed analysis, see McCormick, *Health and Medicine in the Catholic Tradition*, 51-59.

[9] McCormick, "The Best Interest of the Baby," 19-20. Emphasis in original.

[10] McCormick, "Theology and Bioethics," *Theology and Bioethics: Exploring the Foundations and Frontiers*, ed. Earl E. Shelp (Dordrecht, Netherlands: D. Reidel, 1985), 101.

[11] McCormick, "The Judaeo-Christian Tradition and Bioethical Codes," *How Brave A New World?*, 17.

[12] McCormick, *Corrective Vision*, 21.

[13] "Pastoral Constitution on the Church in the Modern World," *The Documents of Vatican II*, no. 11, 209.

[14]McCormick, *Corrective Vision*, 40.

[15]Ibid., 21.

[16]For example, McCormick has written that "if concrete actions promote a value, they are prescribable. If they generally attack a value, they are generally proscribed. If they always attack a value, they are always proscribed." McCormick, *The Critical Calling*, 14.

[17] "Physicalism" refers to the tendency in moral analysis to emphasize or even absolutize the physical and biological aspects of the human person and human actions independently of the function of reason and freedom. An example of what McCormick means by "faculty finality" would be that "the faculty of speech was given to us for the purpose of communicating true information. To use it in a way contradictory of this purpose (*locutio contra mentem*) was morally wrong." Ibid.

[18]For a detailed discussion of historical consciousness, refer to Chapter One, Richard A. McCormick, S. J.—Moral Theologian section above.

[19] "Pastoral Constitution on the Church in the Modern World," *The Documents of Vatican II*, no. 51, 256.

[20]McCormick, *The Critical Calling*, 14. See also *Schema constitutionis pastoralis de ecclesia in mundo huius temporis: Expensio modorum partis secundae* (Vatican Press, 1965), 37-38.

[21]Ibid., 339-340. See also *Schema constitutionis pastoralis de ecclesia in mundo huius temporis: Expensio modorum partis secundae*, resp. 104. McCormick believes the person "integrally and adequately considered" has its origin in Aquinas. McCormick writes: "It is interesting to note that St. Thomas wrote that 'we do not wrong God unless we wrong our own good.'" For McCormick, "our own good" is identical with the person "integrally and adequately considered." Ibid., 16.

[22] For example, the classicist analysis viewed the faculty of speech for the purpose of communicating true information. Thus, to use it contradictory to this purpose was morally wrong. However, if "we view speech in broader perspective (historical consciousness) and see it not simply as an informative power, but as an endowment meant to promote the overall good of persons in community, we have altered our basis for our definition of a lie." Ibid., 14.

[23]Lisa Sowle Cahill, "On Richard McCormick," *Theological Voices in Medical Ethics*, 84.

[24] McCormick cites Janssens' concept of person and his eight essential aspects of person in several of his writings: *The Critical Calling*, 14-15; *Corrective Vision*, 15; *Health and Medicine in the Catholic Tradition*, 16-18; and "Past, Present and Future of Christian Ethics," in *Called*

to Love: Toward a Contemporary Christian Ethic, ed. Francis Eigo (Villanova, PA: Villanova University Press, 1985): 1-19 at 4.

[25]The following is the summary of Janssens' definition of the human person that McCormick incorporates into his understanding of the human person: "The human person is (1) a subject (normally called to consciousness, to act according to conscience, in freedom and in a responsible way); (2) a subject embodied; (3) an embodied subject that is part of the material world. (4) Persons are essentially directed to one another (only in relation to a Thou do we become I). (5) Persons need to live in social groups, with structures and institutions worthy of persons. (6) The human person is called to know and worship God. (7) The human person is a historical being, with successive life stages and continuing new possibilities. (8) All persons are utterly original but fundamentally equal." McCormick, *The Critical Calling*, 14. See also Louis Janssens, "Artificial Insemination: Ethical Reflections," 3-29.

[26]McCormick, *Health and Medicine in the Catholic Tradition*, 17. McCormick believes that the Church has not integrated successfully the notion of the person "integrally and adequately considered" into our moral decision-making. McCormick writes: "Our failure to take Vatican II seriously and flesh out the significance of *persona integre et adequate considerata* has left a vacuum and made it possible for certain authority figures to reduce scientific data to 'mere polls' and dismiss them, or to collapse scientific studies into 'scientism.' Janssens' study has helped to fill the vacuum and overcome the false alternatives." McCormick, *Notes on Moral Theology 1981 through 1984*, 52.

[27]McCormick notes that "Janssens' insistence on the 'person adequately considered' as a normative criterion is absolutely correct, and his elaboration of what that means is very helpful." Ibid., 51. Paulinus Odozor believes that McCormick relies on Janssens' eight aspects of personhood but questions whether McCormick is dependent on Janssens. Odozor writes: "McCormick exhibits a tendency to downplay his own original contribution and to give credit to some other person whose work on the issue he believes to be more encompassing. Sometimes this obscures the fact that he may in fact have been the originator of the idea under discussion or at least that he himself had previously held the same or similar views. Therefore, on the issue of the definition of personhood, it is difficult to distinguish what McCormick appropriates from Louis Janssens from his own original insights." Odozor, *Richard A. McCormick and the Renewal of Moral Theology*, 204. Throughout this chapter I will show how McCormick has incorporated Janssens' eight aspects of the human person.

[28]McCormick, *Corrective Vision*, 64. See also Thomas Clarke, S.J., "Public Policy and Christian Discernment" in *Personal Values and Public Policy*, ed. John C. Haughey, S.J. (Mahwah, NJ: Paulist Press, 1979).

[29]The following are some of the key elements of the Christian mysteries that McCormick isolates: God is the creator and preserver of human life; human persons are on a pilgrimage and thus have no lasting home in this world; in Jesus' life, death, and resurrection humans have been totally transformed both personally and communally; human persons remain subject to sin, although both sin and death have met their victor; the ultimate significance of human lives consists in developing a new life; the ultimate destiny of the combined journeys of human persons is the coming of the Kingdom; all humans are offered eternal life in and through Jesus Christ and the chief and central manifestation of this new life in Christ is the love for each other that manifests in concrete forms of justice, gratitude, forbearance, and chastity. For a more detailed analysis, see McCormick, *Health and Medicine in the Catholic Tradition*, 49.

[30]Ibid., 106-107.

[31]To clarify the position that the human person is the crown of creation, McCormick writes: "The fact that the universe antedated human life by millions of years and will be around after life as we know it has disappeared can be read as God's lavish way of presenting human life precisely as the crown of the universe. The actor remains central even though and when the stage is empty and when the show is, so to speak, over. We have seen such lavishness throughout the natural kingdom. Lavishness may be viewed as highlighting rather than decentralizing human life." Richard A. McCormick, S.J., "Gustafson's God: Who? What? Where? (ETC.)," *Journal of Religious Ethics* 13 (1985): 57.

[32]The models and metaphors for viewing and interpreting our experience that correspond to the triad of creation-fall-redemption have their roots in scripture, especially in St. Paul and St. John. Some of these models and metaphors are the following: light-darkness-enlightenment, freedom-bondage-liberation, integrity-brokenness-reintegration, health-sickness-healing, and peace-estrangement-reconciliation. The secular variants of these models are: "ship-shape," "down-and-out," "on-the-mend." McCormick, *Corrective Vision*, 64-65.

[33]Ibid., 65.

[34]Ibid.

[35]Ibid., 66.

[36]McCormick, "Theology and Bioethics," *Theology and Bioethics*, 100.

[37]McCormick agrees with James Gustafson that God is not only the creator and preserver of order; God is the enabler of our possibilities. Earlier theologians put more emphasis on the creator-preserver perspective of God, which leads to a notion that God is directly and immediately involved in human causality, a kind of creationism. McCormick follows the analysis originally proposed by Karl Rahner which conceived of God as the transcendental ground of all created reality causally active only through created secondary causes. This will have a profound influence on how McCormick shapes moral arguments. For a more detailed analysis of this perspective, see McCormick, "Moral Arguments in Christian Ethics," *Journal of Contemporary Health, Law, and Policy*, 1 (1985): 7-8. See also James Gustafson, *The Contributions of Theology to Medical Ethics* (Milwaukee, WI: Marquette University Press, 1975).

[38]Richard A. McCormick, S.J., "Biomedical Advances and the Catholic Perspective," in *Contemporary Ethical Issues in the Jewish and Christian Traditions*, ed. Frederick E. Greenspahn (Hoboken, NJ: Ktav Publishing House, Inc., 1986), 41.

[39]Richard A. McCormick, S.J., "Who or What is the Pre-embryo?" *Kennedy Institute of Ethics Journal* 1 (March 1991): 12.

[40]Odozor writes that for McCormick, "In these circumstances therefore, good and evil are closely intertwined, and the good we achieve often comes at the price of deprivation and imperfection. Thus, we must kill to preserve life and freedom; we protect one through the pain of another; our education must at times be punitive; our health is preserved at times by pain and disfiguring mutilation; we protect our secrets by misstatements and our marriages and population by contraception and sterilization. Every choice is therefore a sacrifice that could bring about mixed and ambiguous results. Furthermore, finitude implies a practical limitation on human capacity to love. Although McCormick believes that the ideal to love one another as Christ loves us must be pursued constantly, he also understands that there are limits to what each finite creature can do. To refuse to accept this limitation is to fail to recognize that to impose perfect love on imperfect creatures is a disproportionate demand capable of turning creatures from God and in fact turns them into God." Odozor, *Richard A. McCormick and the Renewal of Moral Theology*, 78; see also McCormick, *Health and Medicine in the Catholic Tradition*, 46; Idem, *Doing Evil to Achieve Good*, 49.

[41]McCormick, "Theology and Bioethics," *Theology and Bioethics*, 102.

[42]McCormick, *The Critical Calling*, 268.

[43]Odozor, *Richard A. McCormick and the Renewal of Moral Theology*, 77.

[44]McCormick's notion of the human person being created in the image and likeness of God corresponds to Janssens' view of the human person as a bodily subject in relationship with God. Janssens argues that human persons are to know and worship God in all they do. The God-relationship is the most profound and ultimate aspect of the person.

[45]McCormick, *The Critical Calling*, 268.

[46]McCormick, "The Judaeo-Christian Tradition and Bioethical Codes," *How Brave a New World?*, 10-11. Emphasis in the original.

[47]Richard A. McCormick, S.J., "The Moral Theology of Vatican II," in *The Future of Ethics and Moral Theology* (Chicago, IL: Argus Communications Co., 1968), 17.

[48]McCormick, *Corrective Vision*, 59. See also Karl Rahner, *Foundations of Christian Faith* (New York: Seabury Press, 1978), 93-97; and Ronald Modras, "The Implications of Rahner's Anthropology For Fundamental Moral Theology," *Horizons* 12 (1985): 70-90. Odozor argues that McCormick's notion of "basic freedom" has six characteristics: "(1) It is free. It is within the power, and it is the responsibility of the moral agent to realize 'the fundamental posture or orientation toward the ultimate good of human life' through object choices and a fundamental option or self-disposition. (2) It is supernatural because the radical disposition of the self characteristic of fundamental option is inconceivable without divine empowerment under the grace of the Spirit. (3) It is obscure. Fundamental freedom is located at the deepest level of human consciousness and thus excludes adequate conceptual and propositional formulation. (4) Although it defies total conceptualization, basic freedom is still conscious without objective formulation. (5) We cannot say with certainty when a moral agent opts for openness toward God and the world or makes a negative commitment against them. (6) Fundamental freedom is a definite and total commitment, which 'excludes the possibility of a series of quickly repeated transitions between life and death.'" Odozor, *Richard A. McCormick and the Renewal of Moral Theology*, 84-85; see also McCormick, *The Critical Calling*, 174-175.

[49]McCormick, "The New Morality," 770.

[50]Odozor, *Richard A. McCormick and the Renewal of Moral Theology*, 83.

[51]Ibid., 78-79; see also McCormick, "The New Morality," 771.

[52]McCormick, *Health and Medicine in the Catholic Tradition*, 17.

[53]McCormick's view of the uniqueness and diversity of the human person corresponds to Janssens' concept of the person as a subject, a historical being, and Janssens' notion of human persons as fundamentally equal.

[54]It should be noted that what McCormick is trying to emphasize here is that we must respect all people. He fears that "diagnostic and eugenic interventions that would bypass, downplay, or flatten these diversities and uniqueness should be viewed as temptations. We have a mixed history in the United States regarding sterilization of the retarded and other 'undesirables.'" Our creation in God's image requires us to treat all people with dignity and respect. For a more detailed analysis, see McCormick, *The Critical Calling*, 268-269.

[55]McCormick, "The Judaeo-Christian Tradition and Bioethical Codes," *How Brave a New World?*, 12. Emphasis in the original.

[56]The social and relational aspect of McCormick's view of the human person is similar to Janssens' view of the human person as living in social groups and the human person as essentially interpersonal.

[57]McCormick, "The Judaeo-Christian Tradition and Bioethical Codes," *How Brave a New World?*, 12.

[58] Further McCormick writes: "Assumption into Christ means assumption into His Body, His People. We cannot exist as Christians except in a community, and we cannot define ourselves except as 'of a Body.' Hence it is Christianly axiomatic that the community of believers (the Church) is the extension of the Incarnation. It is similarly axiomatic that those actions wherein we initiate into, fortify, restore, and intensify the Christlife (the Christian sacraments) are at once Christ's actions and the actions of the community." Ibid.

[59]McCormick, "Biomedical Advances and the Catholic Perspective," 44.

[60]McCormick, "The Judaeo-Christian Tradition and Bioethical Codes," *How Brave a New World?*, 12-13.

[61]McCormick, "Bioethical Advances and the Catholic Perspective," 44-45.

[62]Ibid. Emphasis in the original.

[63]McCormick, "The Judaeo-Christian Tradition and Bioethical Codes," *How Brave A New World?*, 14.

[64]McCormick, "Man's Moral Responsibility for Health," 17.

[65] Rahner writes: "Christian love of neighbor is both in potency and in act a moment of the infused supernatural theological virtue of *caritas* by which we love God in his Spirit for his own sake and in direct community with him. This means, therefore, that the love of neighbor is not merely the preparation, effect, fruit and touchstone of the love of God but is itself an act of this love of God itself; in other words, it is at least an act within that total believing and hoping surrender of man to God which we call love and which alone justifies man, i.e., hands him over to God, because, being supported by the loving self-communication of God in the

uncreated grace of the Holy Spirit, it really unites man with God, not as He is recognized by us but as He is in Himself in His absolute divinity." Karl Rahner, "Reflections on the Unity of the Love of Neighbor and the Love of God," *Theological Investigations* vol. 6 (Baltimore, MD: Helicon, 1969), 236.

[66]McCormick, *Health and Medicine in the Catholic Tradition*, 54. Emphasis in the original.

[67]McCormick, *The Critical Calling*, 12.

[68]This refers to 1 Corinthians 15: 28—"And when everything is subject to him, then the Son himself will be subject in his turn to the One who subjected all things to him, so that God may be all in all."

[69]I have stated earlier that because McCormick cites Janssens' eight essential aspects of the human person, it is fair to conclude that they reflect his own anthropology.

[70]The transformation of the natural order is referring to the positive and negative uses of science and technology. Vatican II notes that "technology is now transforming the face of the earth and is already trying to master outer space." "Pastoral Constitution on the Church in the Modern World," no. 5, 203.

[71]Ibid., no. 34, 232.

[72]McCormick, *Health and Medicine in the Catholic Tradition*, 16. McCormick also quotes John Macquarrie to reinforce his position. Macquarrie writes: "The doctrines of creation and providence make possible an ultimate trust but at the cost of imposing an ultimate responsibility. We are not only creatures, but co-creators with God who 'have a share in shaping an as yet fluid and plastic world—a world in which the most fluid entity is human nature itself.'" McCormick, "Bioethics and Method," 310. See also John Macquarrie, in *Christian Theology: A Case Study Approach*, eds. Robert A. Evans and Thomas D. Parker (New York: Harper and Row, 1976), 94.

[73]McCormick, "Bioethics and Method," 310.

[74] "ADA deficiency syndrome is a purine salvage pathway enzyme that converts adenosine and deoxyadenosine to inosine and deoxyinosine, respectively. ADA deficiency results in elevated quantities of deoxyadenosine triphosphate, which inhibits DNA synthesis. These children may be normal at birth but develop progressive immunologic impairment as deoxyATP accumulates." For a detailed analysis, see *The Merck Manual*, 315.

[75]McCormick, *The Critical Calling*, 262.

[76]McCormick, *The Critical Calling*, 50. See also Denzinger-Schonmetzer, *Enchiridion Symbolorum* (Barcelona: Herder, 1963), no. 2853.

[77]Odozor argues that for McCormick, sin is not the only cause of ambiguity in human choice. Odozor states: "Ambiguity is primarily a result of the human condition, a result of human creaturehood and finitude. To argue otherwise would be to imply that sin is the cause of human finitude and creaturehood and to suggest that but for sin, all constraints to human knowing and doing would be nonexistent. McCormick does not subscribe to such a view. Because he acknowledges ambiguity he also acknowledges conflicts in moral decision-making." Odozor, *Richard A. McCormick and the Renewal of Moral Theology*, 171.

[78]McCormick, *Health and Medicine in the Catholic Tradition*, 46.

[79]McCormick, "The Moral Theology of Vatican II," 16.

[80]McCormick, *Corrective Vision*, 57-58.

[81]McCormick, "The Moral Theology of Vatican II," 14.

[82]Ibid.

[83] Richard A. McCormick, S.J., "Personal Conscience," *Chicago Studies* 13 (Fall 1974): 248-250. McCormick continues: "It is the rupture of a covenant relationship with the God of salvation and therefore also with His people, the Church. Since mortal sin is a denial of charity, it bespeaks the death of the life of friendship with God. If such a mortal illness becomes one's final option, it effects eternal death. But as long as it is not final and definitive conversion is possible, but only with the grace of Christ." This type of personal upheaval does not usually occur except in matters that are sufficiently grave. For McCormick, "serious matter is that concrete human disorder likely to provoke an individual to the use of basic freedom in the rejection of God. It is that peak moment in which a person can embody and seal a disintegrating relationship with the God of salvation. Whether an individual does sever his relationship with God (commit mortal sin), we generally cannot say with certainty." Ibid.

[84]Ibid., 249. McCormick writes: "Venial sin, committed as it is at a less central level of person, is compatible with love of God (charity) alive in the depths of the soul. But it undermines the fervor of charity and, over a period of time, can dispose one for the commission of mortal sin." Ibid.

[85] McCormick writes: "The power of sin in the world, even the redeemed world, remains virulent and manifests itself in oppressive and enslaving structures, both individual and social, that touch us all. Individually we are anxious, neurotic, physically ill, selfish, emotionally crippled, instinctively limited. Socially our structures prevent equality of opportunity, reinforce poverty and greed, discriminate. All these things isolate and divide us and inhibit our growth as loving persons." McCormick, *The Critical Calling*, 307.

[86]McCormick, *Corrective Vision*, 18.

[87]Ibid., 65.

[88]McCormick, *The Critical Calling*, 307.

[89]McCormick's phrase "new creatures" appears to come from 2 Corinthians 5:17—"And for anyone who is in Christ, there is a new creation, the old creation has gone, and now the new one is here." In referring to the love commandment McCormick writes: "This is the new law (John 13:34) since it is internal, 'natural' to the new creature (2 Cor. 5:17), . . ." McCormick, "Theology and Bioethics," *Theology and Bioethics*, 103.

[90]McCormick, *Health and Medicine in the Catholic Tradition*, 49.

[91]Ibid.

[92]McCormick, *Corrective Vision*, 57.

[93]McCormick, "Theology and Bioethics," *Theology and Bioethics*, 106-107.

[94]When McCormick speaks of Jesus as the standard of our love he means "that Jesus' love was that of absolute righteousness or purity of heart. That is, it was a love shaped by the absoluteness and ultimacy of the God-relationship." Ibid., 106.

[95]McCormick, *Health and Medicine in the Catholic Tradition*, 46.

[96]For a more detailed analysis of the categorizing of McCormick's writings into three distinct periods, refer to Chapter One, Richard A. McCormick, S.J.—Moral Theologian. It is interesting to note that in the first period of his writing, 1957-1967, McCormick was still operating within the classicist mentality. During this time he wrote his dissertation (510 pages) entitled, "The Removal of a Fetus Probably Dead to Save the Life of the Mother." The word "God" is used only five times and there are no references to "Jesus" or "Christ." It is in the third period, from 1983 to 1999, when McCormick decides to write primarily in the area of bioethics from a theological perspective that he introduces theological notions such as: "new creature," Christology, incarnation, and eschatology. However, he fails to fully develop them.

[97]McCormick, *Health and Medicine in the Catholic Tradition*, 27.

[98]Ibid., 28.

[99]McCormick, *Corrective Vision*, 66. It should be noted here that while McCormick utilizes much of Karl Rahner's anthropology Rahner would not agree with McCormick's notion of "being transformed totally." Freedom, for Rahner, entails the "whole self" making a decision. But because the human person can never fully integrate all aspects of his or her self, one can never give one's self totally over to either good or evil. See Rahner, *Foundations of Christian Faith*, 97-106; and Idem, "The Fundamental Option," *Theological Investigations* vol. VI, 181-188.

[100]McCormick, "Theology and Bioethics," *Theology and Bioethics*, 107. Emphasis in the original.

[101]McCormick, "Moral Theology of Vatican II," 17.

[102]McCormick, *The Critical Calling*, 12.

[103]Ibid., 12-13.

[104]Ibid., 308.

[105]McCormick, "Gustafson's God: Who? What? Where? (ETC.),"59. Emphasis in the original.

[106]McCormick, "Theology and Bioethics" *Theology and Bioethics*, 100.

[107]McCormick, *Health and Medicine in the Catholic Tradition*, 51.

[108]McCormick, "The Judaeo-Christian Tradition and Bioethical Codes," *How Brave a New World?*, 9.

[109]McCormick, "The Moral Theology of Vatican II," 11.

[110]McCormick, *Corrective Vision*, 25.

[111]Ibid., 25-26.

[112]According to Robert Krieg: "A Christology 'from above,' or a 'descending Christology,' starts with an understanding of the triune God and the mystery of God's self-disclosure within creation and history and then moves to reflection upon God's entering into history in Jesus Christ (the Incarnation), his ministry, and his suffering, death, and resurrection. A Christology 'from below,' or an 'ascending Christology,' begins with the humanity of Jesus and/or a historical recollection of Jesus' message, ministry, and destiny and then proceeds to consider Jesus' Resurrection and relationship with God." For a more detailed analysis, see Robert E. Krieg, "Christology," *Encyclopedia of Catholicism*, 311.

[113]See Charles E. Curran, "The Person as Moral Agent and Subject in Light of Contemporary Christology,"in *Called to Love: Toward A Contemporary Christian Ethic*, 24-25.

[114]McCormick, "Theology and Biomedical Ethics," 315.

[115]McCormick, "Moral Arguments in Christian Ethics," *Journal of Contemporary Health Law and Policy*, 1 (1985): 23.

[116]McCormick, "Gustafson's God: Who? What? Where (ETC.)," 60. To clarify this view McCormick quotes Joseph Sittler and writes: "As a result of God's concrete act in the Incarnation, 'human life has available a new relation to God, a new light for seeing, a new fact and center for thinking, a new ground for giving and loving, a new context for acting in this world.'" McCormick, *Corrective Vision*, 26. See also Joseph Sittler, *The Structure of Christian Ethics* (New Orleans, LA: Louisiana State University Press, 1958), 18.

[117]McCormick, *Health and Medicine in the Catholic Tradition*, 49.

[118]McCormick, "The Primacy of Charity," 21.

[119]Ibid., 25.

[120]Michael E. Allsopp, "Deontic and Epistemic Authority in Roman Catholic Ethics: The Case of Richard McCormick," *Christian Bioethics* 2 (1996): 102.

[121]McCormick, *Health and Medicine in the Catholic Tradition*, 49. For an excellent account of eschatology (the study of last things), individual eschatology (the study of the final condition of individual human beings), and universal eschatology (the study of the final state of the universe, the total goal toward which God is moving all creation), see John H. Wright, "Eschatology," *Encyclopedia of Catholicism*, 476-477.

[122]Charles E. Curran, *Politics, Medicine, and Christian Ethics: A Dialogue with Paul Ramsey* (Philadelphia, PA: Fortress Press, 1973), 201.

[123]McCormick, "The Judaeo-Christian Tradition and Bioethical Codes," *How Brave a New World?*, 16.

[124] Theologian Peter C. Phan of the Catholic University of America elaborates on this notion by stating: "Eschatology is an aetiological account from the present situation of sin and grace forward into its final stage of final fulfillment and not an anticipatory description of what will happen at the end of time and beyond. Eschatology is anthropology conjugated in the future tense on the basis of Christology." I believe that McCormick would agree with this evaluation. Peter C. Phan, "Contemporary Contexts and Issues In Eschatology," *Theological Studies* 55 (September 1994): 515-516.

[125]Harvey Cox articulates three distinct views of eschatology—apocalyptic, teleological, and prophetic. Cox writes: "Classical apocalyptic imagery included both a vision of catastrophe and holocaust (the *dies irae*) and a celebration of the restored and glorious new world it would usher in. . . . It also breeds a fantasy of an elect who will be saved from the catastrophe and who will be called to rule the new world." The teleological view "sees the world and the human person evolving, but the evolutionary process proceeds toward a state which will be identical with that from which it began. The *telos* is the recapitulation of the *arche*." Harvey Cox, "Evolutionary Progress and Christian Promise," *Concilium*, vol. 26, ed. Johannes Metz (New York: Paulist Press, 1967), 35-47.

[126]Ibid., 45-47.

[127]McCormick, *Corrective Vision*, 6.

[128] I believe this also serves as the basis for McCormick's notion of development of doctrine in the Church. The development of doctrine involves both continuity and change. That means that the formulations of its moral convictions are also *in via*, never finished and always in need of improvement, updating, and adjustment to changing circumstances. For a

more detailed analysis, see McCormick, *The Critical Calling*, 339-340; and Idem, *Corrective Vision*, 76-81.

[129]McCormick, *Health and Medicine in the Catholic Tradition*, 107.

[130]McCormick, "Biomedical Advances and the Catholic Perspective," 38.

[131]McCormick levels this criticism against Paul Ramsey. McCormick writes: "This is the crux of my problem with Paul Ramsey's 'medical indications policy' with regard to dying—as if such judgments were exclusively scientific in character." Ibid.

[132]Ibid.

[133]Ibid., 39.

[134]For a more detailed analysis, see McCormick, "Theology and Bioethics," *Corrective Vision*, 141-148; and Cahill, "On Richard McCormick," 88.

[135]McCormick, "Theology and Bioethics," *Theology and Bioethics*, 97.

[136]Lisa Sowle Cahill states: "McCormick identifies the good 'higher' than human life as the capacity for relationships of love. This good is related to religious commitment because love of God is accomplished through love of neighbor, a claim made with particular force by contemporary Catholic neo-Thomists such as Karl Rahner and Josef Fuchs." Lisa Sowle Cahill, "On Richard McCormick," 92. See also Josef Fuchs, S.J., "Christian Existence and Love of Neighbor," *Personal Responsibility and Christian Morality* (Washington, DC: Georgetown University Press, 1983), 28-31; and Karl Rahner, "Reflections on the Unity of the Love of Neighbor and the Love of God," 231-249.

[137]McCormick, "Theology and Bioethics," *Theology and Bioethics*, 97.

[138]McCormick writes: "Thus the death of the Christian is viewed as the fulfillment of the life of grace, the completion of the sacraments, as a step toward the coming of God's kingdom, as a sharing of one side of Christ's paschal mystery. As such, it is clearly a decisive moment in each person's life. For it is viewed as fixing for all eternity a person's intention. At this moment the soul ceases to act in fundamentally changeable ways. The 'period of probation' is over." McCormick, *Health and Medicine in the Catholic Tradition*, 121.

[139]McCormick, "Theology and Bioethics," *Theology and Bioethics*, 97. McCormick writes: "Life is indeed a basic and precious good, but a good to be preserved precisely as a condition of other values. It is these other values and possibilities that found the duty to preserve physical life and that also dictate the limits of this duty. In other words, life is a relative good, and the duty to preserve it is a limited one. These limits have

always been stated in terms of *means* required to sustain life." McCormick, "To Save or Let Die," *How Brave a New World?*, 345. Emphasis in the original.

[140]Pope Pius XII, "The Prolongation of Life," *Acta Apostolicae Sedis* 49 (1957): 1,031-1,032.

[141]McCormick, "Theology and Bioethics," *Theology and Bioethics*, 97-98.

[142]McCormick, "To Save or Let Die," *How Brave a New World?*, 347.

[143]McCormick, "In the Best Interests of the Baby,"24. Necrotizing enterocolitis is a condition predominantly seen in premature neonates, which is characterized by partial- or full-thickness intestinal ischemia, usually involving the terminal ileum. This neonatal anomaly will be examined in depth in Chapter Five.

[144]McCormick, "Health and Medicine in the Catholic Tradition," *Acta Hospitalia* 26 (1986): 57.

[145]McCormick, "The Judaeo-Christian Tradition and Bioethical Codes," *How Brave a New World?*, 14.

[146]Ibid.

[147]McCormick, "Biomedical Advances and the Catholic Perspective," 43. See also James Gustafson, *The Contribution of Theology to Medical Ethics*, 85-86.

[148]McCormick, "The Quality of Life, the Sanctity of Life," *How Brave a New World?*, 405.

[149]McCormick writes: "One can say and, I believe, should say that the *person* is always an incalculable value, but that at some point continuance in physical life offers the person no benefit. Indeed, to keep 'life' going can easily be an assault on the person and his or her dignity." Ibid., 406. Emphasis in the original.

[150]McCormick argues that the well-being of human persons is interdependent. McCormick writes: "It cannot be conceived of or realistically pursued independently of the good of others. Social insertion is part of our being and becoming. As Joseph Sittler words it, 'personhood is a social state.'" McCormick, "Biomedical Advances and the Catholic Perspective," 44-45. See also Joseph Sittler, *Grace Notes and Other Fragments* (Philadelphia, PA: Fortune Press, 1981), 98.

[151]McCormick, "Some Neglected Aspects of Moral Responsibility for Health," *How Brave a New World?*, 42.

[152]McCormick's notion of personhood will also have implications for the pre-embryo. He will draw a distinction between genetic individuality and developmental individuality. Genetic individuality occurs at the union of sperm and ovum at fertilization that yields a new hereditary con-

stitution called a zygote. It is a unique genetic individual with the potential to become an adult, but it is a theoretical and statistical potential because only a small minority actually achieve this in the natural process. Developmental individuality occurs when there is a source of only one individual. This does not occur until a single body axis has begun to form, near the end of the second week post fertilization when implantation is underway. McCormick's point is that developmental individuality (singleness) is essential to personhood. The pre-embryo is viewed as a "potential person" because it has the potential for relationality and therefore should be treated with dignity and respect. For a more detailed analysis, see Richard A. McCormick, S. J., "The First 14 Days," *The Tablet* 10 March 1990, p. 301-304; Idem, "Who or What is a Preembryo?," 1-15; and Idem, "The Embryo as Potential: A Reply to John A. Robertson," *The Kennedy Institute of Ethics Journal* 1 (December 1991) 303-305.

[153]An example of a handicapped neonate whose potential for human relationships is simply nonexistent would be one with anencephaly (the neonate lacks a cerebrum and skull). An example of a handicapped neonate whose life is utterly submerged and undeveloped in the mere struggle to survive would be one with a Grade IV massive intraventricular hemorrhage (an untreatable neurological condition that leads to death). A more detailed analysis of both anomalies will be given in Chapter Five.

[154]McCormick, "To Save or Let Die?" *How Brave A New World?*, 348-349.

[155]Ibid., 350. Emphasis in the original.

[156]Sparks, *To Treat or Not To Treat?*, 168.

[157]McCormick, *The Critical Calling*, 268.

[158]McCormick, "The Judaeo-Christian Tradition and Bioethical Codes," *How Brave a New World?*, 10-11.

[159]McCormick, *The Critical Calling*, 268.

[160]McCormick writes: "Quality-of-life assessments ought to be made within an over-all reverence for life, as an extension of one's respect for the sanctity of life. However, there are times when preserving the life of one with no capacity for those aspects of life that we regard as *human* is a violation of the sanctity of life itself. Thus to separate the two approaches and call one *sanctity of life*, and the other *quality of life*, is a false conceptual split that very easily suggests that the term 'sanctity of life' is being used in an exhortatory way." McCormick, "The Sanctity of Life, The Quality of Life," *How Brave a New World?*, 407. Emphasis in the original. It should be noted that this assessment will be discussed in more depth in Chapter Four.

[161]Ibid. Emphasis in the original.

[162]McCormick, "Man's Moral Responsibility for Health," 9.

[163]Palliative care is aimed at controlling pain, relieving discomfort, and aiding dysfunction of various sorts.

[164]McCormick, "The Judaeo-Christian Tradition and Bioethical Codes," *How Brave a New World?*, 12-13.

[165]Ibid., 13.

[166]See Richard A. McCormick, S.J. and John Paris, S.J., "Saving Defective Infants: Options for Life or Death," *How Brave a New World?*, 352-361.

[167]Pope Pius XII, "The Prolongation of Life," *The Pope Speaks* 4 (1958): 394. Emphasis added.

[168]McCormick, "To Save or Let Die," *How Brave a New World?*, 347. McCormick also quotes Gerald Kelly, S.J., to help substantiate his position: "One need not spend money or incur a debt which would impose a very great hardship on himself or his family, because this kind of hardship would be more than 'reasonable' or 'moderate' care of health and therefore more than God would ordinarily demand." Gerald Kelly, S.J., *Medico-Moral Problems* (St. Louis, MO: The Catholic Health Association of the United States and Canada, 1957), 132.

[169]Odozor, *Richard A. McCormick and the Renewal of Moral Theology*, 80.

[170]McCormick, "The Judaeo-Christian Tradition and Bioethical Codes," *How Brave a New World?*, 13. According to social ethicist David Hollenbach: "Recent official Catholic teaching has presented two complementary interpretations of the meaning of the classical concept of the common good. First, *Gaudium et Spes* stated that humans were created by God not for life in isolation but for the formation of social unity (*Gaudium et Spes*, no. 32). The communitarian character of human existence means that the good of each person is bound up with the good of the community. . . . Second, the common good is defined as 'the sum total of conditions of social living, whereby persons are enabled more fully and readily to achieve their own perfection'" (*Mater et Magistra*, no. 65; and *Gaudium et Spes*, no. 26). David Hollenbach, S.J., "Common Good," in *The New Dictionary of Catholic Social Thought*, ed. Judith A. Dwyer (Wilmington, DE: Glazier, 1994), 192-197. Odozor believes that McCormick's position on "the common good" is highly nuanced. There are things that we all, children included, have to do in virtue of social justice. Involvement in non-therapeutic experimentation (even in the case of children and other incompetent subjects) is an issue of social justice if it does not involve undue burden. Odozor, *Richard A. McCormick and the Renewal of Moral Theology*, 81. Lisa Sowle Cahill points out that the concept of the common good from which McCormick argues "is distinc-

tive in its comprehension of all persons equally and by its ordering to a transcendent communion, that of persons in God. McCormick defines justifiable experimentation on the premise that communal interaction is an essential component of the realization of values, and proposes it with the conviction that those values persons 'tend towards' or seek are common ones." Lisa Sowle Cahill, "Within Shouting Distance: Paul Ramsey and Richard McCormick On Method," *Journal of Medicine and Philosophy* 4 (December 1979): 402.

[171]This category would include choices involving notable risk, discomfort, inconvenience. McCormick argues that such works are done based on "individual generosity and charity." This shows that McCormick is aware of the possibility of abuse by sacrificing the rights of the individual to the welfare of the entire community. See McCormick, "Proxy Consent in the Experimentation Situation," *How Brave a New World?*, 67; see also Idem, "Public Policy and Fetal Research," *How Brave a New World?*, 72.

[172]McCormick, *Corrective Vision*, 145.

[173]Leonard Weber elaborates on the difference between causing suffering and enduring suffering. Weber writes: "To cause suffering is something that we should always try to avoid when possible. But to endure suffering is not always evil. Suffering is a little like death: it is terrible to bring it about unnecessarily, but one can often act nobly in accepting it." Leonard Weber, *Who Shall Live?*, 100.

[174]McCormick, *Health and Medicine in the Catholic Tradition*, 116-117.

[175]Ibid., 118.

[176]McCormick's view on suffering as a form of dependence on God is influenced by Drew Christiansen's theology of dependence. Suffering is a form of dependence on God where Christians enter more deeply into the paschal mystery. McCormick writes: "Dependence is an opportunity, a call to let ourselves go, to open up to God, to cling in trust to a power beyond our control, to see more clearly than ever the source and end of life, much as Christ did in his dying dependence on the Father. Suffering leads to dependence on others. Dependence on others should be a sign of a more radical dependence on God. Since our freedom is intended to lead us to a deeper union with God, it is an interesting paradox that our deep dependence on God establishes our own radical independence: independence in dependence." McCormick, *Corrective Vision*, 145. See also Drew Christiansen, S.J., "The Elderly and Their Families: The Problems of Dependence," *New Catholic World* 223 (1980): 100-104.

[177]See Paul Ramsey, *Ethics on the Edges of Life*, 212-227; and Weir, *Selective Nontreatment of Handicapped Newborns*, 168-169.

[178]See Joseph Fletcher, "Infanticide and the Ethics of Loving Care," in *Infanticide and the Value of Life*, 15-20; and Idem, "Ethics and Euthanasia," *American Journal of Nursing* 73 (April 1973): 670-675.

[179]McCormick, "New Medicine and Morality," 316.

[180]McCormick borrowed the phrase "virtually exceptionless norm" from Donald Evans. It means that the theoretical possible exceptions are virtually zero in the practical probability. For a more detailed analysis, see Donald Evans, "Paul Ramsey on Exceptionless Moral Rules," *The American Journal of Jurisprudence* 16 (1971): 184-214. Lisa Sowle Cahill states: "In an earlier article on death and dying McCormick (referring to the work of Germain Grisez and John Finnis) locates life—at least that of the innocent—among the 'basic values' that may never be sacrificed directly. He agrees that although occasionally good reasons may exist for omitting life-sustaining measures, the proposition that there is no proportionate reason for directly dispatching a terminal or dying patient has yet to be refuted. Weighing against direct euthanasia are the possible short- and long-term effects of accepting acts of commission. The 'presumption of a common and universal danger' establishes at least a 'virtually exceptionless' norm against it. This is a social consideration that obviously moves beyond—though not necessarily making obsolete—the older Catholic approach that upholds the 'individual's right to life' in any consideration of direct killing." Lisa Sowle Cahill, "On Richard McCormick," 96-97.

[181]McCormick, "Public Policy on Abortion," *How Brave a New World?*, 197.

[182]It should be noted that God's gifts to humankind also refer to animals. Medical advances, including transplantation techniques have been developed thanks to the sacrifice of a variety of animals. Due to animal research and the use of animal organs, a young infant born with a hypoplastic left ventricle heart (an infant missing the major pumping chamber of the heart), an affliction that caused death for most infants only a few years ago, now has the possibility of being saved. The use of animals for research has caused a great controversy with animal rights groups. McCormick would argue that animals can be used in research as long as the experiments are well designed and are for the good of humanity. For a more detailed analysis, see John D. Aquilino, "Life or Death?: A Parent's Plea for Civility and Reason," *Chicago Tribune*, 26 July 1995, 15.

[183]McCormick, "Bioethics and Method," 310.

[184]McCormick writes: "In relating to the basic human values, several images of man are possible, as Callahan has observed. First, there is the power-plasticity model. In this model, nature is alien, independent of man, possessing no inherent value. It is capable of being used, domi-

nated, and shaped by man. Man sees himself as possessing an unrestricted right to manipulate in the service of his goals. Death is something to be overcome, outwitted. Second, there is the sacral-symbiotic model. In its religious forms, nature is seen as God's creation, to be respected and heeded. Man is not the master; he is the steward and nature is a trust. In secular forms, man is seen as part of nature. If man is to be respected, so is nature. We should live in harmony and balance with nature. Nature is a teacher, showing us how to live with it. Death is one of the rhythms of nature, to be gracefully accepted." McCormick, "The Judaeo-Christian Tradition and Bioethical Codes," *How Brave a New World?*, 7. See also Daniel Callahan, "Living with the New Biology," *Center Magazine* 5 (1972): 4-12.

[185]McCormick, "Some Neglected Aspects of Moral Responsibility for Health," *How Brave a New World?*, 43.

[186]Richard A. McCormick, S.J., "Technology and Morality: The Example of Medicine," *New Theology Review* 2 (November 1989): 32.

[187]McCormick, *The Critical Calling*, xi.

[188]This is in contrast to a theologian like Charles E. Curran, who is quite explicit about the content of his theological stance. It includes the five mysteries of faith: creation, sin, incarnation, redemption, and resurrection/destiny. See Richard Grecco, *Theology of Compromise: A Study in the Ethics of Charles E. Curran* (New York: Peter Lang Publishers, 1991), 1-53.

[189]See McCormick, "Gustafson's God: Who? What? Where? (ETC)," 58.

[190]McCormick, *The Critical Calling*, 67.

[191]Allsopp, 101.

[192]McCormick, "Gustafson's God: Who? What? Where? (ETC)," 59.

[193]Kenneth R. Himes, O. F. M., "The Contribution of Theology to Catholic Moral Theology," in *Moral Theology: Challenges for the Future*, 64.

[194] One contemporary theologian who has expressed the notion of "relation" in the Trinity in a coherent and relevant manner is Leonardo Boff. Boff writes: "The fact that the Son proceeds from the Father and the Spirit from the Father and the Son as from one beginning, means that there are mutual relationships between the three Persons. 'Relationship' means an ordering of one Person to another, a connection between each of the divine Three. . . . As already inferred, the relationships constitute the Persons; in other words, it is through relationship that one Person is situated in relation to the others and differentiated from them, each essentially supposing and requiring the others. So the Father supposes the Son; the Son necessitates the Father; the Holy Spirit can be understood

only in the breathing-out by the Father and the Son. The Persons are mutually distinguished (one from another) and required (one situating the others)." Leonardo Boff, *Trinity and Society* (New York: Orbis Books, 1988), 91-92. See also Jurgen Moltmann, *History of the Triune God: Contributions to Trinitarian Theology* (London: SCM, 1991); and Idem, *The Trinity and the Kingdom: The Doctrine of God* (San Francisco, CA: Harper and Row, 1981).

[195]McCormick's interpretation of the social nature of the human person also comes from the Documents of Vatican II. The fathers at Vatican II argue that being created in the image and likeness of God means creation for community, not isolation. See "Pastoral Constitution on the Church in the Modern World," nos. 12, 32.

[196]See Pius XII, "The Prolongation of Life," *The Pope Speaks*, 394.

[197]See Kelly, *Medico-Moral Problems*, 132.

[198]Sparks, *To Treat or Not to Treat?*, 198.

[199]Ibid.

[200]McCartney is referring to Richard A. McCormick, S.J., and John J. Paris, S.J., "Saving Defective Infants: Options for Life or Death," *America* 148 (April 23, 1983): 313-317.

[201]McCormick and Paris, "Saving Defective Infants," *How Brave a New World?*, 358-359.

[202]James McCartney, "Issues in Death and Dying," in *Moral Theology: Challenges for the Future*, 279.

[203]The articles referred to are: McCormick, "Proxy Consent in the Experimentation Situation," *How Brave a New World?*, 51-71; and Idem, "Sharing in Sociality: Children and Experimentation," *How Brave a New World?*, 87-98.

[204]Sparks, *To Treat or Not to Treat?*, 199.

[205]McCormick, "To Save or Let Die," *How Brave a New World?*, 347. See also M. Zalba, *Theologiae Moralis Summa* 3 (Madrid: *La Editorial Catolica*, 1957), II, 71.

[206]Sparks cites two other reasons for why McCormick fails to apply social and familial factors in a broader manner. First, if social and familial factors are allowed to overrule a relationally able infant's presumed interest in therapy, the subsequent nontreatment would indeed harm the patient left untreated. Death or a more burdened quality of life seem inevitable. Therefore, contrary to the pain-free experimentation premise, incorporation of social factors in these cases cannot help but harm the patient, at least if nontreatment and foreseen death are considered not in the infant's best interest. Second, it is not clear that McCormick and Paris absolutely exclude all social burden factors. In their joint *America* article they assert that familial factors ought not dictate an infant's access

to treatment, since behind one's nuclear family there is a second line of social support or defense, the society. They decline to speculate whether the cost of handicapped care exceeds a society's (finite) resources or the demands in justice for its equitable distribution. See Sparks, *To Treat or Not to Treat?*, 199-200.

[207]Himes, "The Contribution of Theology to Catholic Moral Theology," in *Moral Theology: Challenges for the Future*, 67.

[208]Ibid., 68.

[209]Ibid.

[210]McCormick, *The Critical Calling*, 144.

[211]McCormick, "Theology and Biomedical Ethics," 312.

[212]McCormick, *Corrective Vision*, 57.

[213]McCormick, *The Critical Calling*, 98.

3

Moral Epistemology

INTRODUCTION

Claims to moral knowledge are always made within specific traditions of thought and practice. To understand McCormick's ethical position on treatment decisions for handicapped neonates, one must first understand his ethical tradition, and then how his moral positions originate and how they are maintained.

Moral epistemology is the systematic and critical study of morality as a body of knowledge. According to Michael J. Quirk:

> It is concerned with such issues as how or whether moral claims can be rationally justified, whether there are objective moral facts, whether moral statements strictly admit of truth or falsity, and whether moral claims are universally valid or relative to historically particular belief systems, conceptual schemes, social practices, or cultures.[1]

Specifically, moral epistemology is concerned with the human ways of knowing values/disvalues and moral obligations. Once discovering these values/disvalues, the task of moral epistemology is to inquire how they may be used in the further investigation of knowing whether a particular action is right or wrong. There exists a basic relationship between the discovery of these values/disvalues and the judgment of rightness and wrongness of a particular action. This relationship is the foundational framework for what McCormick means by moral epistemology.

The Roman Catholic tradition, at least since the time of Thomas Aquinas, has always made a distinction between the discovery of values/disvalues and the judgment of rightness and wrongness of a particular action. Aquinas refers to this distinction by using the terms *synderesis* and *conscience*. For Aquinas, synderesis refers to the natural habit of moral knowledge which operates with regard to the first principles of practical reason, in the same way that understanding or intuition does for Aristotle with regard to the principles of theoretical reason.[2] Aquinas writes:

> Synderesis is not a power but a habit; though some held that it is a power higher than reason; while others (Alexander of Hales) said that it is reason itself, not as reason, but as nature. . . . [M]an's act of reasoning, since it is a kind of movement, proceeds from the understanding of certain things—namely, those which are naturally known without any investigation on the part of reason, as from an immovable principle—and ends also at the understanding, inasmuch as by means of those principles naturally known, we judge of those things which we have discovered by reasoning. Now it is clear that, as the speculative reason argues about speculative things, so that practical reason argues about practical things. Therefore we must have, bestowed on us by nature, not only speculative principles, but also practical principles. Now the first speculative principles bestowed on us by nature do not belong to a special power, but to a special habit, which is called *the understanding of principles*, as the Philosopher explains (*Ethics*, vi, 6). Wherefore the first practical principles, bestowed on us by nature, do not belong to a special power, but to a special natural habit, which we call synderesis.[3]

For Aquinas, all persons of good will are aware of these most fundamental principles in their most general form.[4] Therefore, all human persons would agree that in some sense good is to be pursued and evil is to be avoided. The basic inclination in human persons is to know and do the good.

On the other hand, for Aquinas, conscience is the act of applying moral principles to particular concrete actions.[5] Conscience produces a judgment of what a person must do and the commitment required to do it. Aquinas writes:

> Properly speaking conscience is not a power, but an act. . . . For conscience, according to the very nature of the word, implies the relation of knowledge to something: for conscience may be resolved into *cum alio scientia*, i.e., knowledge applied to an individual case. But the application of knowledge to something is done by some

> act. . . . Conscience is said to witness, to bind, or incite,
> and also to accuse, torment, or rebuke. And all these
> follow the application of knowledge or science to what
> we do: which application is made in three ways.[6]

If our conscience tells us that we ought to perform a particular act, then it is our moral duty or moral obligation to perform it. On this subject Aquinas writes: "Every conscience, whether right or wrong, whether it concerns things evil in themselves or things morally indifferent, obliges us to act in such a way that he who acts against conscience sins."[7] Aquinas does not mean to suggest that there is no such thing as right reason and no such thing as an objectively correct moral conscience. For him, ignorance and mistakes are possible in moral matters, and the nearer a person comes to particulars the greater is the field for error.[8] Aquinas argues that "although there is necessity in the general principles, the more we descend to matters of detail, the more frequently we encounter defects."[9]

Since McCormick is a "revised" natural law ethicist who draws heavily upon the Roman Catholic ethical tradition, it is reasonable to situate his moral epistemology within the Thomistic tradition.[10] He states clearly that "every theologian comes from a tradition and is deeply influenced by it."[11] Being part of the Roman Catholic moral tradition, McCormick cannot escape reflecting and theorizing as a member of this tradition. However, as a "revised" natural law ethicist, McCormick will also reformulate the tradition. Instead of restricting moral knowing to a function of the will or the intellect, McCormick understands moral knowing as a function and expression of the person "integrally and adequately considered."[12] In McCormick's view, moral epistemology is the whole person's commitment to values and the moral judgment one makes in light of that commitment to apply these values.

This chapter will examine McCormick's moral epistemology both at the level of how human persons know values and disvalues, which herein after will be referred to as synderesis, and at the level of how human persons know the rightness and wrongness of an action, which herein after will be referred to as normative moral judgment. On the one hand, from this investigation it appears that McCormick operates with a dual moral epistemology, at least at the level of synderesis. This means that at one point in time it appears that a significant shift may have occurred in his moral epistemology at the level of synderesis. This may also be true at the level of normative moral judgment. On the other hand, McCormick's moral epistemology may in fact be a synthesis, which is the product of development and maturity in his thought process. This chapter will articulate, examine, and analyze both moral epistemologies. The first moral epistemology is operative in McCormick's writing up until 1983. The second moral epistemology corresponds to McCormick's decision in 1983 to write primarily in the area of bioethics from a theological perspective. Since the year 1983 seems to be the pivotal time when these two moral epistemologies converge, I will refer to the first moral epistemology as "prior to 1983" and I will refer to the second moral epistemology as "after 1983."[13] An analysis of each moral epistemology will demonstrate how and why the discernment of values and judgments is objective and will examine the sources of moral knowledge for each. This chapter will also attempt to specify the practical implications of McCormick's moral epistemology as they pertain to treatment decisions for handicapped neonates. Finally, this chapter will consider the various criticisms of this part of McCormick's ethical methodology.

MCCORMICK'S DUAL MORAL EPISTEMOLOGY

McCormick's moral epistemology has been the subject of much criticism, especially by his peers. The lack of clarity and the sense of ambiguity surrounding McCormick's moral epistemology stems from the fact that he never articulated it in a systematic manner. Before examining each moral epistemology, a general overview of how McCormick understands synderesis, normative moral judgment, and the sources of moral wisdom will help clarify his two basic epistemological positions.

As a "revised" natural law ethicist, McCormick, following Aquinas, argues that since every agent acts for an end, then the end manifests the notion of the good. The good is that which all things seek.[14] On this is based the first judgment of the practical reason: the good is to be done and pursued, and evil is to be avoided.[15] For Aquinas, the human person knows the good and avoids evil through a reflection on his or her natural inclinations.

For McCormick, at the level of synderesis, all human persons have an innate grasp of the good. His anthropology specifies that all human persons know the basic goods that define human flourishing by reason reflecting on the natural inclinations.[16] Corresponding to each natural inclination is a basic good. In other words, our basic needs direct us toward basic goods. Therefore, the natural inclinations guide the human person's discernment of objective goods. For McCormick, normative moral judgment or conscience is "neither a dictator nor a slave. It is a discerning guide."[17] Normative moral judgment is the specific judgment of the rightness or wrongness of a human action and has its roots in the depths of the person innately inclined toward the good, to love of God and love of neighbor. This inclination takes more concrete form in general moral knowledge and becomes utterly concrete and personal when a person judges about the loving or unloving, selfish or unselfish—briefly, about the moral quality—of his or her own actions.[18] Normative moral judgment is the act of applying principles to concrete situations. The human person apprehends basic goods and then applies normative theories to gain insight into whether an action is right or wrong.[19] The concrete judgment of what a person must do in a particular situation is based on personal perception and the grasp of goods or values. In order to understand McCormick's moral epistemology, it is essential to determine how he believes that we discover objective goods or values in each situation. Further, one must also identify the sources of moral wisdom that help and guide McCormick to perceive and appropriate the truth.

Based on his theory of knowing, it is possible to classify McCormick as a realist, an epistemological position originating out of the "absolutist school" or what is also called the "critical cognitivist school."[20] Adhering to the natural law tradition, McCormick recognizes the objectivity of the moral order rooted in the nature of reality, which can be known through human reason. Such knowing requires more than a simple reading of the physical order. From McCormick's perspective, the world of human meaning can only be known through a critical epistemology of realism.[21]

To perceive and appropriate the truth, McCormick relies on various sources of moral wisdom. In general, these sources are multiple, with the purpose to guide, direct, and illuminate the knowledge of the human person. Without the aid of these multiple sources, the human person risks the possibility of error and ignorance in regard to decision-making. Along similar lines, Karl Popper argues:

> If we must speak of our sources of ignorance it has to be said that the main source of our ignorance lies in the fact that we are human. Our knowledge can only be finite, while our ignorance must necessarily be infinite. . . . There are all sorts of reasons why we remain ignorant; we may be insufficiently inquiring or critical, the problem may be too difficult, we may not have the requisite tools at our disposal, and so on. But there is no insurmountable obstacle to a theoretical kind of knowledge. There may be practical difficulties and perhaps impossibilities in certain areas, but there cannot be theoretical obstacles of the kind the skeptics present.[22]

To overcome such sources of ignorance, McCormick underscores that human persons are members of a believing community, an *ecclesia*. He writes:

> Just as we cannot exist except in community, so also we
> cannot know except as members of a community. Our
> knowledge of God's being and actions, dim and imper-
> fect as it is, is shared knowledge. So is our knowledge of
> its implications for behavior. In other words, we form
> our consciences in community, not in isolation. It is that
> communitarian aspect that is suggested in the words "in
> the Catholic tradition."[23]

For McCormick, there are three main sources of moral knowledge for the
Christian: scripture,[24] the magisterium of the Church,[25] and human reason.[26] However, as part of human reason he will also include: human experience, personal reflection and prayer, the sciences, reflection and discussion with other Christians and non-Christians, etc. These sources of
moral knowledge are not mutually exclusive. Rather, they may be understood as complementary. McCormick argues that, for the Christian,
moral knowledge is, above all and always, shared or communal knowledge—knowledge mediated to the person by the community of believers.
Christians are members of a community and form their consciences in a
community. This is a community of experience, memory, and reflection.[27]

McCormick recognizes the controversial state of moral epistemology
in our time. The world is daily becoming more complex, and situations
facing humankind are more diverse, technical, confusing, and controversial. For him, the current problems facing the world can no longer be
solved or confined satisfactorily within the normative grammar of the
classicist view. Christians today are confronted by difficult ethical problems and they want to be able to apply their faith to these issues within
the cultures in which they live. A mere repetition of past formulas is no
longer adequate. There is a need for innovation, imagination, and creativity, but also faithfulness to the Catholic theological tradition.

McCormick contends that Vatican II addressed this need by giving
the Church a new foundation for examining moral problems when it
centered on a more personalist approach to moral reasoning. The criterion of morality is the human person viewed in his or her totality.
Change, development, and revision are now viewed as ways of coming
to the moral knowledge. Human actions are now interpreted from within
this context. The historically conscious worldview, advanced at Vatican
II, does not absolutize any one particular culture or any one particular
moment in history as having grasped the whole truth, i.e., values, judgments of rightness and wrongness, or moral obligation. For McCormick,
"if there is one thing that is clear about human understanding it is that it
is a process—subject to limitations of partial insight, historical change,

limited philosophical concepts and language, and the intransigence and unpredictability of concrete reality."[28]

The changes proposed at Vatican II, especially the emphasis on the human person as central to moral reflection, have had a significant impact on McCormick's moral epistemology.[29] He will accord more epistemic authority to the *"sensus fidelium"* and the *"scola theologorum"* than he did prior to Vatican II. As a result, "the people of God" are viewed as "the repository of Christian wisdom and truth."[30] McCormick positions himself as a moral theologian who seeks comprehensive knowledge, recognizes the distinctive roles of faith and reason in moral decision-making, and has a great love for the truth wherever found. Grounded in the Catholic theological tradition, McCormick writes:

> The Catholic tradition from which I come has held, at least since the time of St. Thomas, that the sources of faith do not originate concrete obligations (thought to apply to all persons, *essential* morality) that are impervious to human insight and reason.[31]

According to McCormick, to write and think as a Catholic moral theologian means three things. He writes:

> First, religious faith stamps one at a profound and not totally recoverable level. Second, this stamping affects one's instincts, sensitivities, imagination, etc. and hence influences one's perspectives, analyses, judgments. Third, analyses and judgments of such a kind are vitally important in our communal deliberations about bioethics.[32]

McCormick believes that the Catholic theological tradition has always treasured—even if it has not always been ultimately guided or determined by—sound moral analysis. The reason for this is found in two convictions that summarize the tradition on the nature of moral argument. McCormick argues:

> First, the concrete moral implications of our being-in-Christ can per se be known by human insight and reasoning. In other words, those concrete and behavioral norms (commands and prohibitions) regarded as applying to all persons precisely as human persons, are not radically mysterious. Thus the traditional concept of the natural law (one based in the very being of persons) is

knowable by insight and reason. Over a period of centuries, therefore, the criterion of right and wrong actions was said to be *recta ratio* [right reason]. Second, the tradition has viewed man as redeemed but still affected by *reliquiae peccati* [remnants of sin]. This means that notwithstanding the transforming gift of God's enabling grace, we remain vulnerable to self-love and self-deception (sin) and that these noxious influences affect our evaluative and judgmental processes.[33]

McCormick believes that the balancing of these twin currents in the Catholic tradition is often summarized by the lapidary phrase "reason informed by faith." He understands this balance to be

tricky and fragile and . . . not always . . . successfully realized. . . . When I say that "I speak out of the Catholic tradition," I mean to suggest an *ideal* mix of these twin currents, that which very few of us probably achieve, try as we may. One of the reasons for this is that the "enlightened" (in reason enlightened by faith) still cries out for penetrating and systematic study.[34]

McCormick believes his moral epistemology is a way of answering the "cry" of how reason is enlightened by faith.

The remainder of this section will examine McCormick's two moral epistemologies both at the level of synderesis and at the level of normative moral judgment. It will show how the historical context in which McCormick is operating has had a profound impact on his moral epistemology. Finally, this section will conclude with an evaluation of whether McCormick has made a significant shift in his moral epistemology or whether his moral epistemology is in fact a synthesis, which is the product of the development and maturity in his thought process.

FIRST MORAL EPISTEMOLOGY—PRIOR TO 1983

McCormick's first moral epistemology is deeply rooted in the neo-scholastic tradition.[35] At the level of synderesis, human persons seek goods that define human flourishing through a reflection on natural inclinations.[36] The basic needs of persons direct them toward basic goods.[37] At the level of normative moral judgment, further reflection by practical reason on the fundamental natural inclinations of human nature dictates what is good and should be pursued and what is evil and should be avoided.

In the early 1970s, McCormick gradually began to be influenced by the school of thought represented by John Finnis, J. de Finance, G. de Broglie, G. Grisez and others, which deals with the concept of basic human goods. Finnis writes:

> These *principia* which are *fines operabilium* are simply the values corresponding to our fundamental inclinations, and they are named by St. Thomas the first and self-evident principles of natural law. What is spontaneously understood when one turns from contemplation to action is not a set of Kantian or neo-scholastic "moral principles" identifying this as right and that as wrong, but a set of values which can be expressed in the form of principles such as "life is a good-to-be-pursued and realized, and what threatens it to be avoided."[38]

These basic goods define the scope of the human person's possibility and appeal to the person for realization.[39] McCormick's attraction to this approach can be attributed to his commitment to the Catholic natural law methodology.[40] Finnis' notion of the origin of moral obligation and the meaning of natural law (reasonableness) was both persuasive and very attractive to McCormick.[41] McCormick understands the natural human inclinations to be the basis for our interest in specific goods at the level of synderesis. McCormick writes:

> What are the goods or values man can seek, the values that define his human opportunity, his flourishing? We can answer this by examining man's basic tendencies, for it is impossible to act without having an interest in the object, and it is impossible to be attracted by, to have an interest in something without some inclination already present.[42]

With no pretense at being exhaustive, McCormick lists the following as the basic inclinations present prior to acculturation:

> the tendency to preserve life; the tendency to mate and raise children; the tendency to explore and question; the tendency to seek out other men and obtain their approval—friendship; the tendency to use intelligence in

guiding action; the tendency to develop skills and exercise them in play and in fine arts.[43]

Significantly, McCormick's list of basic inclinations is almost identical with those advanced by Finnis.[44]

McCormick argues that "in these inclinations our intelligence spontaneously and without reflection grasps the possibilities to which they point, and prescribes them. Thus we form naturally and without reflection the basic principles of practical or moral reasoning."[45] This shows the origins of both our knowledge of goods and moral obligation. The basic goods toward which these inclinations lead us lay the foundation for whether concrete actions are morally right or wrong. Like Finnis, McCormick argues that these basic goods are "equally basic and irreducibly attractive."[46] By "equally basic" Finnis means:

> First, each is equally self-evidently a form of the good. Secondly, none can be analytically reduced to being merely an aspect of any of the others, or to being merely instrumental in the pursuit of any of the others. Thirdly, each one, when we focus on it, can reasonably be regarded as the most important. Hence there is no objective hierarchy amongst them.[47]

McCormick appears to agree with Finnis, at least initially, that these basic goods are incommensurable.[48] For McCormick, "each of these values has its self-evident appeal as a participation in the unconditioned Good we call God. The realization of these values in intersubjective life is the only adequate way to love and attain God."[49] What it means to remain open and to pursue these basic goods comes at the level of normative moral judgment.

In McCormick's first moral epistemology, at the level of normative moral judgment, there appear to be two formulations for determining the rightness and wrongness of an action. The first formulation is based on Finnis' position, and seems to derive from the fact that the basic goods are "equally basic and self-evidently attractive."[50] For Finnis, these goods or values do not present themselves as what we call "moral values," as rules of right and wrong. Finnis writes:

> Just as all reasoning, even false reasoning, is recognizable as reasoning because it draws on self-evident principles of coherent thought, so all human activity and practical thinking and choosing, even the most vicious and wrongful, draws on and is directed by the natural

law, that is, values (and the principles expressing those
values) which appeal to our intelligence with the glow,
the self-evidence, of innate intelligibility.[51]

These basic goods appeal to human intelligence and will. The moral
choice is that which realizes or suppresses the basic goods in particular
concrete situations. Thus, the morally right act is the one that maximizes
these basic goods to the extent concretely possible.[52] In Finnis' view,
these goods are equally fundamental, for each, when focused upon, can
be regarded "reasonably" as the most important. Since there is no objective priority among them, it is never right to sacrifice one for another.
Further, it is never right to act directly against them. Each act must retain
"openness" to each of these goods and so "remain open to the ground of
all values."[53] Lisa Sowle Cahill argues:

> The essential truth of Finnis' proposal lies in his percep-
> tion that at the heart of natural-law theory is a commit-
> ment to certain basic goods which in themselves are at-
> tractive to human freedom and intelligence and to which
> human nature inclines. McCormick certainly concurs in
> this insight.[54]

For McCormick, the rightness and wrongness of an action is determined by further reflection of practical reason on the basic goods. Such
reflection informs the human person about what it means to remain open
to and pursue these basic human goods. McCormick writes:

> First, we must take them into account in our conduct.
> Simple disregard of one or the other shows we have set
> our mind against this good and, in the process, against
> both the unconditioned Good who is its source and our-
> selves. Immoral action is always self-destructive in its
> thrust. Secondly, when we can do so as easily as not, we
> should avoid acting in ways that inhibit these values, and
> prefer ways that realize them. Thirdly, we must make an
> effort on their behalf when their realization in another is
> in extreme peril. If we fail to do so, we show that the
> value in question is not the object of our efficacious love
> and concern. Finally, we must never choose directly
> against a basic good. For when one of the irreducible
> values falls immediately under our choice, to choose
> against it in favor of some other basic value is arbitrary;
> for all the basic values are equally basic and self-

evidently attractive. What is to count as "turning against
a basic good" is, of course, a crucial moral question. It
need *not* be discussed here. My only point is that particular moral judgments (e.g., about sustaining life and
health, or taking life, what is morally legitimate or ille-
gitimate in dealing with life and health, etc.) are incar-
nations of these basic normative positions, positions that
have their roots in spontaneous, pre-reflective inclinations.[55]

Finnis and McCormick maintain that these goods hold together and
that a person can never directly act against a basic good.[56] When conflict
arises, Finnis and McCormick argue that this is only an apparent conflict.
McCormick writes:

[O]ne does not suppress one basic good for the sake of
another one *equally* basic. The only way to cut the Gor-
dian knot when basic values are conflicted is to only indirectly allow the defeat of one as the other is pursued.[57]

As a result of the incommensurabilty of the basic goods, certain acts are
always intrinsically evil in and of themselves.[58]

The second formulation in McCormick's first moral epistemology, at
the level of normative moral judgment, came as a result of Vatican II, the
birth control debate that surrounded the promulgation of *Humanae Vitae*
in 1968, and the proportionalism debate. Due to the influence of these
three events, McCormick separated himself from the school of Finnis
and Grisez. McCormick writes:

The problem centers around the matter of choice "directly and positively against a basic value." Finnis admits that there is room for dispute about whether a
choice actually is directly against a basic value or not.
But he does not pursue the matter and ask why there is
room for dispute, and what the methodological implications of this fact might be. The crucial question one must
raise with both Grisez and Finnis is: What is to count for
turning against a basic good, and why? At this point I
find them both unsatisfactory.[59]

Following this, McCormick began to reevaluate the genuine objectivity
required in ethics. Moral significance does not only refer to mere physical acts. Rather, it is an assessment of an action's relation to the order of

persons, that is, to the hierarchy of personal value.[60] McCormick does not totally disagree with Finnis and Grisez, especially at the level of synderesis. However, at the level of normative moral judgment, McCormick finds their theory unpersuasive and inconsistent. He states in a personal interview that:

> I learned personally from Germain Grisez, whom I think has many good things to say. I like his views on the development of moral obligation—his understanding and interpretation of St. Thomas, the basic inclinations toward certain basic goods. I found that as satisfying as anything else I have ever encountered. However, I do not think his applications of his moral theory are persuasive. 'You never turn against a basic good.' What does that mean? I think that doesn't make sense. All the same, I find his basic understanding of moral obligation very helpful and enlightening.[61]

This marked a significant shift in how McCormick determines the rightness and wrongness of a moral act. To understand this shift, one must examine it further within its historical context.

Vatican II introduced a historically conscious worldview and stressed the centrality of the human person "integrally and adequately considered" in moral thought. Physicalism gave way to personalism. McCormick writes:

> In an earlier period, significance was drawn from an analysis of faculties and finalities . . . *Gaudium et Spes* asserts that the "moral aspect of any procedure . . . must be determined by objective standards which are based on the nature of the person and the person's acts."[62]

McCormick now believes the Council encourages not only tentativeness in moral judgments, but also leaves room for dissent.[63]

During this time period, Peter Knauer, S.J., published his first of several articles in which he argued that the four conditions of the principle of double effect could properly be reduced to the requirement of proportionate reason. In other words, Knauer believed that an evil effect would be either direct or indirect according to the presence or absence of proportionate reason.[64] McCormick's initial reaction to this article was critical.[65] He argued that Knauer's interpretation would destroy the notion of intrinsic evil *ex objecto*. However, by 1970, Joseph Fuchs, McCormick's mentor, had endorsed Knauer's view on proportionate reason. McCormick at this point is writing "Moral Notes" for *Theological Studies* and has become deeply involved in the proportionalism debate.

By 1970, Knauer has published two additional articles on this topic.[66] Knauer applies the general theory of double effect to the question of contraception. In response McCormick writes:

> It hardly needs to be recalled that Paul VI taught in *Humanae Vitae* that each conjugal act must remain open to the transmission of life. Knauer questions whether this conclusion follows from the general principle that married love must remain open to the transmission of life.[67]

Knauer's basic thesis is that moral evil, i.e., moral wrongness, consists in the permission or causing of a physical evil which is not justified by commensurate reason. For Knauer, it is with this in mind that ethicists must understand the terms direct and indirect. In the past these terms have been tied too closely to physical causality. Knauer stresses that reason is not commensurate because it is sincere, meaningful, or even simply important. Reason is commensurate if the value realized here and now, by measures involving physical evil in a premoral sense, is not in the long run undermined or contradicted by these measures but supported and maximized.[68] Influenced by Knauer's articles and also by an article by Bruno Schüller concerning the "direct/indirect" distinction,[69] McCormick concluded the following:

> First, there is evidence to suggest that our contemporary notion of direct intent of evil, with its very close reliance on direct physical causality, may have narrowed and distorted rather than advanced the original Thomistic analysis. . . . Second, I believe Schüller has convincingly argued that behind our formulated norms in control of concrete conduct is a more general preference-principle from which these norms derive. If this is true, we must approach some traditional conclusions to see if they square with this derivation.[70]

Following these three events, McCormick soon became a leading proponent of proportionalism in the United States[71] and declared his objection to the central thesis of *Humanae Vitae*. From within this historical context, it is now possible to understand why McCormick made this significant shift at the level of normative moral judgment.

In this second formulation (of his first moral epistemology), at the level of normative moral judgment, McCormick believes there is room for commensuration even in situations involving apparently incommensurable and indeterminate goods. Further, he argues that indeterminacy and incommensurability can be overcome by means of a hierarchy of values.[72] He holds that the basic goods exist in a hierarchy that he referred to as the "association of basic goods."[73] This means that the basic goods are associated to each other in such a way that harm to or protection of one will probably or necessarily harm or enhance others.[74] The basic goods are commensurable because they can conflict with one another, thus the human person is forced to compare and choose between them. For McCormick, it is prudence that dictates which of these goods should be chosen in times of conflict. McCormick uses the example of how human persons are willing at times to sacrifice lives to protect their political freedom.[75] McCormick justifies this by arguing:

> Because we are finite, all our acts are metaphysically imperfect. They do not and cannot embody all values. This radical metaphysical limitation will obviously manifest itself at the level of concrete external activity.[76]

The human person can realize only certain limited values, and in doing so must at times do so to the neglect of other values or at the expense of associated disvalues. In this light every choice represents the resolution of a conflict. McCormick writes:

> This means that the concrete moral norms that we develop to guide human conduct and communicate human convictions and experience to others are all conclusions of and vehicles for a larger, more general assertion: in situations of conflict, where values are copresent and mutually exclusive, the reasonable thing is to avoid what is, *all things considered*, the greater evil or, positively stated, to do the greater good. This means, of course, that we may cause or permit evils in our conduct only when the evil caused or permitted is, all things considered, the lesser evil in the circumstances. In other words, we may cause a premoral evil only when there is a truly proportionate reason.[77]

From this, it is clear that McCormick establishes his stress on proportionate reason through his theory of associated goods.[78]

In the second formulation at the level of normative moral judgment, McCormick agrees with Finnis *et al* that there exist basic goods that define human well-being and give rise to moral obligations and value commitments. However, McCormick disagrees with the methodological implications of this starting point. Whereas Finnis *et al* regard directly turning against a basic good to be intrinsically morally evil, McCormick regards turning against a basic good to be a premoral evil,[79] which requires the justification of proportionate reason.[80] For example, McCormick writes that

> causing certain disvalues (ontic, nonmoral, premoral evils) in our conduct does not *ipso facto* make the action morally wrong. The action becomes morally wrong when, all things considered, there is no proportionate reason to justifying it.[81]

For McCormick, moral wrongness occurs when a premoral evil is caused without proportionate reason. Thus, the notion of premoral evil is an admission of imperfection and conflict of values.[82] Before an action can be determined to be intrinsically morally evil, an individual must now assess morally relevant factors, which include the action itself, the intention, circumstances, consequences, values and norms. In conflict situations, the rule of Christian reason, if we are governed by the *ordo bonorum*, is to choose the lesser evil. McCormick's use of proportionate reason is to determine when premoral evil can be allowed and when an action that contains premoral evil can only be permitted.[83] Furthermore, McCormick's point of proportionate reason is to prove that the traditional notion of intrinsic moral evil cannot be sustained in the way it has been formulated.[84] Proportionate reason becomes McCormick's criterion of determining moral rightness and wrongness.[85]

McCormick offers three modes of knowing to determine whether his criteria for proportionate reason have been fulfilled and that a proportionate reason exists. The first way of knowing whether a proper relation exists between a specific value and all other elements of an act is through human experience. For example, human experience tells us that private property is essential to the overall well-being of persons and their social relations, therefore, robbery is counterproductive or disproportionate. Second, McCormick maintains we can know prediscursively through a sense of profanation, outrage, or intuition that some actions are disproportionate. The examples of torture and forms of fanatical human experimentation fall within this category. Third, he believes that a person can come to know some actions to be disproportionate only gradually by the methods of trial and error. This mode of knowing pertains to areas where we have little experience as yet and should proceed cautiously, such as whether recombinant DNA research should be permitted.[86] In conclusion, McCormick now rejects Grisez's deontological interpretation of the meaning of direct and indirect voluntariety. For McCormick, proportionate reason is the criterion for determining objective moral rightness and wrongness.

In this second formulation at the level of normative moral judgment, McCormick draws upon the various sources of moral wisdom to perceive and appropriate the moral truth (i.e., judgments of rightness and wrongness or moral obligations) in any situation. McCormick's renewed awareness of the human person's historicity affects his understanding of the traditional sources of moral wisdom. For him, this means

> taking our culture seriously as soil for the "signs of the times," as framer of our self-awareness. That means a fresh look at how Christian perspectives ought to read the modern world so that our practices are the best possible mediation of gospel values in the contemporary world.[87]

Scripture, tradition, and the magisterium must now be sensitive to changing historical and cultural factors.

For example, scripture, as a source of moral wisdom, nourishes the overall perspectives of the human person. Where in the past, scripture was used in the form of proof-texting, now scripture identifies various insights and key perspectives that help inform human reasoning. The magisterium can no longer mean the "hierarchical issuance of authoritative decrees."[88] As the articulated wisdom of the community, the magisterium enlightens the conscience instead of replacing it. McCormick writes:

> This renewed awareness of man's historicity will affect our understanding of the Church's non-infallible magisterium and our reading of its past teachings. The magisterium will realize that its teachings must be developed out of an ever increasing range of competences. Furthermore, an enlightened sensitivity to changing historical and cultural factors will recommend to the magisterium great caution in descending to detailed specifications of the demands of radical Christian love.[89]

As the *Pastoral Constitution on the Church in the Modern World* observes:

> Let the layman not imagine that his pastors are always such experts that to every problem which arises, how-

> ever complicated, they can readily give him a concrete
> solution, or even that such is their mission. Rather, en-
> lightened by Christian wisdom and giving close attention
> to the teaching authority of the Church, let the layman
> take on his own distinctive role.[90]

The magisterium will assist persons in moral deliberations by being
broadly consultative, questioning, critical, open, and appropriately tentative.[91] Therefore, if the magisterium is to be a confirming source of
moral wisdom for the human person in determining the moral rightness
or wrongness of an action, it must have the competence to understand
and judge the many factual dimensions involved in modern complex
ethical problems.[92] Thus, it is necessary for the magisterium to be in
dialogue with the other sciences.[93] More attention must be given to evidence and analysis in evaluating moral teachings. Only persuasive reasons will command assent. McCormick believes that a human person
with a well-formed conscience, that is, one formed in community and
one that draws upon the diverse sources of moral wisdom, can use proportionate reason to determine concretely and objectively the moral
rightness and wrongness of a particular action.

McCormick utilizes this moral epistemology up until 1983. At the
level of synderesis, the human person seeks the goods or values that define human flourishing by reflecting on the natural inclinations. At the
level of normative moral judgment, it is proportionate reason that determines the rightness and wrongness of a human action. In 1983, McCormick makes a significant epistemological shift, at least at the level of
synderesis, thus formulating a new moral epistemology.

SECOND MORAL EPISTEMOLOGY—AFTER 1983

In 1983, McCormick began to write primarily in the area of bioethics,
and it appears that he made a conscious effort to approach bioethics from
a theological perspective. One reason for this move may be McCormick's involvement in the question of the distinctiveness of Christian
ethics discussion.[94] This discussion appears to have provoked in him the
need to articulate what Christian faith adds to the essential level of ethics. From this point onward, McCormick continues to rely on right reason, but he incorporates the Christian story both at the level of synderesis
and at the level of normative moral judgment.[95] In this way, McCormick
can show what relation his natural law commitments bear to more specifically Christian ones. He argues that "the Christian story will influence
not only personal dispositions, but also moral judgments—but in a rather

general way."[96] The Christian story will help guide the human person's discernment of objective morality.

Another impetus for the inclusion of the Christian story in his moral epistemology appears to be Vatican II's appeal to show the relation of religious belief to concrete areas of human behavior.[97] The *Pastoral Constitution on the Church in the Modern World* states clearly that "Faith throws a new light on everything, manifests God's design for man's total vocation, and thus directs the mind to solutions that are fully human."[98] McCormick makes a conscious effort to explore, to clarify, and to make more persuasive how faith enlightens and directs the mind to solutions, especially in the concrete area of bioethics.[99] Right reason remains at the center of McCormick's second moral epistemology, but it is right reason informed by faith.

To understand McCormick's second moral epistemology (after 1983) one must analyze how he interprets "reason informed by faith." McCormick understands human reason to mean

> all those dimensions of human understanding that play a role in our evaluation of actions as morally right or wrong. Among those dimensions are: experience, the sense of profanation, trial and error, discursive reasoning, long-term consequences, the experience of harmony and guilt over our actions. There is always the danger that the term *recta ratio* will be impoverished by collapsing it into a barren rationalism that overlooks the affective richness of human understanding.[100]

The incorporation of the Christian narrative can help overcome the problem of barren rationalism. For McCormick, reason informed by faith is neither reason replaced by faith or reason without faith. It is reason shaped by faith and this shaping takes the form of perspectives, themes, and insights associated with the Christian story that help the human person construe the world.[101] In discussing how reason informs faith, McCormick writes:

> I am suggesting that the stories and symbols that relate the origin of Christianity and nourish the faith of the individual affect our perspectives by intensifying and sharpening our focus on the human goods definitive of our flourishing. It is persons so informed, persons with such "Christian reasons" sunk deep in their being, who face new situations, new dilemmas and reason together as to what is right and wrong. They do not find concrete

answers in their tradition, but they bring a worldview
that informs their reasoning—especially by allowing the
basic human goods to retain their original attractiveness
and not be tainted by cultural distortions.[102]

For McCormick, the sources of faith do not originate concrete moral obligations that are impervious to human insight and reasoning. However,
they do confirm them.

Christian morality, while theological at its core, is not isolationist or
sectarian. Isolating accounts of the Christian story would repudiate a
constant of the Catholic theological tradition: that God's self-revelation
in Jesus Christ does not obliterate the human but illuminates it.[103] For
McCormick, Christian commitment shapes human perspectives, motivation, and processes of reasoning, but only in a general way. In the process faith encourages certain insights, which are inherently intelligible and
commendable. What McCormick emphasizes is that a Christian's conclusions will not be substantively different from those yielded by objective and reasonable but nonreligious analysis. For McCormick, "Christian emphases do not immediately yield moral norms and rules for decision-making, nor do they conduce to concrete answers unique to that tradition."[104] Human reason, unaided by explicit faith, can come to the same
judgments about rightness and wrongness.[105]

McCormick's understanding of "reason informed by faith" is the
foundation upon which he constructs his second moral epistemology. In
order to understand this second moral epistemology, an in-depth analysis
will be given at both the level of synderesis and at the level of normative
moral judgment.

At the level of synderesis, McCormick introduces the idea that the
basic goods that define human flourishing are discovered and known by
the human person's prediscursive reason informed by the Christian story.
McCormick explains that this type of knowledge is prereflective or
prethematic, or connatural.[106] Prediscursive knowledge is prior to cultural
differentiations, although its judgments can be affected by cultural distortions. To explain the meaning of prediscursive reason, McCormick
considers the example of slavery. He writes:

We find this demeaning and immoral not because of rational (discursive) argument—which is not to say that
rational arguments will not support the conclusion.
Rather, over time our sensitivities are sharpened to the
meaning and dignity of human persons. We then experience the out-of-jointness, inequality and injustice of
slavery.[107]

To clarify further his meaning of prediscursive reason, McCormick quotes Nobel laureate Peter Medawar, who discusses the difference between a humanizing and dehumanizing use of technology. Medawar states that the answer we give in practice

> is founded not upon abstract moralizing but upon a certain natural sense of the fitness of things, a feeling that is shared by most kind and reasonable people even if we cannot define it in philosophically defensible or legally accountable terms.[108]

Therefore, it seems for McCormick that prediscursive reason is the inner structure of the heart that can know human moral reality. For McCormick, prediscursive reasoning appears to be similar to what Aquinas meant by connatural knowledge.

After reviewing McCormick's writings, it becomes evident that his understanding of prediscursive reason is ambiguous. The basis of McCormick's view of prediscursive reason can be traced to Aquinas, but it also appears that McCormick relies on Rahner's notion of the "moral instinct of faith" and Daniel Maguire's understanding of the affections. McCormick agrees with Rahner that there is a "moral instinct of faith." He writes:

> This instinct can be called by any number of different names; but the point is that there is a component to moral judgment that cannot be adequately subject to analytic reflection. But it is this component that is chiefly responsible for one's ultimate judgments on concrete moral questions. In this sense these ultimate judgments are not simply the sum of the rational considerations and analyses one is capable of objectifying and no adequate understanding of proportionate reason implies this.[109]

McCormick argues that if human moral sensitivities are outraged, for example, by the sheriff who would frame and execute one innocent man to pacify a riot-prone mob bent on indiscriminate killing, then he is "prepared to trust this instinctive reaction."[110] For McCormick, even though a person's spontaneous and instinctive moral judgments can be affected by cultural distortions and can be confused with deeply ingrained conventional fears and biases, they still remain a more reliable test of the humanizing and dehumanizing, than that of our discursive reasoning.[111]

Unfortunately, even with this explanation one is still left with a sense of ambiguity in regard to what McCormick means by prediscursive reasoning.

McCormick's understanding of prediscursive reason has also been influenced by Daniel Maguire's notion of the affections. Maguire is convinced of the natural moral instinct. Maguire presents the thesis that there is "an intellectualistic fallacy rampant in contemporary ethical deliberation, an analytic and rationalistic approach that assumes that morality becomes intelligible in the same way that mathematics and logic do."[112] Maguire argues that *recta ratio* in Aquinas is profoundly shaped by an affective component. Maguire writes: "While Aquinas does not systematize this notion, it is undeniably present in many of his treatises: on prudence, wisdom, the gifts of the Holy Spirit, delight, and faith."[113] For Maguire, "moral knowledge is born in the awe and affectivity that characterizes the foundational moral experience—the experience of the value of persons and their environment."[114] Maguire concludes that human persons can know much of what is right or wrong but that they should be a bit more modest about the claims of reason.[115]

McCormick agrees with Maguire's contention that the affections shape moral knowledge. On this subject McCormick writes:

> Maguire's insistence on the affective shaping of moral knowledge is certainly correct. It suggests many things. One thing I want to highlight is the expansive and deepening role of affect in moral knowledge. From the Christian point of view, faith creates sensitivities in the believer beyond the reach of natural vitalities. It bestows sensitivity to dimensions of possibility not otherwise suspected, or what Thomas Clarke, S.J., refers to as "distinctive habits of perception and response." This is no call to true obscurantism, nor is it an invitation to authority to press unsupportable claims. It is simply an acknowledgment of the depth and beauty of the spiritual life, the complexity of reality, and therefore of the many-faceted ways of discovering moral truth.[116]

Maguire suggests that Aquinas understood that the affections are implicated in the work of practical reason, in the deliberation of reasonableness. Being Thomistic in his approach, it seems to follow that McCormick would agree with Maguire's approach drawing some of his understanding of prediscursive reasoning from Aquinas. However, what McCormick means precisely by "prediscursive reason" is still not clear. It is clear that McCormick believes that moral sensitivities—affections and feelings—and even intuition play a distinctive role in discovering the basic goods that define human flourishing and moral obligations. McCormick writes: "Judgments of the moral 'ought,' have deep roots in our sensitivities and emotions."[117] Therefore, one might well conclude that, for McCormick, prediscursive reason in one respect is another name for the affections. Not only does the human person discover the basic goods through the affections, but they also ground and animate McCormick's ethical positions.

The influence of the Christian narrative on the affections is such that it is much more a value-raiser than an answer-giver.[118] It affects basic human goods at the spontaneous, prethematic level. The Christian story sensitizes the believer beyond the reach of natural vitalities. It bestows sensitivity to "dimensions of possibility" not otherwise suspected.[119] McCormick writes:

> One who has accepted in faith God's stupendous deed in Christ, one who sees in Christ God's self-disclosure and therefore who sees (and *accepts*) in the Christ-event the central fact of human history, will come to be (by God's healing grace) stamped by the dispositions associated with that event. Some are putting others' needs ahead of our own; seeking God's will in hard times; carrying one's cross in imitation of Christ; giving one's life for one's friends; turning the other cheek; seeking Christ in the neighbor; subordinating everything to the God-relationship; trusting in God's providential care. Such dispositions do not, of course, solve problems. They do however incline us to seek out and discern the morally right. *Good* people will strive to do morally *right* things.[120]

The Christian story sinks deep into the person and sensitizes the human person to the meaning of life and to the goods that are definitive of human flourishing. Even though the human person can know the basic goods prior to acculturation, McCormick argues that they can still exist as culturally conditioned. For McCormick, the Christian story attends to and lifts out those cultural leanings and biases that may distort our grasp of the basic goods.[121] It is the person of Jesus Christ who sensitizes the human person to the meaning of persons. For example, McCormick writes:

> Faith in the Christ-event, love and loyalty to Jesus Christ, yields a decisive way of viewing and intending

the world, of interpreting its meaning, of hierarchizing
its values. In this sense the Christian tradition only illumines basic human values, supports them, and provides
a context for their reading at given points in history. It
aids us in staying human by underlining the truly human
against all cultural attempts to distort the human.[122]

The way the person perceives and relates to the basic human goods is
shaped by how he or she views the world. The Christian story brings
about a worldview that informs human reasoning—especially as this reasoning touches the basic goods. McCormick argues that:

This worldview is a continuing check on and challenge
to our tendency to allow cultural enthusiasms to sink
into and take possession of our prediscursive selves.
Such enthusiasm can reduce the good life to mere adjustment in a triumph of the therapeutic, collapse an individual into his functionality, exalt his uniqueness into
a lonely individualism or crush it in a suffocating col-
lectivism. In this sense it is true to say that the Christian
story is much more a value-raiser than an answer-
giver.[123]

At the level of normative moral judgment, the moral rightness and
wrongness of an act is determined by the discursive reason informed by
the Christian story. At this level, McCormick no longer speaks about the
"association of basic goods." He will continue to use proportionate reason in determining the rightness and wrongness of a human action. However, it should be noted that McCormick introduces a new criterion of
morality, that is, the person "integrally and adequately considered." Proportionate reason becomes a tool for establishing what is promotive or
destructive of the whole person. This criterion will be examined in detail
in the next chapter.

After the affections discover and identify the basic human goods,
discursive moral reason is concerned with rational analysis and the
adoption of a hierarchy of goods. For McCormick, in order to determine
the moral rightness and wrongness of an action, a person must take these
apprehensions discovered intuitively and test them by critical rational
analysis within a larger community, to determine what is more promotive
of the human person "integrally and adequately considered." This critical
analysis occurs by discursive reason informed by the Christian story.

At the level of normative moral judgment, the Christian story influences moral judgments in a rather general way. The Christian story does

not yield moral rules and norms for decision-making, but it does influence and affect them. The stories and symbols provide both the perspectives from which choices can be made and the confirmatory warrant for testing their validity.[124] McCormick writes:

> The Christian story tells us the ultimate meaning of ourselves and the world. In doing so, it tells us the kind of people we ought to be, the goods we ought to pursue, the dangers we ought to avoid, the kind of world we ought to seek. It provides the backdrop or framework that ought to shape our individual decisions. When decision-making is separated from this framework, it loses its perspective. It becomes a merely rationalistic and sterile ethic subject to the distortions of self-interested perspectives and cultural fads, a kind of contracted etiquette with no relation to the ultimate meaning of persons. Indeed, even when our deliberations are nourished by the biblical narratives, they do not escape the *reliquiae peccati* [remnants of sin] in us.[125]

The Christian story serves as a "corrective" for the human person. Because of the human condition, we have a tendency to make idols, to pursue the basic goods as ends in themselves.[126] This is what McCormick refers to as secularization. It is discursive reason informed by the Christian story that assists the human person in radically relativizing all human goods. Imitating Christ, means, negatively, never pursuing human goods as final ends, and positively, pursuing them as subordinate to the God-relationship.[127] For McCormick, the Christian story informs discursive reason and helps to shape the human person's moral vision. The very meaning, purpose, and value of a person is grounded in and ultimately explained by this story. When it informs the discursive reason, it gives shape to a person's ethical deliberations. For McCormick, "[T]he Christian story itself is the overarching foundation and criterion of morality. It stands in judgment of all human meaning and actions. Actions which are incompatible with this story are thereby morally wrong."[128]

The Christian story furnishes the Christian with a knowledge of the human person's integral vocation. For McCormick, the Christian story is mediated through the believing community by tradition, the magisterium, personal reflection and prayer, reflection and discussion with other Christians and non-Christians, and theological scholarship. However, if Christian knowledge is to take concrete meaningful form, it must also draw upon and integrate the insights and experiences of a variety of disciplines that study the world and provide the context of decision and choice. These include: economics, medicine, psychology and psychiatry, sociology, law, cultural anthropology, etc. For McCormick, these sources of knowledge are not mutually exclusive, but are complementary. This variety of sources aid moral reasoning and insight.[129] The Christian story in "confrontation with human experience will be the source of ever fresh insights into the meaning and challenge of being a Christian in the modern world."[130] Although discursive knowledge is communal in its sources, judgment of rightness and wrongness is a personal judgment.[131] Discursive reason informed by the Christian story determines objectivity and reasonableness. It is an objectivity that is structured, but not held captive, by a person's subjectivities.[132]

In conclusion, because of developments in his career as a moral theologian, there has been a significant shift in McCormick's moral epistemology at least at the level of synderesis. In his first moral epistemology (prior to 1983), one apprehends the basic goods through the experience of and reflection on our natural inclinations. After 1983, McCormick makes a conscious decision to write primarily in the area of bioethics from a theological perspective. Because of this development in his career there is now a significant shift in his moral epistemology. In his second moral epistemology, one apprehends the basic values though one's affections influenced by the Christian story. The Christian story plays an integral role by both sensitizing the person and maintaining his focus on the basic values. The affections influenced by the Christian story represent a major shift at the level of synderesis in McCormick's moral epistemology.

At the level of normative moral judgment, it appears that McCormick's moral epistemology is the product of a developing synthesis. In his first moral epistemology, McCormick moved from the basic goods being incommensurable, following the school of Finnis *et al.*, to the position that these basic goods can, in fact, conflict with one another. This conflict is due to the fact that, for McCormick, there is an association of basic goods. Proportionate reason became the principle to determine concretely and objectively the rightness and wrongness of acts and the various exceptions to behavioral norms. In his second moral epistemology, the discursive reason informed by the Christian story can know the objective moral rightness and wrongness of an act by determining what constitutes the good of the human person "integrally and adequately considered." Proportionate reason continues to play a vital role in determining the rightness and wrongness of an action, but it does so in association with the criterion of the whole human person.

McCormick's moral epistemology, which has developed over the years, has much to offer Christian ethics. He argues that his epistemological foundation, which is based on reason informed by faith, leads to sound moral analysis. His emphasis on the affective component in moral conviction, he believes, has particular application in the area of bioethics. McCormick writes:

> Judgments of the moral "ought," what I as a Christian should do or avoid, and actions upon such conclusions, originate not simply in rational analysis, book learning or exposure to sociological facts. They have deep roots in our sensitivities and emotions. This has particular relevance where health needs of the elderly and *dependent* (fetuses, *infants*, retarded, the poor) are concerned.[133]

McCormick's moral epistemology, both at the level of synderesis and normative moral judgment, specifies practical implications as applied to treatment decisions for handicapped neonates. The following section will examine what we know from McCormick's moral epistemology and will apply it to treatment decisions for handicapped neonates.

PRACTICAL IMPLICATIONS OF MCCORMICK'S MORAL EPISTEMOLOGY (AFTER 1983) AS APPLIED TO TREATMENT DECISIONS FOR HANDICAPPED NEONATES

McCormick's moral epistemology guides the human person toward becoming more humane by informing our reasoning about what it means to be fully human. He writes: "It is only against such understandings that our concrete deliberations can remain truly humane and promote our best interests."[134] For the human person, reason informed by faith results in various enlightening perspectives, insights, and themes that have a direct bearing on bioethics.[135] McCormick does caution that there are five aspects that need to be noted about these themes and perspectives. He writes:

> First, they are by no means an exhausting listing . . . Second, these themes do not immediately yield concrete moral judgments about the rightfulness or wrongfulness of human actions. Rather, they direct and inform our view of the world. Third, they are not ultimately mysterious. They find resonance in broad moral experience and in this sense are not impervious to human insight. Fourth, they are capable of yielding different applications in different times and circumstances. Finally, they are themes or perspectives that stem from the Christian

story in a dynamic sense: as the story is continuously appropriated in a living tradition.[136]

With these qualifications, this section will examine three specific insights or perspectives that inform human reasoning in regard to treatment decisions for handicapped neonates.

Human Life Is a Good But Not an Absolute Good

At the level of synderesis, McCormick has determined that human life is a basic good, but not an absolute one. According to McCormick, there is a hierarchy of goods that is teleological in nature. Each good exists in an interrelationship that consists in a single scale. The ultimate good, the highest good, the End of ends, is God. Therefore, human life is a relative good, because there are higher goods for which life can be sacrificed.[137] At the level of normative moral judgment, discursive reason informed by the Christian story determines if the presence of proportionate reason exists to determine if one value can be sacrificed for another in a conflict situation, for the good of the whole person.

For McCormick, the Christian story influences both personal dispositions and moral judgments. He writes: "In the Christian story we are baptized into the mysterious drama of Christ's passion, death and resurrection. Just as he rose from the dead and lives, so too will we."[138] The belief that we are pilgrim people with no lasting home here on earth yields an immediate value judgment on the meaning of life: human life is a good but not an absolute good. McCormick will rely upon both scripture and the magisterium to confirm this value judgment.[139]

In McCormick's view, human life is a relative good, and the duty to preserve it is a limited one. Therefore, human life need not be preserved at any cost and with every means if there is a proportionate reason for not prolonging it. McCormick bases this in the Catholic theological tradition. On this subject McCormick writes:

> Life is not a value to be preserved in and for itself. To maintain that would commit us to a form of medical vitalism that makes no human or Judaeo-Christian sense. It is a value to be preserved precisely as a condition for other values, and therefore insofar as these other values remain attainable. [140]

For the Christian, reason informed by faith knows that death is a natural part of the rhythm of life. It is not the absolute end for the Christian. It is a transition, the end of one stage—physical life—and the beginning of another—eternal life. McCormick writes:

> Excessive concern for the temporal is at some point a neglect of the eternal. An obligation to use all means to preserve life would be a devaluation of human life, since it would remove life from the context or story that is the source of its ultimate value.[141]

The practical implications of this reasoning are significant regarding treatment decisions for handicapped neonates. Since human life is a relative good, then under certain circumstances, all things considered, not all means need to be used to preserve the physical life of a handicapped neonate.[142] McCormick argues that it is within this context that prevents the absolutization of life that decision-makers are prepared intellectually and psychologically to say at some point "enough." McCormick explains:

> Without such a context (established by the informing faith), we are in constant danger of falling prey to merely technological judgments. Such judgments can push us to either of two extremes: (1) If it can be done, it ought to be done (thus people are kept on respirators in a permanent vegetative state when they can benefit not a whit from such continuance). (2) The dying process is abbreviated by active euthanasia. The notion of the patient's "best interests" is collapsed into what medical technology and expertise can do.[143]

This suggests that the basic value of human life can call forth different obligations at various stages or phases of existence. He argues that to say there is a proportionate reason for not using all means to preserve this particular life in this particular situation, all things considered, is to say simply that there is a point where one judges it to be in the best interests of this handicapped neonate and all concerned to allow death to occur naturally. What is judged to be the good of this neonate and all concerned is rooted in Christian attitudes concerning the meaning of life and death, attitudes that value life without absolutizing it, and that fear and avoid death without absolutizing it.[144] If a handicapped neonate's bodily existence represents a value that conflicts with another more important and even preferred value, such as personal dignity and eternal life, then one may sacrifice bodily existence for this higher value.

HUMAN LIFE IS SACRED AND CANNOT BE DIRECTLY TERMINATED

At the level of synderesis, McCormick argues that since human life is a basic good on which many other basic goods depend, and since human life is created by God, then human life is also sacred. Created in the image and likeness of God, every human life is sacred and therefore should be treated with dignity and respect.[145] The human affections informed by the Christian story discover human life to be not only a basic good, but a basic good that carries the qualification of being sacred.

At the level of normative moral judgment, McCormick uses discursive reason informed by the Christian story to determine that human life may not be directly terminated. Drawing on the doctrine of creation and the lordship of God over all creation, McCormick writes: "If all persons are equally the creatures of the one God, then none of these creatures is authorized to play God toward any other. And if all persons are cherished by God, regardless of merit, we ought to cherish each other in the same spirit."[146] This means that even the most handicapped neonates, those who experience extreme pain and suffering, can never be denied their dignity and respect. Adhering to the Catholic theological tradition, McCormick argues that pain and suffering have a special place in God's saving plan. Without glorifying pain and suffering, the Catholic theological tradition has viewed suffering and even death within a larger perspective, that of the redemptive process. In suffering, Christians participate in the paschal mystery.[147] For McCormick, grave illness is to be seen as an intensifying conformity to Christ. The Catholic theological conviction is that grave illness should be a time of grace, of the gradual shedding of the sinful self.[148]

Based on the Catholic ethical tradition, the magisterium confirms McCormick's rejection of the direct termination of a handicapped neonate. The magisterium has always made a distinction between allowing to die and direct termination of human life. The direct termination of one's life is morally wrong

> because such an action on the part of a person is to be considered as a rejection of God's sovereignty and loving plan . . . However, one must clearly distinguish suicide from that sacrifice of one's life whereby for a higher cause, such as God's glory, the salvation of souls or the service of one's brethren, a person offers his or her own life or puts it in danger (cf. John 15:14).[149]

Epistemologically, McCormick finds unsatisfying the two central positions taken on whether an irreversibly dying life may be terminated directly. Concerning the first, he writes:

> Those who argue the immortality of positive euthanasia by appeal only to the inherent value of human life, even dying life, and therefore to the general disproportion at the heart of the prohibition of killing and suicide in general, forget that they have already abandoned this evaluation when they have provided for passive euthanasia. They have already said of the basic value of human life that it need not be supported while dying in the same way and with the same means as it need be while in a non-dying condition. In other words, they have evaluated dying life differently but then return to and appeal to the evaluation of non-dying life where direct intervention is concerned. This is inconsistent.[150]

This is the position that McCormick held in the first formulation at the level of normative moral judgment in his first moral epistemology (prior to 1983). The second position is held by Joseph Fletcher and those who see no difference between direct termination and allowing to die.[151] McCormick writes: "For them, if there is a truly proportionate reason to allow to die, then there is also thereby a proportionate reason to end life by positive direct intervention."[152] For the proponents of this position there is no moral difference between direct termination and allowing to die, therefore, a reason that justifies one justifies the other. Once death is imminent and inevitable, then it makes no difference how it occurs. McCormick disagrees with both positions.[153] McCormick argues, what is "proportionate for allowing a terminal patient to die is not proportionate for directly causing death."[154] For McCormick, "proportionate reason, if it is adequately developed must include all the effects of a proposed course of action, its relationship to all the values. In this sense, it is not the end that justifies the means, as Fletcher contends, but the ends."[155] McCormick states his moral position quite clearly: "there is no proportionate reason for directly dispatching a terminal or dying patient."[156] Not only would the direct termination of a handicapped neonate's life show a complete utter disrespect for the dignity of that life, it would also involve dangers for the living.[157] McCormick is once again pushing in the social direction, stressing the inevitability of human interdependence. Therefore, McCormick argues that the harm involved in direct termination is disproportionate to the benefits, not only for the neonate but for society as a whole. For McCormick, human life is sacred and the direct killing of an innocent life is a virtually exceptionless norm.[158]

MEDICAL TECHNOLOGY IS A GOOD, BUT A GOOD
THAT IS LIMITED AND TO BE USED RESPONSIBLY

At the level of synderesis, medical technology is the result of the basic inclination or "tendency to explore and question."[159] Created in the image and likeness of God and graced with free will and reason, the human person has been enabled by God to use these gifts in creative ways that can help transform self, others, and the world. As a gift from God, medical technology has given neonatologists the ability to save the lives of many handicapped neonates. However, as a good, it also has the potential to be abused.

At the level of normative moral judgment, McCormick's use of discursive reason informed by the Christian story helps him remain focused on the basic goods. Therefore, medical technology must be used in a responsible manner that will advance the good of humankind. Like Daniel Callahan, McCormick is concerned that humanity today has become corporately *homo technologicus*. In this situation, some believe the best situation to the dilemmas created by technology is more technology. McCormick argues that we tend to eliminate the maladapted condition (defectives, retardates, and so on) rather than adjust the environment to it.[160] Because of this model of the human person, cultural biases have affected how persons view the meaning of life and thus, how persons view the meaning of death. McCormick believes there is a virtual consensus in America today that individuals have successfully conspired to suppress death into the realm of the unreal. Death has become the enemy to be defeated at all costs. However, it is the Christian story informing reason that allows the individual to identify these cultural biases and to overcome them. McCormick writes:

> Only when this task is accomplished will we be able to make quality-of-life decisions without forfeiting true quality. Only then will we be able to avoid both a demeaning vitalism that canonizes physiological processes and an Orwellian interventionism that collapses the physical as meaningless. Only then will we be able to view death as both a rhythm of nature and yet as the inimical wages of sin, as both choice and yet submission. Only then will the physician grow tolerably comfortable with the paradox at the heart of his profession: the commitment to preserve life and health, yet acceptance that ultimate defeat is inevitable.[161]

The responsible use of medical technology must consider the good of the whole person and the common good of society, not just a particular problem.

As finite creatures, the goods of creation are limited. Therefore, these goods must be allocated in a responsible way. In considering the good of society, McCormick argues that we must examine the escalating costs of health care. This is due to many factors, such as increasing sophistication of services, higher wages, more personnel, cost pass-along systems, and inflation. These cost factors have forced allocation questions and decisions of the most painful kind. Are we using neonatal intensive care units effectively? Must we begin to exclude some categories of handicapped neonates from these sophisticated services?[162] Cost factors raise very difficult questions and demand even more difficult decisions regarding treatment decisions for handicapped neonates.

McCormick is concerned that both the human and the moral good will be identified with what is technologically possible and affordable, with the result that technology will create its own morality regarding treatment decisions for handicapped neonates. For McCormick, discursive reason informed by the Christian story determines when there is proportionate reason to either use or not use specific medical treatments for handicapped neonates. The Christian story provides a framework by which the Christian can reasonably determine what is truly in the "best interests" of the handicapped neonate against any cultural attempts to distort it.

In conclusion, when McCormick's moral epistemology is applied to treatment decisions for handicapped neonates, various moral judgments can be derived that are not only reasonable but firmly grounded in the Catholic theological tradition. However, not all of McCormick's ethicist colleagues concur with this evaluation. Various criticisms have been directed at McCormick's moral epistemology that must be addressed in order to have a comprehensive view of how he makes moral decisions regarding treatment for handicapped neonates. To complete the analysis of McCormick's moral epistemology the next section will articulate, analyze, and evaluate some of these criticisms.

CRITICISM

Serious criticisms have been directed at McCormick's moral epistemology at both the foundational and structural levels. These criticisms range from questions concerning the shift in his moral epistemology to inconsistency in regard to language. Further, others question the ambiguity in McCormick's moral epistemology and whether he is a critical or naive

realist. McCormick has stated on a number of occasions that "theologians should become more critical of one another—in a courteous and dis-
ciplined way."[163] This section will respond to McCormick's invitation by
examining a number of major criticisms directed at his moral epistemology.

First, as we have seen, McCormick made a significant shift in his
moral epistemology at the level of synderesis. In the first moral epistemology (prior to 1983), the human person knows the basic goods that
define human flourishing by reason, reflecting on the human person's
basic tendencies or inclinations. McCormick writes: "For it is impossible
to act without having an interest in the object, and it is impossible to be
attracted by, to have an interest in, something without some inclination
already present."[164] In the second moral epistemology (after 1983), it is
through one's feelings or affections, informed by the Christian story, that
one becomes aware of the basic goods. At the level of synderesis, there
has been a significant shift from reason reflecting on the basic inclinations to the affections informed by the Christian story discovering the
basic goods.

The problem with this movement from the first to the second moral
epistemology is that McCormick failed to articulate or give a systematic
explanation for why he made this epistemological shift. Literally,
McCormick creates a second moral epistemology at the level of synderesis and proceeds to apply it to the area of bioethics without any acknowledgment that he has made an epistemological change. From 1983 onward, it will be the affections informed by the Christian story that discover the basic goods, not reason reflecting on the basic inclinations.
This creates serious methodological questions and has been the source of
much confusion. McCormick's many contributions to Christian ethics
could have benefitted greatly from a systematic analysis of his moral
epistemology, by himself or a third party, especially at the level of synderesis. The problem is that McCormick never saw himself as a "system-
builder." He basically approaches moral problems as they arise in life.[165]
This has far-reaching ramifications for him as a moral theologian and for
his ethical positions. McCormick was looked to by his colleagues and by
the Catholic Church for his moral evaluations on bioethical issues affecting the faithful. Unless his moral epistemology is clearly articulated
and systematically presented, his moral positions on bioethical issues can
become suspect and open to a wide range of criticisms.

Second, both of McCormick's moral epistemologies have inconsistencies in language and ambiguities in application. For example, in one
of his earliest articles, published in 1974, he writes that the basic values
are *"equally basic and irreducibly attractive."*[166] In a reprint of the same
article published in 1981, this section of the original article was elimi-

nated.[167] In 1981, McCormick published an article in which he argues that the basic values are now *"equally underivative and irreducibly attractive."*[168] In the 1974 article, "Proxy Consent in the Experimentation Situation," McCormick appears to be closely aligned with Finnis' theory of equally fundamental basic goods. The fundamental change of terminology in the later article, "Bioethics and Method," reveals a shift in formulation at the level of normative moral judgment in his first moral epistemology. Regrettably, this is done without any explanation or justification. On this subject, Lisa Sowle Cahill has observed:

> In a personal communication (8/18/81), McCormick has indicated that the basic goods are to be spoken of properly as "equally underivative" rather than "equally basic." He notes that this shift in language might imply conclusions about the goods other than those drawn by Finnis. A systematic exposition by McCormick of the quality of being "underivative" would no doubt have a significant impact upon the critique that follows in the present essay, inasmuch as the latter is premised precisely on the hypothesis that Finnis' conclusions do not find adequate warrants in McCormick's general perspective.[169]

McCormick never provided a systematic exposition of the quality of being "underivative." This example demonstrates not only inconsistencies in McCormick's use of terminology, but also indicates a shift in formulation in his first moral epistemology at the level of normative moral judgment. This fundamental shift demands a systematic explanation and analysis, or an admission that the author has in fact changed his mind. Unfortunately, he never addressed these issues before his death.

It is possible to point out additional examples of inconsistency in terminology and ambiguity in application. For example, McCormick writes: "Thus I see 'association of basic values,' 'proportionate reason,' and 'adoption of a hierarchy of values' as attempting to say the same thing, or at least very closely related."[170] Again McCormick writes:

> In summary, then, proportionate reason as I understand it can be explained in several different ways, no one of which need reduce to 'greatest net good.' Namely, one can speak of association of basic goods (rather than commensuration); one can speak of corporate *adoption* of a hierarchy; or one can speak of a certain equivalence

(aggression against liberty is tantamount to aggression against life).[171]

Each of these terms needed to be more clearly defined.[172] A further example is McCormick's response to an article written by Sanford Levy. McCormick writes:

> Levy makes some worthwhile points, particularly in reference to my proposal of a "theory of associated goods." He does not think much of it, and I would add that *I am not wedded to it*. However, I am convinced that our assessments of proportion and disproportion are destined to remain somewhat intuitive without our full ability to state them adequately in reasoned analysis.[173]

Important questions remain: what did McCormick mean that he was not wedded to the theory of associated goods? Did he not formulate his hierarchy of goods through the theory of associated goods? Why does he no longer refer to the "association of basic goods" after 1983?

McCormick is also ambiguous in his second moral epistemology concerning the meaning of prediscursive reason or the affections. Unfortunately, throughout the entire discussion he never clearly articulates what is meant by this term. McCormick argues that human affectivity plays a major role in discovering the basic goods. However, McCormick fails to elaborate on what is meant by feelings or the affections. McCormick states that "judgments of the moral 'ought' have deep roots in our sensitivities and emotions. This has particular relevance where the health needs of the elderly and dependent (fetuses, infants, retarded and poor) are concerned."[174] If this is true, then McCormick needs to be clear on what he means by the affections. After reviewing McCormick's views on feelings, affections, aspirations, etc., questions remain: what does McCormick mean by prediscursive reason? Are connatural knowledge and "moral instincts of faith" the same? Or, does McCormick have two different senses of the idea of prediscursive reason?

Ethicist James J. Walter believes that various terms used by McCormick to describe prediscursive reason appear to create two slightly different senses of the idea. Walter argues:

> In his discussion of natural inclinations, which are the basis for our interest in specific values, he [McCormick] claimed that our intelligence spontaneously and without reflection grasps the possibilities to which they point . . . As a moral instinct of faith, this latter aspect of moral

knowing cannot be adequately subjected to analytic reflection, but it is responsible for one's ultimate judgments on concrete moral issues.[175]

Odozor responds to Walter's criticism by observing that:

Ultimately we are not speaking of two distinct realities.
Prediscursive knowledge described as connatural knowledge or as the "moral instinct of faith," "cannot be adequately subject to analytic reflection." In spite of possible distortions due to personal or cultural biases they
remain, "a more reliable test of humanizing and dehumanizing, of the morally right and wrong, of proportion,
than our discursive arguments."[176]

While these two aspects may not be two distinct realities in McCormick's mind, they can certainly cause confusion in the minds of others. If
sensitivities and emotions have "particular relevance" in treatment decisions for handicapped neonates, then McCormick should have clarified
what he meant by prediscursive reasoning.

These examples present both inconsistencies in terminology and ambiguities in application throughout McCormick's first and second moral
epistemologies. McCormick never adequately addressed these criticisms.
It is possible to speculate that the cause for these inconsistencies and ambiguities might be the direct result of his writing the "Notes on Moral
Theology." While he was writing these "Notes on Moral Theology," he
was called upon to address a wide range of topics, and to offer his critique of these issues. He was challenged to reflect on and respond to new
ideas that were being presented in various articles. He articulated these
new ideas and at times responded to them in a rather offhanded manner.
In the process he would accept new ideas and principles or reject old
ones without providing any sustained justification.[177] On a broader scale,
his lack of clarity has added to the confusion surrounding such fundamental issues as proportionalism, premoral evils, etc. One could speculate that the conflicts that have developed between the magisterium and
proportionalists might have been lessened if the language used to explain
notions such as proportionate reason and premoral evils were consistent
and precise. Much of the criticism directed at many of McCormick's
ethical positions may not have been necessary if his moral epistemology
were more systematically presented.

Third, there are many critics of McCormick's hierarchy of values.
James J. Walter writes:

I think McCormick's original intuitions, if I may call
them that, were correct about the need for a hierarchy of
values; however, I remain relatively unconvinced of the
way in which he has demonstrated this hierarchy and
how he has construed the conflicts between the associated goods.[178]

Finnis *et al.* do not believe there is a hierarchy of values, because the
basic goods are equally basic and irreducibly attractive. Ronald McKinney, S.J.,[179] and Garth Hallett, S.J.,[180] both argue that it is not only unnecessary but impossible analytically to develop a hierarchy of values.
Walter believes that these latter assessments are important not only in
themselves but because these authors are known proportionalists.[181]
Walter's criticism appears to be well-founded. McCormick spends a
great deal of time talking about the hierarchy of values and in fact, the
hierarchy of values is the one consistent element that underlies both of
his moral epistemologies. However, he never clearly articulates how this
hierarchy is established. Odozor argues that

McCormick assumes a hierarchy of values (*ordo bonorum*). Prudence dictates which of these goods should be
chosen in times of conflict. This choice is not made ar-
bitrarily, because some obligations are certain in all circumstances, even if there is a doubt of fact, because the
good to be protected and secured, "prevails over any
good which can be adduced as *incommodum*." Prudence
merely dictates what is proportionate reason according to
this prevalence of goods.[182]

Odozor further states:

I do not share Cahill's view that the difficulty in discerning and agreeing on a hierarchy of values constitutes
"an undeniable shortcoming" in McCormick's teleology.
Instead, it indicates that there is no other route to ethics
but through responsible teleology. This is because the
difficulty she points out stems from the human condition—our individual, social, and cultural differences as
well as our finiteness. Although determining a hierarchy
of values might involve "an intricate conceptualization
of relative values and disvalues," it is not foreign to any
normal adult. Nor is it something "theoreticians" instead
of "decision-makers" do.[183]

To say that the virtue of prudence plays an integral role in determining the hierarchy of values unfortunately provides little clarity. McCormick refers to prudence a number of times in both of his moral epistemologies, but he never defines the virtue or explains how he uses it.[184]

Odozor attempts to clarify further McCormick's understanding of the hierarchy of values as he writes: "McCormick's casuistry is, in a way, a constant search for the order in this value system. This search is conducted, not in spite of, but in accord with human experience."[185] Again, Odozor's explanation lends little clarity. Instead, more questions remain: Does this mean that in the hierarchy of values, the values are constantly in flux? Is proportionate reason the tool for determining the placement of the values within the hierarchy? Or is it human experience? There is a need for a hierarchy of values, as McCormick contends. However, because he never articulated how this hierarchy is formed, one is left to mere speculation on how the values are placed within the hierarchy.

A further criticism with respect to the hierarchy of values has to do with confusing premoral and moral values within the hierarchy. McCormick has claimed that the basic values can, in fact, conflict. In this case, the human person must compare and choose among them. Walter believes that one of the possible difficulties in McCormick's position may be related not to his claim that the basic goods are associated, but rather to the fact that he might have included both premoral and moral values into his category of basic goods.[186] There are two distinct examples in McCormick's writings that support this criticism. The first centers on the example McCormick uses of the sheriff in the southern town who is faced with two alternatives in a rape case of either framing a black suspect (whom he knows to be innocent) or carrying on a prolonged search for the real culprit. The immediate indictment and conviction of the suspect would save many lives and prevent other harmful consequences. There seem to be two different types of values being weighed in this conflict situation—freedom (political liberty) and the protection of life.[187] James Walter has written:

> One might argue that life is a premoral value but that liberty (political freedom) is a moral value because the latter value describes a quality of moral persons as they confront various situations. If my suggestion is correct, then the conflict is not between values as associated but between values of a *different* kind.[188]

Walter's position is further clarified by ethicist Timothy O'Connell who argues that moral values describe qualities of moral persons themselves as they confront and correctly deal with their situations.[189]

The second example centers on the basic values that McCormick takes from Finnis *et al.*[190] Included is the basic value of friendship which many critics argue is a moral value and thus should be reclassified. On this subject Cahill writes: "Friendship, as distinct from mere social interaction, connotes moral virtues such as love, justice, honesty, and fidelity."[191] Cahill argues that friendship is distinct from the basic value of procreation and life. Cahill views both of these values as being premoral. Each of these examples demonstrates that McCormick has mixed premoral and moral values within his hierarchy of values. McCormick is unable to explain not only how he forms the hierarchy of values, but how the values are construed and how conflicts are understood. It appears that McCormick's understanding of basic values entails both premoral and moral values. Since the hierarchy of values is foundational to both forms of McCormick's moral epistemology, a more systematic analysis and justification of how he forms the hierarchy is required.

Fourth, it appears that McCormick identifies himself as a critical realist. It is possible to question if this has always been the case. A naive realist knows human reality on the model of taking a look at what is already out there to be looked at. Reaching an objective judgment is just verifying that something is true or real or valuable by using the standards of empirical observation based on one's sensory faculties. The critical realist, on the other hand, acknowledges that the facts of human knowing and judging values are related to the appropriation of our own operations of self-transcendence. The real world is the world mediated by meaning and motivated by value, and it is constituted by its reference to the invariant process of experiencing, understanding, judging, and deliberating.[192] One could question whether McCormick is a naive realist in regard to the basic goods. For McCormick, are the basic goods something "out there to be looked at?" In McCormick's first moral epistemology, at the level of normative moral judgment, is physicalism and its deductive method a form of naive realism? A number of ethicists, including Charles E. Curran, suggest that physicalism reflects a naive realism.[193] If this is true, then McCormick has not always been a critical realist.

Finally, McCormick places emphasis on scripture as a traditional source of moral wisdom. He believes the renewal of moral theology entails using scripture more effectively. Unfortunately, this is not clear in his own moral epistemology. Odozor writes:

> Although McCormick is aware of the importance of
> scripture for ethics, he is not inclined to use particular

texts to buttress his points or even ask questions about the meaning of particular texts for contemporary society. It is not that this does not matter. For him, scripture is a "moral reminder," and a privileged articulation of what everyone can know through human reason. Apart from the danger that this attitude may fail to see that sacred scriptures command us to love our neighbor in a particular way, it makes McCormick's work no more scriptural than the theology of the manuals.[194]

McCormick stresses the important need for theologians to follow the guidelines suggested at Vatican II, especially its insistence that morality's scientific exposition should be more thoroughly nourished by scriptural teaching.[195] He states: "Scripture nourishes our overall perspectives, tells us through Christ the kinds of people we ought to be and become, the type of world we ought to create."[196] It is possible to ask that, if scripture is so integral to his moral epistemology, then why does he use it so sparingly and selectively? Cahill observes that McCormick appears to limit himself to the gospel of John and the epistles of Paul.[197] If the stories of the Christian narrative nourish the faith of the individual and affect perspectives, and if they sharpen and intensify our focus on the human goods that are definitive of our flourishing, then McCormick ought to allow scripture to nourish his moral epistemology in a more comprehensive manner. With an emphasis on scripture, McCormick can show his critics that he is not presenting some radically new morality. Instead, he can show that he is only trying to recapture the sources of a quite old one and hence represent a healthy exercise in Christian memory.[198]

McCormick has always underscored the primacy of method. In the conclusion to his review of Joseph Fletcher's book on situation ethics, McCormick argues that Fletcher has not made up his mind on how moral judgments are made. He adds:

As long as this remains unclear, he can squeeze out of any epistemological corner, because he has none he calls his own. And as long as he has none he calls his own, one can say that he has adopted a method (and its content-conclusion) without first solving the problem of methodology.[199]

McCormick criticizes Fletcher for excessive ambiguity. This same criticism might also be leveled against McCormick and his moral epistemology. There is a critical need for McCormick's moral epistemology to be systematically explained so that any ambiguity that exists can be clarified. Since he never did this, it is up to future theologians to undertake this task. Unless this is done, there could be dire consequences in many diverse areas of bioethics, but in particular, in regard to treatment decisions for handicapped neonates.

CONCLUSION

Daniel Maguire believes that "moral theology would benefit tremendously from a full statement of method from McCormick."[200] This critical analysis of McCormick's moral epistemology certainly reinforces Maguire's criticism. McCormick made a significant shift in his moral epistemology at the level of synderesis. At the level of normative moral judgment, it appears that McCormick's moral epistemology is a synthesis, which is the product of development and maturity in his thought process. Because of the numerous criticisms that surround McCormick's moral epistemology, and the ambiguity that it entails, McCormick needed to articulate his theoretical foundations clearly and develop them systematically and coherently. Numerous moral theologians have called for him to do this, yet he never responded.[201] A systematic understanding of McCormick's moral epistemology is not only necessary but crucial in determining treatment decisions for handicapped neonates. It is necessary because it is the basis of moral decision-making. It is crucial because the life and death of handicapped neonates may hang in the balance.

Once McCormick establishes how a person knows, it becomes important to determine the criteria, that is, norms or tests, by which one may judge what is true and certain in human reasoning. Criteriology is the science of true and certain knowledge and complements moral epistemology. If McCormick's moral epistemology is the basis for life and death decisions regarding handicapped neonates, then the moral criteria one uses to determine life and death decisions are equally important. The next chapter will focus on substantive issues, that is, what McCormick believes are the appropriate standards or criteria for making treatment decisions for handicapped neonates.

NOTES

[1]Michael J. Quirk, "Ethics: Moral Epistemology," *Encyclopedia of Bioethics*, rev. ed., vol. 2, 727.

[2]John Langan, S.J., "Beatitude and Moral Law in St. Thomas," *The Journal of Religious Ethics* 5 (Fall 1977): 189.

[3]Thomas Aquinas, *Summa Theologica* Ia, 79, 12; see also Idem, *Summa Theologica* Ia-IIae, 94, 1; Idem, *Truth*, 16, 1. Emphasis in the original. Thomas further states: "Whence synderesis is said to incite to good, and to murmur at evil, inasmuch as through first principles we proceed to discover, and judge of what we have discovered. It is therefore clear that synderesis is not a power, but a natural habit." Idem, *Summa Theologica* Ia, 79, 12.

[4]John Langan argues that Thomas is not clear on what are the things we know through this intuitive grasp of first principles. He believes there are several candidates proposed in the *Summa Theologica* Ia-IIae, 94. The first is "good is to be sought and done, evil to be avoided" (*Summa Theologica* Ia-IIae, 94, 2). Secondly, Thomas speaks of the precept that "we should act intelligently (*ut secundum rationem agatur*)" in ways which make it clear that this is a first principle of practical reason; for it is accepted by all persons and from it he holds we can derive more specific conclusions (*Summa Theologica* Ia-IIae, 94, 40). Thirdly, Thomas also says that this precept is equivalent to the precept that we should act virtuously (*ut secundum virtutem agatur*) (*Summa Theologica* Ia-IIae, 94, 3). See Langan, "Beatitude and Moral Law in St. Thomas," 189.

[5]Thomas refers to conscience, but more contemporary theologians in the Thomistic tradition would use the term normative moral judgment.

[6] For Thomas the application would be as follows: "One way in so far as we recognize that we have done or not done something; *Thy conscience knoweth that thou hast often spoken evil of others* (Eccles. vii. 23), and according to this, conscience is said to witness. In another way, so far as through the conscience we judge that something should be done or not done; and in this sense, conscience is said to incite or to bind. In the third way, so far as by conscience we judge that something done is well done or ill done, and in this sense conscience is said to excuse, accuse, or torment. Now, it is clear that all these things follow the actual application of knowledge to what we do. Wherefore, properly speaking, conscience dominates an act." Aquinas, *Summa Theologica* Ia, 79, 13. Emphasis in the original.

[7]Thomas Aquinas, *Quaestiones Quodlibetales*, 3, 27 (Rome, Italy: Marelli Publishers, 1956), 64.

[8]F. C. Copleston, *Aquinas* (London: Penguin Books, 1955), 228.

[9]Aquinas, *Summa Theologica* Ia-IIae, 94, 4. This position of Aquinas will serve as the basis for McCormick's distinction between the substance of a teaching and its formulation.

[10]Lisa Sowle Cahill lists three main initiatives of Richard McCormick as a revised natural law ethicist. For a more detailed analysis of these three initiatives, refer to Chapter One, Bioethical Methodologies section, Natural Law Methodology sub-section above.

[11]McCormick, "Theology and Biomedical Ethics," 311.

[12]For a detailed discussion of the person "integrally and adequately considered," refer to Chapter Two, McCormick's Theological Anthropology, above. McCormick argues: "The basic thrust of the natural law was and is that man's being is and must be the basis for his becoming. Catholic theologians are more keenly aware of the fact that in many respects this being is changeable and changing. . . . On the other hand, in retreating from the unhistorical orthodoxies and instant certainties of the past and allowing full range to man's historical existence and creativity, we must retain the courage to be concrete." McCormick, "The New Morality," 771.

[13]For a more detailed analysis of the categorizing of McCormick's writings into three periods, refer to Chapter One, Richard A. McCormick, S.J.—Moral Theologian section above.

[14]Aquinas writes: "Everything—whether it has knowledge or not—tends toward the good. Whatever is oriented or inclined to something by another is inclined to whatever is intended by the one inclining or orienting. Therefore, since all natural things have been directed by a certain natural inclination toward their ends by the First Mover, God, whatever is willed or intended by God is that to which everything is naturally inclined. But inasmuch as God's will can have no other end than Himself, and God is essentially goodness, everything must be naturally inclined toward good. To desire or have a tendency is only to yearn for something, tending as it were toward whatever is suitable for oneself. Hence because all things are destined and oriented by God toward a good, and this is done so that in each one there is a principle whereby it tends toward good as though seeking good itself, we must admit that all things naturally tend toward good. If everything tended toward good while lacking within itself any principle of inclination, they might be spoken of as being led to good but not tending toward good. But through an innate principle everything is said to tend to good as self-inclining. Hence we read in Wisdom 8:1 that divine wisdom 'ordered all things sweetly' because each by its own action tends toward that to which it has been divinely directed." Thomas Aquinas, *De Veritate*, 22, 1, c, trans. Mulligan-McGlynn Schmidt (Chicago, IL: Regnery, 1952-54); see also Mary T. Clark, *An Aquinas Reader* (Garden City, NY: Image Books, 1972), 257.

[15]Thomas writes: "All things which should be done or which should be shunned pertain to precepts of the natural law insofar as practical reason naturally apprehends them to be human goods." Aquinas, *Summa Theologica* Ia-IIae, 94, 2.

[16]McCormick's point is that one cannot move from synderesis to the natural inclinations without reference to anthropology.

[17]McCormick, "The New Morality," 771.

[18]McCormick, "Personal Conscience," 243-244.

[19]Normative theories formulate and defend a system of fundamental principles and rules that determine which actions are right and which are wrong. See Tom L. Beauchamp and James F. Childress, *Principles of Medical Ethics*, 3rd ed., 9.

[20]James J. Walter and Stephen Happel state that there are three main theories or schools of thought that attempt to explain the grounding of moral knowledge and the cognitive status of the moral interpretations that emanate from moral apprehensions. They write: "First, there is the relativist school, which can be divided into the social-relativist wing and the personal-relativist wing. For the social relativist, moral evaluations are governed by the culturally available categories of a given society. . . . For the personal relativist, moral evaluations must find their ground in personal feelings or emotions. Accordingly, an action is right or wrong by reference to whether one approves or disapproves of the action and feels happy or sad when the action is performed. The second main theory of moral knowledge is found in the noncognitivist school. . . . Moral statements are simply emotional utterances. The third school or theory is known as the absolutist. Briefly stated, those in the absolutist school argue that moral standards are about objective common human reality, and thus, that in principle there can be universal agreement about the truth and falsity of any particular claim. . . . The central reason there should be universal agreement is that all humans are looked on as attempting, however imperfectly, to determine a judgment that comes from a *single source*." For a more detailed analysis, see James J. Walter and Stephen Happel, *Conversion and Discipleship: A Christian Foundation for Ethics and Doctrine* (Philadelphia, PA: Fortress Press, 1986), 104-105. Emphasis in the original.

[21]Kenneth R. Himes suggests that McCormick is a critical realist. As he puts it: "this epistemology accepts the nature of the real as a basis for moral judgment but demands a process of critical questioning that takes the subject beyond the world of sense data to the world of meaning. Objectivity in the world of sense data requires functional sensory organs. Objectivity in the world of meaning asks of us to wed sense data with

intelligence and reason. Thus, to obtain moral meaning it is insufficient to rely upon the immediacy of sense data alone. Meaning comes to be in the encounter of the subject with the object of the world of immediacy. The criteria for an authentic encounter are the transcendental precepts: Be attentive! Be intelligent! Be reasonable! Be responsible!" Himes, "The Contribution of Theology to Catholic Moral Theology," *Moral Theology: Challenges for the Future*, 56. The classic texts for describing an epistemology of critical realism are Bernard Lonergan's *Insight: A Study of Human Understanding* (London: Longmans, Green, & Co., 1957); and *Method In Theology* (New York: Herder and Herder, 1972).

[22]Karl Popper, "A Complete Theory of Knowledge?" in *The Theory of Knowledge* ed. D. W. Hamlyn (Garden City, NY: Doubleday & Company, 1970), 284-285; see also K. R. Popper, *Conjectures and Refutations* (New York: Harper and Row, 1968).

[23]Richard A. McCormick, S.J., "Health and Medicine in the Catholic Tradition," *Acta Hospitalia* 1 (1986): 55.

[24]Scripture (as reread and continually reappropriated by the community: tradition) is a "moral reminder," and a privileged articulation of what all people of good will can know through human reason. For McCormick, "scripture does not immediately yield moral norms and rules. But it affects them. The stories and symbols that relate the origin of Christianity and nourish the faith of the individual affect one's perspectives. . . . [Persons] do not find concrete answers in the sources of faith, but they bring a worldview that informs their reasoning—especially by allowing the basic human goods to retain their attractiveness and not be tainted by cultural distortions. This worldview is a continuing check on and challenge to our tendency to make choices in light of cultural enthusiasms which sink into and take possession of our unwitting, pre-discursive selves." McCormick, "Health and Medicine in the Catholic Tradition," 58.

[25]For McCormick, "the magisterium in our time gives us the enlightenment of the whole Church. However, it also imposes on us the responsibility of being critical Catholics. In this sense, it is both privilege and responsibility. If we are to enjoy the privilege, we must incur the responsibility." McCormick further argues that "an effective magisterium necessarily involves a teaching-learning process in which teachers learn and learners teach. Dissent is an integral part of this process. . . . Viewing the magisterium as involving a processive dialogue is particularly important in medico-moral matters." Ibid., 61.

[26]For McCormick, human reason refers to "all those dimensions of human understanding that play a role in our evaluation of actions as mor-

ally right or wrong. Among these dimensions are: experience, the sense of profanation, trial and error, discourse reasoning, long-term consequences, the experience of harmony or guilt over our actions. There is always the danger that the term *recta ratio* will be impoverished by collapsing it into a barren rationalism that overlooks the affective richness of human understanding." Ibid.

[27]McCormick, "Personal Conscience," 243. McCormick continues: "However, if the Christian's knowledge of the morally good or bad is to take concrete meaningful form, it must also draw upon and integrate the insights and experience of a variety of disciplines that study the world and provide the context of decision and choice: economics, medicine, psychology and psychiatry, sociology, law, cultural anthropology, etc. Thus the light of the Gospel in confrontation with human experience will be the source of ever fresh insights into the meaning and challenge of being a Christian in the modern world." Ibid.

[28]McCormick, *The Critical Calling*, 35.

[29]For a more detailed analysis of the changes proposed at Vatican II that emphasize the human person as central to moral reflection, see "Pastoral Constitution on the Church in the Modern World," *The Documents of Vatican II*, ed. Walter M. Abbott.

[30]Allsopp, 105. See also, McCormick, *The Critical Calling*, 54.

[31]McCormick, "Theology and Biomedical Ethics," 311. Emphasis in the original. McCormick argues that there are four levels at which the term "ethics" is to be understood. Those levels are: essential ethic, existential ethic, essential Christian ethics, and existential Christian ethics. For McCormick, an essential ethic means "those norms that are regarded as applicable to all persons, where one's behavior is but an instance of a general, essential moral norm. Here we could use as examples the rightness and wrongness of killing actions, of contracts, of promises and all those actions whose demands are rooted in the dignity of the person." It is at this level where explicit faith does not "add new content at the material or concrete level. However, revelation and our personal faith do influence ethical decisions at the other three levels." For a more detailed analysis, see Idem, "Does Religious Faith Add To Ethical Perception?," *Readings in Moral Theology No. 2: The Distinctiveness of Christian Ethics*, eds. Charles E. Curran and Richard A. McCormick, S.J. (New York: Paulist Press, 1980), 156-173; and Idem, *The Critical Calling*, 196.

[32]McCormick, "Theology and Biomedical Ethics," 312.

[33]McCormick, "Moral Arguments in the Catholic Tradition," 5.

[34]Ibid. Emphasis in the original.

[35]Neo-scholasticism provided Catholic theology with a common philosophical language that facilitated teaching and dialogue; it offered clarity in definition and argumentation; and it provided some metaphysical grounding for those natural truths that prepare one for Christian faith, namely the existence of God, the spirituality of the human soul, and the natural moral law. The weaknesses of neo-scholasticism were its lack of historical perspective; its eclectic confusion of Thomism with the alien doctrines of Francisco de Suárez, Duns Scotus, René Descartes, G. W. Leibniz, Immanuel Kant and idealism; its failure to deal adequately with the findings of modern science and to recognize human historicity and subjectivity; and its teaching methods, which tended toward conceptualism, while neglecting to ground principles and definitions in experience. For a more detailed analysis, see *The Encyclopedia of Catholicism*, 911; refer also to Chapter One, Richard A. McCormick, S.J.—Moral Theologian section, above.

[36]Thomas argues that there are certain natural impulses that humans share with all created things, for example, the impulse to preserve oneself in being. There are other inclinations that we share with other animals, for example, the urge to mate and raise offspring. Finally, there is an inclination to the good according to the nature of reason, peculiar to humans. For example, human persons have the natural inclination to seek the truth and live in society. See Aquinas, *Summa Theologica* Ia-IIae, 94, 2.

[37]It should be noted that throughout McCormick's writings he uses "basic goods" and "basic values" to mean the same thing. I will attempt to be consistent by referring to them as "basic goods," however, there will be certain times when I will quote McCormick and he will refer to the basic goods as "basic values." It should also be noted that John Finnis and Lisa Sowle Cahill will also use "basic goods" and "basic values" to mean the same thing.

[38]John Finnis, "Natural Law and Unnatural Acts," *Heythrop Journal* 11 (1970): 373.

[39]McCormick, *Notes on Moral Theology: 1965 through 1980*, 451.

[40]For a more detailed analysis of the Catholic natural law methodology, refer to Chapter One, Bioethical Methodologies section, Natural Law Methodology subsection above.

[41]Ibid., 453. Finnis writes: "Natural law is not a doctrine. It is one's permanent dynamic orientation towards an understanding grasp of the goods that can be realized by free choice, together with a bias (like the bias in one's 'speculation' towards raising questions that will lead one on from data to insight and from insight to judgment) towards actually

making choices that are intelligibly (because intelligently) related to the goods which are understood to be attainable, or at stake, in one's situation." Finnis, "Natural Law and Unnatural Acts," 366.

[42]McCormick, "The Judaeo-Christian Tradition and Bioethical Codes," *How Brave a New World?*, 5.

[43]Ibid.

[44]Finnis claims that: "Now besides life, knowledge, play, aesthetic experience, friendship, practical reasonableness, and religion, there are countless objectives and forms of good. But I suggest that these other objectives and forms of good will be found, on analysis, to be ways or combinations of ways of pursuing (not always sensibly) and realizing (not always successfully) one of the seven basic forms, or some combination of them." John Finnis, *Natural Law and Natural Rights* (Oxford: Clarendon Press, 1980), 90. Lisa Sowle Cahill notes that: "The basic inclinations mentioned by McCormick are roughly equivalent to these (though not so definitively enumerated), with the addition of 'the tendency to mate and raise children.' Procreation is called a basic value by Finnis in an article on sexual morality but is not included in the list in his later volume on natural rights." Lisa Sowle Cahill, "Teleology, Utilitarianism, and Christian Ethics," 622. See also John Finnis, "Natural Law and Unnatural Acts," 385.

[45]McCormick, "The Judaeo-Christian Tradition and Bioethical Codes," *How Brave a New World?*, 5.

[46]Ibid.; see also McCormick, "Proxy Consent in the Experimentation Situation," in *Love and Society: Essays in the Ethics of Paul Ramsey*, eds. James Johnson and David Smith (Missoula, MT: University of Montana Press, 1974), 217. It should be noted that in a reprint of this same article in *How Brave a New World?*, published in 1981, the section of the article where McCormick states that "these basic values are equally basic and irreducibly attractive" has been eliminated.

[47]Finnis, *Natural Law and Natural Rights*, 92.

[48]The incommensurability of the basic goods means that they cannot be measured. One cannot choose directly against a basic good. Finnis writes: "To choose directly against it in favour of some other basic value is arbitrary, for each of the basic values is equally basic, equally irreducibly and self-evidently attractive." Finnis, "Natural Law and Unnatural Acts," 375.

[49]McCormick, "Proxy Consent in the Experimentation Situation," in *Love and Society*, 217.

[50]Finnis, "Natural Law and Unnatural Acts," 375.

[51]Ibid., 368.

[52]Finnis writes: "What is (what we call) 'morally' right and wrong, virtuous and vicious, emerges only as the product of a *further* understanding (which may of course be spontaneous or reflective) of what particular forms of pursuit and realization of these values do represent, in concrete types of situation, an adequate openness to and tension towards the God who is the source of the irreducible *claritas* of each of the fundamental values of human living." Finnis, "Natural Law and Unnatural Acts," 373. Emphasis in the original.

[53]Ibid., 375.

[54]Cahill, "Teleology, Utilitarianism, and Christian Ethics," 622.

[55]McCormick, "Proxy Consent in the Experimentation Situation," in *Love and Society*, 217-218. Emphasis mine.

[56]Finnis writes: "So where one of these irreducible values falls immediately under our choice directly to realize it or spurn it, then, in the Christian understanding, we remain open to that value, that basic component of the human order, as the only reasonable way to remain open to the ground of all values, all order. To choose directly against it in favour of some other basic value is arbitrary . . ." Finnis, "Natural Law and Unnatural Acts," 375.

[57]McCormick, *Notes on Moral Theology 1965 through 1980*, 717. Emphasis in the original. McCormick goes on to quote Paul Ramsey who writes: "My own view is that the distinction between direct and indirect voluntariety is pertinent and alerts our attention as moral agents to those moral choices where incommensurable conflicting values are at stake, where there is no measurable resolution of value conflicts on a single scale, where there are gaps in any supposed hierarchy of values, and therefore no way to determine exactly the greater or lesser good or evil. . . . Where there is no single scale or common denominator, or where there is discontinuity in the hierarchy of goods or evils, one ought not to turn against any human good." McCormick, *Doing Evil to Achieve Good*, 85.

[58]Traditional moralists have claimed that certain actions (such as masturbation, artificial contraception, direct sterilization, artificial insemination, direct killing of the innocent, divorce and remarriage) were intrinsically morally evil. These actions were regarded as such either by being contrary to nature (following the "order of nature" interpretation of natural law) or by defect of right. To qualify any action as intrinsically morally evil means that no intention or set of circumstances could ever justify it. Its moral quality is already determined before the person does it in whatever circumstances. For a more detailed analysis, see Richard M. Gula, *Reason Informed by Faith*, 268.

[59]McCormick continues his discussion by stating: "Finnis argues that whenever one positively suppresses a possible good, he directly chooses against it. And since one may never do this, he argues, there are certain actions that are immoral regardless of the foreseeable consequences. This is a sophisticated form of an older structuralism. A careful study of Christian moral tradition will suggest that an action must be regarded as 'turning directly against a basic good' only after the relation of the choice to all values has been weighed carefully." McCormick, *Notes on Moral Theology: 1965 through 1980*, 453.

[60]McCormick writes: "There are two facts that profoundly affect the significance of human activity. First, we are changing beings. Our self-experience and self-definition emerge from a consciousness in contact with a rapidly changing world. Secondly and consequently, our assessment of significance is conditioned by a host of personal and social factors whose limitations we are incapable of perceiving with the clarity we would like. We swim in the historico-cultural stream. Thus we analyze ourselves, our world, our actions, out of the limitations of philosophical systems, out of changing cultural conditions, as well as out of our own only partial personal maturity. These two facts suggest that our grasp of significance is always partial and imperfect." McCormick, "The New Morality," 771.

[61]Odozor, *Richard A. McCormick and the Renewal of Moral Theology*, 160.

[62]McCormick, *The Critical Calling*, 14; see also "The Pastoral Constitution on the Church in the Modern World," no. 51, 256.

[63]McCormick writes: "Two influences have combined to lead us to a renewed awareness of the necessary tentativeness of our formulations: the complexity and changeability of reality and a knowledge of the cultural influences that went into past formulations. This suggests powerfully to us that our grasp of significance is at any time limited, rooting as it does in limited self-awareness and imperfect formulations. This tentativeness was explicitly recognized by the Vatican Council. Following John XXIII, it states, 'The deposit of faith or revealed truths are one thing; the manner in which they are formulated without violence to their meaning and significance is another.' Here we have a clear distinction between the substance of a teaching and its formulation." Ibid., 16; see also, John XXIII, "Speech delivered on October 11, 1962, at the beginning of the Council," *Acta Apostolicae Sedis* 54 (1962): 792.

[64]James J. Walter, "The Foundation and Formulation of Norms," in *Moral Theology: Challenges for the Future*, 125. See also Peter Knauer,

S.J., *"La détermination du bien et du mal moral par le principe du double effet," Nouvelle Revue Théologique* 87 (1965): 356-376.

[65] McCormick, *Notes on Moral Theology: 1965 through 1980*, 8-13. It is interesting to note that Odozor believes McCormick, in his doctoral dissertation, was already engaged in the reinterpretation of the principle of double effect. Odozor argues that, McCormick, without saying it, had already decided to consider moral evil as a premoral disvalue sanctioned or caused without proportionate reason while still operating out of the manual tradition. Odozor writes: "McCormick located proportionate reason in a hierarchy of values (*ordo bonorum*). He claimed that the distinction between direct and indirect killing cannot be determined by cause and effects relationship alone. He only insinuated but did not claim clearly that this intentionality (that is, direct and indirect) also hinges on proportionate reason. McCormick's use of proportionate reason represents not only a radical departure from the position of the manuals, but it also anticipates Peter Knauer's efforts to reinterpret the principle of double effect." Odozor does state that McCormick may not have been aware of this fact, and, even if he had been aware of it, he could not have articulated it. "For if he even questioned the objectively evil nature of exposing an innocent life to danger of death, on the grounds that there can be proportionate reasons for doing so, he would have been in conflict with the tradition." McCormick was not yet prepared to question the notion of intrinsic evil. For a more detailed analysis, see Odozor, *Richard A. McCormick and the Renewal of Moral Theology*, 17-24.

[66]See Peter Knauer, S.J. *"Überlegungen zur moraltheologischen Prinzipienlehre der Enzyklika 'Humanae Vitae,'" Theologie und Philosophie* 45 (1970): 60-74; and Idem "The Hermeneutic Function of the Principle of Double Effect," *Natural Law Forum* 12 (1967): 132-162.

[67]McCormick, *Notes on Moral Theology: 1965 through 1980*, 311.

[68]Ibid., 312-314.

[69]See Bruno Schüller, S.J., *"Zur Problematik allgemein verbindlicher ethischer Grundsätze," Theologie und Philosophie* 45 (1970): 1-23.

[70]McCormick, *Notes on Moral Theology: 1965 through 1980*, 318.

[71]This became apparent with the publication of his Père Marquette Theology lecture "Ambiguity In Moral Choice" in 1973. Like the other proportionalists, McCormick began to view the human act as a structural unity. Therefore, one cannot isolate the object of an act and morally appraise it apart from the other components of the unified action. James Walter states: "Once one denies that the object (*objectum actus*) can be abstracted from the total act and judged separately, the theory of intrinsic evil *in the way* that the tradition has established this notion deontologi-

cally is denied. Revisionists do not deny the notion of intrinsic evil alto-
gether, but for them it can only be determined *concretely* not abstractly,
after considering all the relevant factors in a situation." Walter, "The
Foundation and Formulation of Norms," 128. Emphasis in the original.
See also McCormick, *Notes on Moral Theology: 1965 through 1980*,
710; and Joseph Fuchs, S.J., "The Absoluteness of Moral Terms," in
Readings in Moral Theology No. 1, eds. Richard A. McCormick and
Charles E. Curran (New York: Paulist Press, 1979), 126. It should also
be stated that proportionalists take into consideration "all the circumstances" of an act. This includes foreseeable consequences. Some critics
have accused McCormick and other proportionalists as being mere con-
sequentialists. This is a misrepresentation of their position. What is true
of proportionalism is that this structure of moral reasoning, appraisal of
human acts, and its grounding of behavioral norms is teleological, i.e., it
always, but not only, looks to and includes an assessment of consequences. Walter, "The Foundation and Formulation of Norms," 129.

[72]To explain this McCormick writes: "We go to war to protect freedom. That means we are willing to sacrifice life to protect this good. If
'give me liberty or give me death' does not involve *some kind* of commensurating, then I do not know what commensurating means. Our tradition allows violent, even, if necessary, lethal, resistance to rape attempts. If this does not mean measuring *somehow or other* sexual integrity against human life, I fail to see what it means. Our tradition allows
(perhaps incorrectly) capital punishment as a protection and deterrent.
That involves weighing one individual's life against the common safety
which he threatens." McCormick, *Doing Evil to Achieve Good*, 227. Emphasis in the original.

[73]McCormick writes: "What I have suggested is that the interrelatedness of human goods, their associatedness, means that in a sense there is
a single scale, but the means of assessing the greater and lesser evil are
more difficult, uncertain, and obscure because the assessment must be
done at times through associated goods. . . . To reword the matter, I
would suggest that the scale is indeed single *in a sense* (through the association of basic goods) but the means of assessing the lesser evil more
difficult and hazardous, a prudent bet if you will. When life is at stake (or
liberty, or what have we) in certain tragic conflict situations, I am not
exactly weighing life *against* other values, but attempting to discover
what is best in the service of life itself in terms of its relationship to other
values." Ibid., 229-230. Emphasis in the original. It should also be noted
that McCormick uses the cluster theory of virtues to add support to his
notion of the association of basic values. But as James Walter notes,

McCormick offers no support for this theory. Walter writes: "McCormick has used the cluster theory of virtues, in which the virtues are
viewed as a kind of seamless fabric, to show that all the basic values are
interrelated. Without offering any proof for this cluster theory of virtues,
he postulated that to weaken any one of the virtues is to weaken all the
others. Now, on the basis of analogy to the virtues he assumed that to
attack any one of the basic values would be to attack all the others associated with it. McCormick's reasoning here appears very close to Finnis'
position on the basic goods, but the associating of these values did give
him the basis on which to show why the direct killing of noncombatants
is morally wrong." Walter, "The Foundation and Formulation of Norms,"
138; McCormick, *Doing Evil to Achieve Good*, 253; and John Langan,
"Augustine on the Unity and the Interconnection of the Virtues," *Harvard Theological Review* 72 (January-April 1979): 81-95.

[74] McCormick, *Doing Evil to Achieve Good*, 228.

[75]McCormick writes: "Do we not go to war (involving killing, the
suppression of a basic human good) to protect our political freedom? Is
there not *some kind* of commensuration there even though the values involved are 'objectively incommensurable'? Have we not corporately
concluded ('adopted a hierarchy') that political freedom is so basic a
value that it is worth sacrificing lives to preserve it? It seems so. It seems
that we might argue that the conclusions of traditional Christian ethics
here (the just-war theory) are the community's adoption of a hierarchy of
values which relates the violence and death involved in war to other basic values." Ibid., 252. Emphasis in the original.

[76]McCormick, *Notes on Moral Theology: 1965 through 1980*, 123.

[77]McCormick, "The New Medicine and Morality," 316. Emphasis in
the original.

[78]Odozor argues that establishing proportionate reason through the
theory of associated goods "helps McCormick to give persuasive answers to critics who charge that proportionate reasoning cannot apply to
cases of justice without employing a utilitarian calculus. In the case of
the sheriff with an innocent black prisoner, this would imply that he must
hand over the innocent black man or risk the 'greater evil' of widespread
rioting, murder, and arson. Applying the principle of associated good,
McCormick insists that the sheriff ought not to give in to the mob demand because to do so would imply that the protection of the human
good, in this case life, property, and so on, by framing an innocent person will undermine that good in the long run 'by serious injury to an associated good (human liberty).'" Odozor, *Richard A. McCormick and the
Renewal of Moral Theology*, 114-115; see also McCormick, *Doing Evil*

to Achieve Good, 229; and Idem, *Notes on Moral Theology: 1965 through 1980*, 720. Odozor also argues that besides the principle of associated goods, McCormick introduces the principle of necessity to explain more clearly the meaning of proportionate reason. He writes: "The principle of necessary connection as an aspect of the notion of proportionate reasoning expresses the conviction that 'it is wrong to do evil when the evil has no necessary connection to the good being sought.' This connection does not exist when evil is done 'to convince a free and rational agent to refrain from evil.'" McCormick writes: "Let us put this in another way and explicitly in Christian terms. It is the Christian's faith that another's ceasing from his wrongdoing is *never* dependent on my doing nonmoral evil. For the Christian believes that we are truly what we are, redeemed in Christ. We are still threatened by *reliquiae peccati* but we are free and powerful in Christ's grace." Odozor, *Richard A. McCormick and the Renewal of Moral Theology*, 115. Emphasis in the original. See also McCormick, *Doing Evil to Achieve Good*, 236; Idem, *Notes on Moral Theology: 1965 through 1980*, 720; and Sanford S. Levy, "Richard McCormick and Proportionate Reason," *Journal of Religious Ethics* 13 (1985): 259.

[79]McCormick refers to premoral evils as, "harms, lacks, pains, deprivations, etc. that occur in or as a result of human agency." McCormick, "Notes on Moral Theology: 1985," *Theological Studies* 47 (1986): 86. There are various terms for premoral evil. Premoral is used by Josef Fuchs; physical evil is used by Peter Knauer; nonmoral evil is used by McCormick and Bruno Schüller; and ontic evil is used by Louis Janssens. All of these terms—physical evil, premoral evil, nonmoral evil, ontic evil, and premoral disvalue—refer to the same reality, and they are used interchangeably in the discussion. Premoral, physical, nonmoral, and ontic evils refer to the lack of perfection in anything whatsoever. As pertaining to human actions, it is the aspect which we experience as regrettable, harmful, or detrimental to the full actualization of the well-being of persons and of their social relations. Since we never get away from these features of our actions, we must learn to live in ways which will keep premoral, ontic, nonmoral, physical evils to a minimum, even though we cannot completely eliminate them in all their forms. For a more detailed analysis of premoral evils, see Gula, *Reason Informed by Faith*, 269.

[80]McCormick in his writings defines proportionate reason as the basic analytic structure of moral reasoning in conflict situations and moral norming. See McCormick, *Ambiguity in Choice*, 76-77; Idem, *Doing Evil to Achieve Good*, 215, 232; and Idem, "Notes on Moral Theology:

1984," *Theological Studies* 46. (1985): 62. James J. Walter argues that this definition advanced by McCormick is really the definition of proportionalism. He writes: "In other words, proportionalism is the general analytic structure of determining the objective moral rightness and wrongness of acts and of grounding concrete behavioral norms. This structure of moral reasoning as such is committed to assessing all relevant circumstances, viz. all aspects of the unified human act, consequences, premoral values/disvalues, institutional obligations, etc. before arriving at a final moral determination of an act. 'Proportionate reason,' on the other hand, is the moral principle used by proportionalists to determine concretely and objectively the rightness and wrongness of acts and the various exceptions to behavioral norms." Walter, "The Foundation and Formulation of Norms," 132.

[81]McCormick, *The Critical Calling*, 134. McCormick writes: "Thus just as not every killing is murder, not every falsehood a lie, so not every artificial intervention preventing (or promoting) conception is necessarily an unchaste act. Not every termination of a pregnancy is necessarily an abortion in the moral sense. This has been called 'proportionalism.'" Ibid.

[82]McCormick, *Notes on Moral Theology: 1965 through 1980*, 317; see also Odozor, *Richard A. McCormick and the Renewal of Moral Theology*, 110.

[83]For McCormick, an action can be regarded as "turning against a basic value" only after the relation of that choice to all values has been considered. This inevitably involves a balancing of values that Finnis *et al.* do not want to make. For McCormick, these values are associated and a direct sacrifice of a particular value may be justified in certain situations. McCormick argues that a premoral value can be sacrificed directly in favor of one which is higher or at least equal.

[84]Odozor, *Richard A. McCormick and the Renewal of Moral Theology*, 110. McCormick writes: "Proportionate reason represents above all a structure of moral reasoning and moral norming, teleological in character, whose thrust is that concrete norms understood as exceptionless because they propose certain interventions dealing with nonmoral goods as *intrinsic evils* cannot be sustained." McCormick, *Doing Evil to Achieve Good*, 232. Emphasis in the original. McCormick goes on to explain that although there cannot be exceptionless moral norms, there can be norms that are "virtually exceptionless." McCormick borrows this notion from Donald Evans. By this McCormick means that the theoretically possible exceptions are virtually zero in their practical possibility. For a more detailed analysis of "virtually exceptionless norms," see

McCormick, *Notes on Moral Theology: 1965-through 1980*, 433; see also Donald Evans, "Paul Ramsey and Exceptionless Moral Rules," 184-214.

[85]McCormick first proposed his criteria for a proportionate reason in his Père Marquette Lecture of 1973, "Ambiguity in Moral Choice," and subsequently reworked them in response to criticisms of his first effort. The substance of the criteria are as follows: First, the means used will not cause more harm than necessary to achieve the value. Second, no less harmful way exists at present to protect the value. Third, the means used to achieve the value will not undermine it. For a more detailed analysis, see McCormick, *Doing Evil to Achieve Good*, 193-267; and Gula, *Reason Informed by Faith*, 273-275.

[86]See McCormick, "Notes on Moral Theology: 1980," *Theological Studies* 42 (March 1981): 74-90. James J. Walter builds on McCormick's foundation and suggests three additional ways of knowing whether a proper relationships exists. He adds the mode of discursive reasoning or rational analysis and argument, long-term consequences, and our experience of harmony and guilt over our actions. For a more detailed analysis, see James J. Walter, "Proportionate Reason and Its Three Levels of Inquiry: Structuring The Ongoing Debate," *Louvain Studies* 10 (Spring 1984): 30-40; see also Gula, *Reason Informed by Faith*, 275-276.

[87]McCormick, *The Critical Calling*, 9.

[88]Ibid., 19.

[89]McCormick, "The New Morality," 771.

[90] "Pastoral Constitution on the Church in the Modern World," no. 43, 244.

[91]McCormick believes after Vatican II a fresh notion of the teaching function of the Church unfolded. This notion has the following three characteristics: "(1) the learning process is seen as essential to the teaching process; (2) teaching is a multidimensional function, of which the judgmental or decisive is only one aspect; (3) the teaching function involves the charisms of many persons." McCormick, *The Critical Calling*, 20.

[92]Ibid., 84.

[93]For example, the magisterium cannot be in full possession of the truth where the ethics of recombinant DNA research is involved. Therefore, many competencies are needed to face the rapidly changing times and the ethical problems these times produce. The magisterium must consult with the sciences and allow for an openness of dialogue.

[94]For a more detailed analysis of this discussion, see McCormick, "Does Religious Faith Add To Ethical Perception?," *Readings in Moral Theology No. 2: The Distinctiveness of Christian Ethics*, 156-173.

[95]McCormick spells out the key elements of the Christian story which are contained in Scripture, the Creed, and the Church's living traditions. He writes: "The Christian story illumines for us that God is author and preserver of life; the human person has a supernatural destiny; God has been disclosed to us in Jesus Christ; in Jesus' life, death and resurrection we have been totally transformed into 'new creatures'—into a community of the transformed; we remain subject to sin, although sin and death have met their victor; we are a eucharistic community and a pilgrim people called to love one another in manifestation of the new life in Christ; and the ultimate destiny of our combined journeys is the coming of the kingdom." For a more detailed analysis, see McCormick, *Health and Medicine in the Catholic Tradition*, 49.

[96]McCormick, "The Best Interests of the Baby," 20.

[97]In addition to the influence of Scripture on moral theology at the time of Vatican II, two other influences may have given Scripture a more visible place in McCormick's epistemology. First was the publication of Bernard Häring's *The Law of Christ*; and the second was the appearance of Josef Fuch's essays on the distinctiveness of Christian morality. See Bernard Häring, *The Law of Christ*, (Westminister, MD: The Newman Press, 1966) and Josef Fuchs "Is There a Specifically Christian Morality," in *Readings in Moral* Theology, No. 2,eds. Richard McCormick and Charles Curran (New York: Paulist Press, 1980), 3-19.

[98] "Pastoral Constitution on the Church in the Modern World," no. 11, 209. McCormick further quotes this document by stating: "But only God who created man to His own image and ransoms him from sin provides a fully adequate answer to these questions. This He does through what He has revealed in Christ His Son, who became man. Whoever follows after Christ, the perfect man, becomes himself more a man." Ibid., no. 41, 240.

[99]This is in response to a statement McCormick made in regard to a self-assessment. He writes: "I think my greatest failing as a moral theologian (others will certainly note many others) has been my failure to explore and make clearer and more persuasive Vatican II's statement: 'Faith throws a new light on everything, manifests God's design for man's total vocation, and thus directs the mind to solutions that are fully human.' But, as I stated at the outset, the body is still warm and twitching." McCormick, "Self-Assessment and Self-Indictment," *Corrective*

Vision, 45; refer also to Chapter One, Richard A. McCormick, S.J.—Moral Theologian section above.

[100]McCormick, "Health and Medicine in the Catholic Tradition," 61. It should be noted that although McCormick does not cite James J. Walter's essay ("Proportionate Reason and Its Three Levels of Inquiry: Structuring the Ongoing Debate," *Louvain Studies* 10 [Spring 1984]: 30-40); nonetheless, he incorporates Walter's three additional ways of knowing—discursive reasoning or rational analysis and argument, long-term consequences, and our experience of harmony and guilt over our actions—into his own dimensions of human understanding in this 1986 article.

[101]McCormick, *Health and Medicine in the Catholic Tradition,* 48.

[102]McCormick, "Bioethics and Method," 310.

[103]McCormick, *Corrective Vision,* 28. McCormick follows the Catholic theological tradition on natural law that implies an understanding that "moral values and obligations are grounded in a moral order known by human reason reflecting on experience." McCormick is convinced that moral order is grounded in the being of the human person as such. Odozor states: "In 1965 [McCormick] wrote that natural law is the law 'inscribed in our being by the creative act of God,' the dictates of reason, 'as historical man confronts his inclinations, drives, tendencies, and potentialities.' Besides being inscribed in our hearts, natural law is natural because it is founded in nature and can, for this reason, be known without supernatural assistance." Odozor, *Richard A. McCormick and the Renewal of Moral Theology,* 26-27; see also Cahill, "On Richard McCormick," 111; and McCormick, "Practical and Theoretical Considerations," in *The Problem of Population: Vol. 3 Educational Considerations* (Notre Dame, IN: University of Notre Dame Press, 1965), 61.

[104]McCormick, "Theology and Biomedical Ethics," 329.

[105]For example, McCormick writes: "Since Christian ethics is the objectification in Jesus Christ of every person's experience of subjectivity, 'it does not add and cannot add to human ethical self-understanding as such any material content that is, in principle strange or foreign to man as he exists and experiences himself in this world.' However, a person within the Christian community has access to a privileged articulation, in objective form, of this experience of subjectivity. Precisely because the resources of Scripture, dogma, and Christian life (the 'storied community') are the fullest available objectifications of the common human experience, 'the articulation of man's image of his moral good that is possible within historical Christian communities remains privileged in its access to enlarged perspectives on man.'" McCormick, "Theology and

Biomedical Ethics," 331. See also James F. Bresnahan, S.J., "Rahner's Christian Ethics," *America* 123 (1970): 351-354.

[106]It should be noted that McCormick refers to this type of knowledge as "prereflective" in McCormick, "The Judaeo-Christian Tradition and Bioethical Codes," *How Brave a New World?*, 4. He refers to it as "prethematic" and "connatural" in McCormick, *Doing Evil to Achieve Good*, 250.

[107]McCormick, "Bioethics and Method," 304.

[108]McCormick, *Doing Evil to Achieve Good*, 250; see also Peter B. Medawar, *The Hope of Progress* (New York: Doubleday & Company, 1973), 84.

[109]McCormick, *Doing Evil to Achieve Good*, 250-251. Rahner uses as an example the rejection of Artificial Insemination by a Donor (A.I.D.). Rahner states explicitly "all the 'reasons' which are intended to form the basis for rejecting genetic manipulation (namely A.I.D.) are to be understood, at the very outset, as only so many references to the moral faith-instinct. . . . For in my view the moral faith-instinct is aware of its right and obligation to reject genetic manipulation, even without going through (or being able to go through) an adequate process of reflection." Karl Rahner, S.J., "The Problem of Genetic Manipulation," *Theological Investigations* Vol. 9 (New York: Herder and Herder, 1972), 243.

[110]McCormick, *Doing Evil to Achieve Good*, 251.

[111]Ibid.

[112]McCormick, *Notes on Moral Theology: 1981 through 1984*, 121; see also Daniel Maguire, "*Recta Ratio* and the Intellectualistic Fallacy," *Journal of Religious Ethics* 10 (1982): 22-39.

[113]Ibid. For example, where prudence is concerned, that virtue perfects reason by being conjoined with the moral virtues. The moral virtues, however, attune a person to the morally good so that it becomes connatural to judge correctly about the good. This connaturalizing effect of virtue affects the manner of knowing and perceiving the good. The way of knowing is affectively qualified. Ibid.

[114]Ibid., 122.

[115]Ibid.

[116]Ibid.; see also Thomas Clarke, S.J. "Touching in Power: Our Health System," *Above Every Name* (Mahwah, NJ: Paulist Press, 1980), 252.

[117]McCormick, "Man's Moral Responsibility for Health," 18.

[118]McCormick, *Notes on Moral Theology: 1965 through 1980*, 638.

[119]McCormick, "Theology and Bioethics," *Theology and Bioethics*, 110.

[120]McCormick, "The Best Interests of the Baby," 20. Emphasis in the original.

[121]McCormick, "Man's Moral Responsibility for Health," 19.

[122]McCormick, "Theology and Biomedical Ethics," 315.

[123]McCormick, *Notes on Moral Theology: 1965 through 1980*, 638.

[124]Odozor, *Richard A. McCormick and the Renewal of Moral Theology*, 156.

[125]McCormick, *Health and Medicine in the Catholic Tradition*, 50.

[126]For a more detailed analysis of why human persons have a tendency to pursue the basic goods as ends in themselves, refer to Chapter Two, McCormick's Theological Anthropology section, Doctrine of the Fall subsection above.

[127]McCormick, "Theology and Bioethics," *Corrective Vision*, 143.

[128]McCormick, "Theology and Biomedical Ethics," 318.

[129]McCormick, "Personal Conscience," 243. One example of the complementarity of the sources of moral knowledge would be the magisterium's reliance on the sciences in regard to discerning its position on complex issues like genetic manipulation, fetal tissue transplants, treatment decisions for handicapped neonates, etc. For McCormick, the teachings of the magisterium are to enlighten the conscience, not replace it. Its teachings are made within the community of experience, reflection, and memory. In this day and age, when science and technology are developing complex new techniques on a daily basis, it is imperative that the magisterium be in consultation with authorities within these fields. The magisterium cannot be expected to be competent in all areas of modern medicine and technology. Therefore, it must rely on and learn from those who have the proper competence in order to help inform and enlighten the faithful. McCormick writes: "Christ did not promise us that as individuals we would always be right when deliberating about practical implications of 'being in Christ.' He did not promise that the ultimate official teaching would always be right. He did say, *in the fact of our being a community of believers,* that there is no better way of walking the narrow path than to walk it together—with the combined eyes and strength and experience of the entire people, all supporting each other's charisms and gifts." McCormick, *The Critical Calling*, 44-45. Emphasis in the original.

[130]McCormick, "Personal Conscience," 243.

[131]Ibid.

[132]Odozor, *Richard A. McCormick and the Renewal of Moral Theology*, 155.

TO TREAT OR NOT TO TREAT

[133]McCormick, "Man's Moral Responsibility for Health," 18. Emphasis mine.

[134]McCormick, "Theology and Biomedical Ethics," 320.

[135]McCormick lists six such themes: "(1) Life as a basic but not absolute value. (2) The extension of this judgment to nascent life. (3) Human relationships as the basic quality of human physical life to be valued as the *conditio sine qua non* for other values. (4) Our essential sociality. (5) The unity of the spheres of life-giving (procreative) and love-making (unitive). (6) Heterosexual, permanent marriage as normative." Ibid., 329.

[136]McCormick, "Bioethics and Method," 311.

[137]For a more detailed analysis of human life as a relative good, refer to Chapter Two, McCormick Theological Anthropology section above.

[138]McCormick, "The Best Interests of the Baby," 20.

[139]For a more detailed analysis of how scripture and the magisterium confirm this value judgment, see Ibid. Refer also to Chapter Two, Practical Implications of McCormick's Theological Anthropology as Applied to Treatment Decisions for Handicapped Neonates section, Human Life Is a Basis But Not Absolute Good subsection above.

[140]McCormick, "To Save or Let Die," *How Brave a New World?*, 349.

[141]McCormick, *Health and Medicine in the Catholic Tradition*, 52.

[142]This statement has its basis in the centuries-long tradition of the Catholic Church on the duty to preserve life. In 1595, Domingo Báñez formulated the distinction between extraordinary and ordinary means, by which was meant measures proportionate to one's condition in life. For a more detailed historical analysis, see Richard McCormick and John Paris, "The Catholic Tradition on the Use of Nutrition and Fluids," *America* 156 (May 2, 1987): 356-361.

[143]McCormick, "The Best Interests of the Baby," 20-21.

[144]McCormick, "The New Medicine and Morality," 317.

[145]For a more detailed analysis of the sacredness of human life as derived from the Christian story, refer to Chapter Two, Practical Implications of McCormick's Theological Anthropology as Applied to Treatment Decisions for Handicapped Neonates section, Human Life As Sacred subsection above. McCormick writes: "Human life is sacred because of its origin and destiny, because of the value God places on it." McCormick, *The Critical Calling*, 268.

[146]McCormick, "Public Policy on Abortion," *How Brave a New World?*, 197.

[147]McCormick writes: "Just as Christ suffered and died for us to enter his glory, so we who are 'in the Lord,' who are inserted into the redemptive mystery, must expect that our growth 'to deeper life' will share the characteristic of God's engendering deed in Christ." McCormick, *Health and Medicine in the Catholic Tradition*, 116-117.

[148]Ibid., 118.

[149]The Congregation for the Doctrine of the Faith, *Declaration on Euthanasia*, (Washington, DC: United States Catholic Conference, 1980), 2-3.

[150]McCormick, "The New Medicine and Morality," 317.

[151]See Joseph Fletcher, "Ethics and Euthanasia," *American Journal of Nursing* 73 (1973): 670-675. This article also appears as a chapter in *To Live and To Die*, ed. Robert H. Williams (New York: Spinger-Verlag, 1973), 113-122.

[152]McCormick, "The New Medicine and Morality," 318.

[153]McCormick writes: "Descriptively different actions may have different short and/or long range implications and effects. And it is these effects, either feared, suspected, unknown, or clearly foreseen that could spell, or at least reveal, the *moral* difference between omission and commission where the dying are concerned. In other words, mere omission may not entail, either logically or factually, the same consequences as direct commission would. And if this is so, a different calculus of proportion may be called for. For proportion must encompass the good of the patient and all concerned." Ibid. Emphasis in the original.

[154]Ibid.

[155]Ibid.

[156]Ibid., 316.

[157]For a more detailed analysis of how positive euthanasia causes dangers for society McCormick refers to two articles: Merle Longwood, "Ethical Reflections on the Meaning of Death," *Dialog* 11 (1972): 195-201; and David W. Louisell, "Euthanasia and Biathanasia: On Dying and Killing," *Linacre Quarterly* 10 (1974): 14-22.

[158]For a more detailed analysis of McCormick's understanding of "virtually exceptionless norms," see McCormick, *Notes on Moral Theology 1965 through 1980*, 433.

[159]This is one of the human person's basic inclinations present, according to McCormick, prior to acculturation. See McCormick, "The Judaeo-Christian Tradition and Bioethical Codes," *How Brave a New World?*, 5.

[160]McCormick, "The Judaeo-Christian Tradition and Bioethical Codes," *How Brave a New World?*, 7.

[161]McCormick, "The New Medicine and Morality," 321.

[162]See Richard A. McCormick, S.J., "Bioethical Issues and the Moral Matrix of U.S. Health Care," *Hospital Progress* 60 (May 1979): 42; See also Idem, "1973-1983: Value Impacts of a Decade," *Hospital Progress* 63 (December 1982): 41.

[163]McCormick, *Notes on Moral Theology: 1965 through 1980*, 667.

[164]McCormick, "Proxy Consent in the Experimentation Situation," *Love and Society*, 217.

[165]Odozor writes: "McCormick himself acknowledged this in my interview with him in this description of how the late Dr. André Hellegers, the founder of the Kennedy Institute of Bioethics at Georgetown University, used to introduce him and others to visitors at the Institute. Dr. Hellegers would show people around the Institute and tell them who was there. He'd say, 'Well, this is Leon Kass over here, he is our Jewish scholar. . . and this is McCormick's office. He puts out fires.' People would say, 'What do you mean?' Hellegers would say, 'McCormick and I put out fires. We respond to problems. We have no eternally valid ten year schemes or methodological revolutions. All we do is respond to fire alarms.'" Odozor, *Richard A. McCormick and the Renewal of Moral Theology*, 23.

[166]McCormick, "Proxy Consent in the Experimentation Situation," in *Love and Society*, 217. Emphasis mine.

[167]See McCormick, "Proxy Consent in the Experimentation Situation," *How Brave a New World?*, 51-71.

[168] McCormick "Bioethics and Method," 305. Emphasis mine.

[169]Cahill, "Teleology, Utilitarianism, and Christian Ethics," 621.

[170]McCormick, *Doing Evil to Achieve Good*, 253.

[171]Ibid. Emphasis in the original.

[172]James J. Walter agrees with this point. Walter writes: "It could be argued, as I have above, that the 'association of basic values' and the 'adoption of a hierarchy of values' more properly relate to the discussion of the general level of how we know that a proportionate reason can be obtained and more particularly to the mode of discursive reasoning." For a more detailed analysis, see James J. Walter, "Proportionate Reason and Its Three Levels of Inquiry: Structuring the Ongoing Debate," 40.

[173]McCormick, "Notes on Moral Theology: 1985," *Theological Studies* 47 (1986): 87. Emphasis mine. See also Sanford S. Levy, "Richard McCormick and Proportionate Reason," 261.

[174]McCormick, "Man's Moral Responsibility for Health," 18.

[175]Walter, "The Foundation and Formulation of Norms," 140.

[176]Odozor, *Richard A. McCormick and the Renewal of Moral Theology*, 86; see also McCormick, *Doing Evil to Achieve Good*, 251.

[177]A prime example would be the Levy article when McCormick states that he is "not wedded" to the theory of associated goods. He simply stated this without any analysis or justification.

[178]Walter, "The Foundation and Formulation of Norms," 145.

[179]Ronald H. McKinney, S.J., "The Quest for an Adequate Proportionalist Theory of Value," *Thomist*, 53 (January 1989): 56-73.

[180]Garth L. Hallett, S.J., *Christian Moral Reasoning: An Analytic Guide* (Notre Dame, IN: University of Notre Dame Press, 1983): 137-143.

[181]Walter, "The Foundation and Formulation of Norms," 145.

[182]Odozor, *Richard A. McCormick and the Renewal of Moral Theology*, 17-18.

[183]Ibid., 108-109; see also Cahill, "Teleology, Utilitarianism, and Christian Ethics," 617.

[184]Throughout both his moral epistemologies McCormick refers to the "prudent person"; a "prudent bet" is used in assessing if there is a proportionate reason in a conflict situation; and "the use of prudence must conform to an objective scale . . ." Prudence obviously plays a major role in how a person determines the measure of proportionate reason. One could assume that because McCormick is a natural law ethicist, albeit revised, in the Catholic Thomistic tradition, that he agrees with Thomas' understanding of prudence. However, this would be speculation at best. For a more detailed analysis of Aquinas' position on prudence, see Aquinas, *Summa Theologica* Ia-IIae, 61.

[185]Odozor, *Richard A. McCormick and the Renewal of Moral Theology*, 158.

[186]Walter, "The Foundation and Formulation of Norms," 145.

[187]McCormick, *Doing Evil to Achieve Good*, 252.

[188]Walter, "The Foundation and Formulation of Norms," 145. Emphasis in the original.

[189]O'Connell writes: "They describe the kind of persons they should *be*. If we name these values by using adjectives (fair, honest, just, chaste, etc.), then the adjectives are most appropriately modifiers of moral agents themselves. They describe their way of *being*, they report their success and failure in maximizing the premoral good and minimizing the premoral evil in a particular area of life. For this reason, again, they are called 'moral values.'" Timothy O'Connell, *Principles for a Catholic Morality* (San Francisco, CA: Harper & Row, 1978), 159. Emphasis in the original.

[190]See McCormick, "The Judaeo-Christian Tradition and Bioethical Codes," *How Brave a New World?*, 5.

[191]Cahill, "Teleology, Utilitarianism, and Christian Ethics," 623.

[192]For a more detailed evaluation of naive and critical realism, see Walter and Happel, *Conversion and Discipleship*, 74-75; 106.

[193]At the level of normative moral judgment, Curran argues that physicalism reflects the naive realism of the classicist wordview. This means that physicalism is based on an essentialist definition of human nature which has no room for change; it views nature as a finished product so that change and historical process are incidental; also, it depends on a moral order that is fixed and undeveloping. See Charles E. Curran "Absolute Norms and Medical Ethics," *Absolutes in Moral Theology?* (Washington, DC: Corpus Books, 1968), 108-153; see also Gula, *Reason Informed by Faith*, 234.

[194]Odozor, *Richard A. McCormick and the Renewal of Moral Theology*, 45-46.

[195]McCormick, "The New Morality," 772.

[196]McCormick, "Health and Medicine in the Catholic Tradition," 56.

[197]Cahill, "On Richard McCormick," 89.

[198]McCormick, "The New Morality," 772.

[199]McCormick, *Notes on Moral Theology: 1965 through 1980*, 77; see also Odozor, *Richard A. McCormick and the Renewal of Moral Theology*, 176-177.

[200]Daniel Maguire, review of *Doing Evil to Achieve Good*, by Richard A. McCormick, S.J., in *Journal of Religion* 61 (1981): 117.

[201]Lisa Sowle Cahill and Daniel Maguire, for example.

4

Moral Criteriology

INTRODUCTION

In philosophical and theological inquiry a criterion is understood as a means or rule of discrimination, whereby a person can distinguish one thing from another.[1] It is a standard or basis for judging quality. The study of such a criterion or set of criteria is called criteriology. In the area of ethics, moral criteriology is frequently used as a synonymous term for moral epistemology.[2] However, in reality, they are two distinct components of an ethical methodology with two distinct purposes. Once the human ways of knowing values/disvalues and moral obligations have been established, there is a need to formulate some criterion or set of criteria, which guides moral reasoning in measuring human actions. Moral criteria span a number of uses. Moral criteria function both as a standard for determining the rightness and wrongness of actions, and in terms of the discernment process. These dual aspects are distinguishable, but there are times when they overlap in the decision-making process. The function of moral criteria in terms of the discernment process is how moral criteriology is linked to moral epistemology.

For McCormick, a moral criterion concerning treatment decisions for handicapped neonates addresses both substantive and procedural issues. The substantive issues focus on the appropriate standard for making treatment decisions and present various options. Aaron L. Mackler argues that these options can be narrowed down to four specific approaches. He writes:

> One basic option would be to treat every newborn as aggressively as possible. A second option is selective treatment based in the balance between direct benefits and burden of care. Another set of approaches, focusing on the best interests of the infant, argues that treatment should be limited only if suffering or a radically dimin-

ished quality of life would make existence a net burden to the infant. The fourth approach considers the personal and financial costs to the family and to society (at least in extreme cases). Alternatively, some argue that there are limitations on personal and societal obligations to help in such cases because the resources used might save or improve the lives of others.[3]

Procedural issues focus on how such treatment decisions are made and by whom. The procedural issues will be articulated and analyzed in chapter five.

Parents and health care professionals are often forced to draw lines between neonates who will be treated and those who will not be treated. If these lines are being drawn, then McCormick argues "it is of public importance that we find out the criteria by which they are being drawn. My attempt is to search our tradition on the meaning of life and so forth and see if we couldn't develop criteria."[4] McCormick will determine where the lines are to be drawn and will establish moral criteria as a "revised" natural law ethicist in the Catholic tradition. In this process he will demonstrate both the suppleness and the commonsense basis of natural law thinking, while stretching it to new applications.[5]

This chapter will focus on McCormick's set of moral criteria as applied to the area of bioethics, specified for never-competent patients. While this set of criteria can also be applied to those who are competent and those who were once competent, the focus of this chapter will be on the never-competent because handicapped neonates fall only within this category. McCormick's moral criteria for treatment decisions for handicapped neonates is based on a patient-centered approach. The structure and individual components that make up McCormick's moral criteria for decision-making are normative; they center on what "ought" to be the case, not what "is" the case. By normative McCormick means what the never-competent patient would want because he or she "ought" to want it. The never-competent patient "ought" to make this choice because it is in his or her "best interests."[6]

It appears that over the years McCormick has used four distinct criteria in moral decision-making regarding treatment decisions for the never-competent patient. The first criterion is the "reasonable person standard." The second is proportionate reason. The third is the person "integrally and adequately considered." Finally, there is his quality-of-life criterion, which is based on a normative understanding of what is in the "best interests" of the handicapped neonate. The fourth criterion evolves out of the previous three criteria. To further specify his moral criteria, in particular the quality-of-life criterion, McCormick uses both guidelines and norms. In addition, McCormick uses various moral principles to assist him in further specifying his moral criteria. The moral principles he uses both implicitly and explicitly are charity, autonomy, justice, beneficence, and nonmaleficence. These moral principles will be highlighted as they impact his moral criteria. McCormick has devoted much time and intellectual energy into specifying the basis of moral norms, guidelines, and principles in order: (1) to better understand them; (2) to strengthen morality; and (3) to develop a morality that is intelligible to Catholics, Protestants, and those of other faiths.[7] He believes this will lead to a more rational approach to resolving moral conflicts. A brief analysis of each of the principles might be helpful in order to understand how McCormick utilizes them.

The primary moral principle is charity, which is the foundation of all the other moral principles. McCormick reiterates the Thomistic dictum: "Charity is the form of the virtues."[8] Charity does not destroy the individuality of virtuous acts, or make them all uniquely and identically acts of charity alone. Rather, McCormick argues that human actions possess ultimate meaning only insofar as they are caught up in the conferred divine life. For the "new creatures" it is charity that expresses this "being caught up in," this "being grasped by God in Christ," this ordering to an end, this animating or forming.[9] Thus, all the other principles are rooted in charity. Autonomy is rooted in the dignity of the human person. For McCormick, "self-determination is a conditional or instrumental good— that is, a good precisely insofar as it is the instrument whereby the best interests of the patient are served by it."[10] The right of autonomy is always rooted in the best interests of the person. In regard to treatment decisions, autonomy is "simply an acknowledgment that treatment is always treatment of a *person* with values and beliefs, and that it must take these into account if it is to remain humane and respectful of human dignity."[11] The third moral principle is justice. Christians maintain that charity enters the very definition of justice. For McCormick,

> if we define justice simply as the habit that inclines one to render to another his or her due, we have disengaged it from the subject and from that which confers its complete Christian intelligibility. We have conceptualized it with no reference to the Christian context.[12]

Created in the image of God, all persons are radically equal before God.[13] As social beings who are interrelated and interdependent, we must realize that decisions we make or that are made for us have a profound impact on family and society. Therefore, justice as the mediation of charity, ought to incorporate both familial and social factors when determining the best interests for a never-competent patient. Finally, there are the moral principles of beneficence and nonmaleficence. Beneficence involves duties to prevent harm, remove harm, and promote the good of another person. Nonmaleficence prohibits the infliction of harm, injury, or death upon others. These are companion moral principles that are derived from the idea that one should maximize the benefits for a patient, and minimize the harms. This is accomplished when both of these principles are rooted in charity.

This chapter will examine and analyze each of McCormick's four moral criteria. However, the bulk of this chapter will center on his quality-of-life criterion based on a normative understanding of the "best interests" of a never-competent neonate, because this criterion has evolved into McCormick's primary criterion for moral decision-making regarding treatment decisions for handicapped neonates. Finally, this chapter will examine and analyze the criticism directed against McCormick's moral criteria. This chapter will deviate from the structure of the earlier chapters by not presenting any practical implications of McCormick's moral criteriology. The reason for this is that chapter five will be a complete examination and analysis of how McCormick's moral criteriology is applied to the five diagnostic treatment categories of handicapped neonates.

MCCORMICK'S ETHICAL CRITERIA

As a "revised" natural law ethicist in the Catholic tradition, McCormick has always sought a balanced middle course between extreme positions—a course which he understands as characteristic of the Judaeo-Christian tradition.[14] This tendency holds true in his understanding of moral criteriology. McCormick believes that few, if any, physicians are willing to make substantive criteria when it comes to treatment decisions for handicapped neonates. On the other hand, moral theologians, in their concern to avoid total normlessness and arbitrariness, can easily become quite dogmatic.[15] Between the two extremes of sheer concretism and dogmatism, McCormick argues that there is a middle course that entails the use of substantive criteria to assist decision-makers regarding treatment decisions for handicapped neonates. For McCormick, a moral criterion is not to be viewed as a slide rule that makes decisions. It is far less than that. He argues:

> It is more like a light in a room, a light that allows the individual objects to be seen in the fullness of their context. Concretely, if there are certain infants whom we agree ought to be saved in spite of illness or deformity, and if there are certain infants whom we agree should be

allowed to die, then there is a line to be drawn. And if
there is a line to be drawn, there ought to be some criteria, even if very general, for doing this.[16]

McCormick's moral criteria for decision-making, functioning both in
terms of the discernment process and the judgment of the rightness and
wrongness of actions, have gone through four distinct stages of development. Each moral criterion will be analyzed generally and, when
McCormick further specifies his criterion, there will be a further analysis
of the appropriate guidelines, norms, and moral principles. The "reasonable person" criterion will be analyzed first, not because it was the first
to be used but because it is the only one of the four that McCormick has
completely abandoned.

The "reasonable person standard" attempts to determine what a reasonable person in a normative sense would want in a particular situation.
It became the basis for how McCormick determined substituted judgments for never-competent patients. McCormick borrowed the notion of
"reasonable person" from ethicist Robert Veatch.[17] Veatch's interpretation of a reasonable person is based on the "reasonable man" standard in
tort law.[18] James Walter argues that McCormick makes several assump-
tions that ground the possibility of constructing and employing the "reasonable person standard." Walter writes:

> First, he assumes a normative social anthropology which
> views our well-being as necessarily linked to the pursuit
> and attainment of fundamental goods for ourselves and
> others. Second, he assumes that we can know the mor-
> ally good and that such insights are available in principle
> to everyone. Third, he assumes that the "reasonable" in a
> normative sense is not arbitrary but objective, i.e., it is
> not concerned with frivolous or eccentric desires or what
> we might desire when we commit sin.[19]

For McCormick, there must be a standard that is objectively reasonable.
He writes, "otherwise there would be no standard against which we could
identify the eccentric, the idiosyncratic, the wrongful."[20] McCormick
makes the assumption that most people are reasonable, and as such they
will choose what is in their or others' best interests.[21] However, he does
recognize that not all people are reasonable, nor do all people always
want to act reasonably. McCormick's understanding of the "reasonable
person standard" is very similar to the tort law understanding of the "reasonable man." This does not mean that the "reasonable person" is an actual person. It is an ideal, not unlike Veatch's ideal observer theory.[22]
McCormick argues that the "reasonable person standard" "is an appeal to

what most of us, in similar circumstances would do—as reasonable people—with healthy outlooks on the meaning of life and death."[23] As reasonable people, persons should act in the same way under similar conditions. For McCormick, this means that there is a normative set of insights that all reasonable persons can know. This mutually-related set of theoretic and practical insights originate in the interplay between concrete experience and thoughtful reflection, and they are constantly open to further correction in this interplay. This set of insights comes closest to an approximation of what any reasonable person can know at any given time of the objective moral order based upon the nature of persons.[24] To determine what is objectively valuable for a person in a particular situation requires some kind of empirical means of evaluation. For McCormick, "that would be asking what is reasonably seen as *objectively valuable by a reasonable person*."[25]

McCormick's understanding of the "reasonable person standard" is grounded in his theological anthropology. As pilgrim people, persons are subject to the human conditions of sinfulness and finitude.[26] Thus, we can never know with absolute or metaphysical certitude what is required of us in any particular situation. But this does not mean that we cannot know, as reasonable persons, the general moral requirements and the limits that all human persons are subject to with probable certitude. James Walter argues that McCormick's notion of the "reasonable person standard" is a

> heuristic way of expressing those moral requirements and their limits which impinge upon us all as persons. Because our moral reasons are historically conditioned, the set of normative insights can fluctuate between advance and decline depending upon our/society's historical-cultural situation.[27]

For McCormick, the "reasonable person standard" is a formal criterion. However, it does not specify the actual guidelines or norms that reasonable people would use in making moral decisions. It is the root of and the justification for both hypothetical substituted judgments and guardian substituted judgments.[28] As a formal criterion, the "reasonable person standard" guides the human person on both the requirements and the limits of moral obligation. McCormick writes: "The judgment of reasonable people is not *constitutive* of the rightness of a decision. It is merely *confirmatory* that the criterion is close to the mark."[29] By this McCormick correctly means that

> if the situation is such that most or very many of us
> would not want life-preserving treatment *in that condi-*
> *tion,* it would be morally prudent (reasonable) to con-
> clude that life-preserving treatment is not morally re-
> quired for this particular patient. But once again, it is not
> the consensus that *constitutes* the reasonableness.
> Rather, reasonable people can be presumed to be draw-
> ing the line on the kind of life being preserved at the
> right place—in the best overall interests of the patient.[30]

As a "revised" natural law ethicist, McCormick presumes that most people will come to the same conclusions, because he has assumed that most
people are reasonable or want to approximate reasonableness. Therefore,
the consensus of reasonable people confirms what would be objectively
valuable for the never-competent patient in a particular condition.

The major problem with McCormick's "reasonable person standard"
is that the actual criterion or standard lacks clarity. The reason for this is
that as a moral criterion its foundation is too general. Both Veatch's interpretation of the "reasonable person standard" and the original interpretation in tort law are vague. After being criticized that the "reasonable
person standard" was too vague and too subjective, McCormick abandoned it as a moral criterion. He did so in a very subtle way without any
explanation or justification, which has become somewhat typical of his
style.[31] Even though he abandoned the "reasonable person standard" as a
moral criterion, McCormick continues to place great emphasis on the
reasonableness of the human person.[32]

McCormick's second moral criterion is proportionate reason. For
him, proportionate reason "is a general term for those characteristics of
an action that allow us to conclude that, even though the action involves
nonmoral evil, it is morally justifiable when compared to the only alternative (its omission)."[33] It refers to both a specific value and its relation
to all elements, including nonmoral evils in the action.[34] The rules for
proportionate reason were first proposed in McCormick's Père Marquette
Lecture in 1973, "Ambiguity in Moral Choice," and subsequently reworked in response to criticisms of his first effort. The substance of the
criterion is as follows: First, the means used will not cause more harm
than necessary to achieve the value. Second, no less harmful way exists
at present to protect the value. Third, the means used to achieve the value
will not undermine it.[35] Proportionate reason defines what a person is
doing in a particular action. One must consider the proportionate relationship of the material action and the intention in the total set of essential circumstances. Like other proportionalists, McCormick began to
view the human act as a structural unity; therefore, one cannot isolate the

object of an act and morally appraise it apart from the other components of the unified action. McCormick writes:

> This means that the concrete moral norms that we develop to guide human conduct and communicate human convictions and experience to others are conclusions of and vehicles for a larger, more general assertion: in situations of conflict, where values are copresent and mutually exclusive, the reasonable thing is to avoid, *all things considered*, the greater evil or, positively stated, to do the greater good. This means, of course, that we may permit evil in our conduct only when evil caused or permitted is, all things considered, the lesser evil in the circumstances. In other words, we may cause a premoral evil only when there is a truly proportionate reason.[36]

For McCormick, causing certain disvalues does not *ipso facto* make a particular action morally wrong. A particular action becomes morally wrong when, all things considered, there is no proportionate reason justifying it.[37] For McCormick, proportionate reason serves as a moral criterion to determine the moral rightness and wrongness of an action.[38]

Proportionate reason became the main moral criterion McCormick used for determining if there is a sufficient reason for treating a never-competent patient. For McCormick, medical treatments should be provided that are proportionate to the patient's condition and are beneficial and promotive of the whole person. Without explanation or justification, this notion of the good of the whole person gradually became central to McCormick's understanding of the moral criterion governing treatment decisions. The criterion of proportionate reason was not abandoned. Rather, it appears to have been synthesized into a new moral criterion, which is the person "integrally and adequately considered."[39]

McCormick's third moral criterion is "integral personalism," or what he refers to as the person "integrally and adequately considered." The move away from neo-scholasticism that characterized so much of Vatican II brought with it this "methodological shift" to personalism.[40] McCormick argues that the importance of this criterion can scarcely be overstated. He writes: "If the person 'integrally and adequately considered' is the criterion for rectitude, it means that a different (from traditional) type of evidence is required for our assessment of human actions."[41] Here again, McCormick is referring to a moral criterion to decide the moral rightness and wrongness of an action. The nature of the whole human person now becomes McCormick's objective criterion. Proportionate reason becomes the "tool" or device for determining what is promotive or destructive of the good of the human person "integrally and adequately considered." The source of this criterion can be found in both Vatican II and St. Thomas Aquinas.[42]

McCormick's understanding of the human person "integrally and adequately considered" builds upon the anthropology of Vatican II, but one can also infer from his writings that he has adopted Louis Janssens'concept of the human person. Janssens'concept of the human person seeks to understand the human person in all his or her essential aspects.[43] To base moral evaluation on the nature of the whole person means to consider not only the individual person, but to consider the person and his or her relations to the world, to others, to social groups, and to God. This will have direct implications for McCormick in regard to treatment decisions for never-competent patients. Not only must he consider the good of the never-competent patient, but he must also consider social and familial factors.[44]

The moral criterion of the human person "integrally and adequately considered" calls for an inductive approach, which is committed to the relevance of human experience, the sciences, and personal reflection. Therefore, actions that undermine the person "integrally and adequately considered" are morally wrong. Actions which are judged to be promotive and supportive of the human person in the sum of his or her essential dimensions are morally right.[45] Gradually this criterion also became translated into a normative understanding of the "best interests" of the patient.

McCormick's fourth criterion of morality in determining treatment decisions for never-competent patients is his quality-of-life criterion, which he identifies with the category of the patient's "best interests." This is a patient-centered, teleological assessment of what is considered to be in the "best interests" of the patient. On initial examination it may appear that the criterion for decision-making is the "best interests" standard. However, after examining the writings of McCormick, it is apparent that his quality-of-life criterion is really a further specification of his normative understanding of a patient's "best interests."[46] Initially,McCormick argued that there are only two test formulations for determining moral decisions for the incompetent: the hypothetical test and the best interests test. For McCormick, these two tests are interrelated. In fact, he argues later that there is really only one test or criterion that can be applied to never-competent patients and that is the "best interests test."[47] McCormick has a normative understanding of "best interests" because, "as social beings, our good, our flourishing (therefore, our best interests) is inextricably bound up with the well-being of others."[48] James Walter believes that two things need to be noted about McCormick's understanding of "best interests." Walter writes:

First, "best interests" are normatively defined in terms of
those fundamental values to which our natural tendencies incline us. As we have seen, our openness to and
pursuit of these values enable us to share in human
flourishing, i.e., the *summum bonum*. Second, McCormick places his definition squarely within the context of
his social anthropology. Thus, "best interests" include, in
part at least, the family's interests, since the newborn's
interests are most intimately bound up with those upon
whom it must rely.[49]

Initially, McCormick's "best interest" standard was determined by
the "reasonable person standard." McCormick writes:

The standard for treating incompetents is to discover
whether the treatment would be *objectively valuable for
a patient in that condition*. In order to determine this, we
have to resort to some empirical means. For me, that
would be asking what is reasonably seen as *objectively
valuable by a reasonable person*. It is the "best interests"
standard controlled by the "reasonable person" standard
that Veatch and I proposed. . . . "Best interests" as controlled by the "reasonable person" standard may permit a
range. But a range is not necessarily subjective.[50]

The construction of the "reasonable person standard" allowed McCormick to understand "best interests" normatively.[51] However, once this
standard was criticized for being subjective and utilitarian in nature,
McCormick abandoned it.[52] Despite this setback, McCormick remained
committed to the possibility of formulating a consensus about what constitutes the "best interests" of patients.

Three factors influenced McCormick to propose his quality-of-life
criterion as a further specification or basis of his normative understanding of a patient's "best interests." The first was a conscious decision on
McCormick's part in 1983 to write in the area of bioethics and to do so
from a theological perspective. After 1983, McCormick introduces a new
moral epistemology at the level of synderesis.[53] The affections informed
by the Christian story create certain dispositions within the Christian person. He argues that "such dispositions will prepare us and incline us to
seek out the best interests of the child."[54] The Christian story influences
not only personal dispositions, but also moral judgments in a rather general way. This new moral epistemology establishes a context in which
human reason and calculation ought to operate.[55] It is a context that pre-

vents the absolutization of life, and allows decision-makers to make treatment decisions for never-competent patients based on "best interests" that will now include some consideration of future quality of life.

The second influence on McCormick's decision to include some consideration of future quality of life in determining the "best interests" of a patient was the controversy that Judge Robert Meade created in the Brother Joseph Charles Fox case.[56] Judge Meade rejected a substituted judgment approach that had been previously accepted in the *Quinlan* case and the *Saikewicz* case.[57] Meade argued that *"by its very nature* the right to decline life-saving treatment can be exercised by the individual alone, for it is a right of the individual to make up his or her own mind."[58] McCormick understood this ruling to have dire consequences for never-competent patients. McCormick points out that:

> If Judge Meade disallows substituted judgment in cases of perpetual incompetency such as *Saikewicz* (he refers to any attempt to discern the actual interests and preferences of *Saikewicz* as "a ritualistic exercise, necessarily doomed to failure"), it is clear *a fortiori* that he would have to do the same for infants. That would imply that no dying infant could ever be withdrawn from life-sustaining equipment if such equipment could continue to keep that life going—regardless of condition or prognosis. This seems to us at odds with humane medical practice and good morality.[59]

McCormick understood Judge Meade's ruling to have "driven a wedge between true best interests and personal desires, favored the latter as the basis of treatment, and left certification of these desires in the hands of the nearest kin."[60] For McCormick, this would leave open the possibility for abuse in determining what are the "best interests" for a never-competent patient. As a result, McCormick proposed a quality-of-life criterion to assist decision-makers in discerning treatment decisions for never-competent patients.

The third influence was McCormick's belief that the quality-of-life criterion best summarizes what the Catholic tradition meant by the ordinary/extraordinary means distinction. Decisions about medical treatment and life-preservation have for years been formulated in terms of what has been called "ordinay" and "extraordinary" means.[61] McCormick argues that the ordinary/extraordinary means distinction has always focused on the means necessary to sustain life, which implies a quality-of-life orientation. McCormick writes:

> But often enough it is the kind of, the quality of the life
> thus saved (painful, poverty-stricken and deprived, away
> from home and friends, oppressive) that establishes the
> means as extraordinary. *That* type of life would be an
> excessive hardship for the individual. It would distort
> and jeopardize his grasp on the over-all meaning of
> life.[62]

The sophistication of contemporary medicine obviates the need to consider the means used to sustain life and places the judgmental burden on
the hope of benefit for the patient or the quality of life involved.[63] For
McCormick, the quality-of-life criterion is a reconceptualization of the
ordinary/extraordinary means distinction in order to address new medical
circumstances so that it can be used to assist the appropriate decision-
makers in determining which treatments are in the "best interests" of
never-competent patients.

Due to the fact that the notion of "best interests" is so central to
treatment decisions for the never-competent, there are three elements of
the notion that McCormick underlines because he believes they can be
easily obscured. These three elements are:

> First, there is the *danger* of the determination. The key
> danger is that the concerns of parent, physician, and
> hospital will be allowed to play too early and too deci-
> sive a role in determining the child's best interests. Sec-
> ond, there is the *difficulty* of the determination of best
> interests. Medical uncertainties and contingencies head
> the list of factors that constitute this difficulty. Decisions
> must be made at the very time when prognoses are most
> problematic. Third, there is the *depth* of the notion of
> best interests.[64]

To make his notion of "best interests" more specific and objective,
McCormick incorporates Edmund Pellegrino's four components of "best
interests" into his own interpretation.[65] McCormick believes that the
most informed moral decision should attend to all four components. The
following is McCormick's interpretation of Pellegrino's four components:

> (1) *Medical good*. This refers to the effects of medical
> intervention on the natural history of the disease being
> treated, to what can be achieved by application of medi-

cal knowledge: cure, containment, prevention, ameliora-
tion, prolongation of life. This good can vary.

(2) *Patient preferences.* The scientifically correct (medically good) decision must be placed within the context
of a patient's life situation or value system. Thus to be
good in this sense a decision must square with what the
patient thinks worthwhile.

(3) *The good of the human as human.* This refers to the
good proper to humans as humans. Pellegrino notes that
this is philosophically debatable: among the various values associated with this good are freedom, rationality,
consciousness, and the capacity for creativity. One thing
is not debated: unique to humans is the very capacity to
make choices, to set a life plan. This capacity is frus-
trated if choice is not free. To be treated as humans includes being accorded the dignity of choosing what we
believe to be good. Therefore, all other things being
equal, a treatment that preserves the capacity to choose
is to be preferred to one that does not. In this sense it is
the patient's best interests.

(4) *The good of last resort.* This is the good that gathers
all others, is their base and explanation. It gives life ultimate meaning. It will or should inform and explain patient preferences and life plans. [66]

The fourth component of McCormick's notion of "best interests" serves
as the foundation for his quality-of-life criterion. McCormick argues:

With the always incompetent (and babies are included
here), it is this good that will undergird the judgment of
best interests simply because the second and third components are irrelevant to babies. And this only compli-
cates matters, for reasonable persons may have differing
theologies, differing conceptions of last resort.[67]

It is the "good of last resort" that should inform the appropriate decision-
makers what the never-competent patient ought to want in a particular
situation. For McCormick, "'best interests,' being a dangerous, difficult,
and profound notion, will involve elements of the intuitive, the imagina-
tive, and the unexplainable. That is because we are dealing with a human
judgment, not a straight-forward scientific one."[68] McCormick under-

stood that the same could also be said about his quality-of-life criterion. Nonetheless, McCormick is committed to the possibility of hammering out some consensus about quality of life.[69] Such a consensus must be both based in reason and rooted in the Christian context.

McCormick's quality-of-life criterion is a synthesis of both the proportionate reason criterion and the criterion of the person "integrally and adequately considered." He understands "quality of life" to be an elusive term whose meaning varies according to context.[70] However, at a more profound level, when the issue is preserving human life, the term assumes a more basic meaning. McCormick writes:

> Just as life itself is a condition for any other value or achievement, so certain characteristics of life are the conditions for the achievement of other values. We must distinguish between two sets of conditions: those that allow us to do things well, easily, comfortably, and efficiently, and those that allow us to do them at all.[71]

To assist McCormick in making quality-of-life judgments, he uses proportionate reason as a "tool" for establishing what is promotive or destructive for the good of the whole person. This synthesis of proportionate reason and the person "integrally and adequately considered" assists McCormick in determining what is an acceptable quality of life on the basis of the never-competent patient's "best interests." For him, "judgments about the preservation of life increasingly are made in terms of quality of life, i.e., procedures are extraordinary or ordinary according to their capacity to give a patient a certain 'level' of life."[72] McCormick's quality-of-life criterion respects not only the value of the whole person, but it affirms that respect for the human person entails considering all the relevant factors and circumstances that are involved in any situation.

McCormick understands the difficulties in trying to establish a perfectly rational criterion for making quality-of-life judgments. However, he believes, "we must never cease trying—in fear and trembling—to be sure. Otherwise we have exempted these decisions in principle from the one critique and control that protects against abuse. Exemption of this sort is the root of all exploitation, whether personal or political."[73] To make his quality-of-life criterion more concrete, McCormick establishes two guidelines and four norms that further specify his criterion.[74] McCormick also utilizes moral principles to help clarify and specify his quality-of-life criterion. These moral principles will be highlighted as they impact the quality-of-life criterion.

The first guideline that specifies McCormick's quality-of-life criterion is the potential for human relationships associated with the infant's condition. The second, which is a further specification of the first, is the benefit/burden calculus. Both guidelines demonstrate the commonsense basis of McCormick's natural law reasoning and how it creatively connects with the Catholic moral tradition, relating it both to religious commitment and to a reasonable hierarchy of values.[75] To understand McCormick's quality-of-life criterion both of these guidelines will be analyzed to show how he has further concretized them throughout the years.[76]

The first guideline developed for dealing with never-competent patients focuses on the potential for human relationships associated with the infant's condition. By relational potential McCormick means "the hope that the infant will, in relative comfort, be able to experience our caring and love."[77] McCormick is proposing a "minimum potential for human relationships" as a specification of what he means by "best interests." Specifically, he proposes that

> if a newborn baby had no potential for such relationships or if the potential would be totally submerged in the mere struggle to survive, then that baby had achieved its potential and further life-prolonging efforts were not mandatory, that is, would no longer be in the best interests of the baby.[78]

Therefore, according to this guideline, when a never-competent patient, even with treatment, will have no potential for human relationships, the appropriate decision-makers can decide to withhold treatment and allow the patient to die.[79] McCormick claims this quality-of-life approach has its foundation in the traditional ordinary/extraordinary means distinction that was later clarified by Pius XII.[80] McCormick has never claimed that this is an easy guideline to apply, especially in the case of never-competent patients. He also understands that some bioethicists will want to continue to use the extraordinary means language to justify not treating particular handicapped neonates. McCormick believes this is fair, but he adds a caution:

> they should realize that the term "extraordinary" has been so relativized to the condition of the patient that it is this condition that is decisive. The means is extraordinary because the infant's condition is extraordinary. And if that is so, we must face the fact head-on—and discover the substantive standard that allows us to say this of some infants, but not others.[81]

To make this point clear, McCormick attaches four caveats to this first guideline. He writes:

> First, this guideline is not a detailed rule that pre-empts
> decisions; for relational capacity is not subject to
> mathematical analysis but to human judgment. However,
> it is the task of physicians to provide some more con-
> crete categories or presumptive biological symptoms for
> this human judgment. Second, because this guideline is
> precisely that, mistakes will be made. Third, it must be
> emphasized that allowing some infants to die does not
> imply that "some lives are valuable, others not" or that
> "there is such a thing as a life not worth living." Every
> human being, regardless of age or condition, is of incal-
> culable worth. Fourth, this whole matter is further com-
> plicated by the fact that this decision is being made by
> someone else.[82]

In essence, this guideline requires that the appropriate decision-makers
must be able to determine if a minimally accepted "quality of life" can be
expected. This determination ought to be made on the basis of the never-
competent's "best interests," understood normatively. This guideline
does not depreciate the value of the never-competent individual but affirms that a genuine respect for the person demands attention to the pros-
pects held out by continued life.[83]

In this first guideline, McCormick argues that the value of the human
person is affirmed by showing how it is rooted in his theological anthropology. The Christian story does not yield concrete answers and fixed
rules, but it does yield various perspectives and insights that inform human reasoning. One such insight is that human life is a "relative" good.
McCormick writes:

> The fact that we are (in the Christian story) pilgrims, that
> Christ has overcome death and lives, that we will also
> live with Him, yields a general value judgment on the
> meaning and value of life as we now live it. It can be
> formulated as follows: life is a basic good but not an ab-
> solute one. It is basic because it is the necessary source
> and condition of every human activity and of all society.
> It is not absolute because there are higher goods for
> which life can be sacrificed.[84]

Human life is not a value to be preserved in and of itself. It is a value to
be preserved as a condition for other values, and therefore, as far as these

other values remain attainable. Since these other values cluster around and are rooted in human relationships, it seems to follow that life is a value to be preserved only insofar as it contains a potentiality for human relationships. When in human judgment this potentiality is totally absent or would be, because of the condition of the individual, totally subordinated to the mere struggle for survival, that life can be said to have achieved its potential.[85]

McCormick bases this potential for human relationships in the Catholic tradition. The Catholic tradition has always maintained that since human life is a relative good, and the duty to preserve it is a limited one, then it is not always morally obligatory to use all means to preserve human life if a person cannot attain the higher, more important good.[86] For McCormick, the higher, more important good is the capacity for relationships of love. The core of this guideline is developed from the love commandment found in the New Testament.[87]

For McCormick, the love of neighbor is in some real sense the love of God. He understands this to mean that:

> The good our love wants to do Him and to which He enables us, can be done only for the neighbor, as Karl Rahner has so forcefully argued. It is in others that God demands to be recognized and loved. If this is true, it means that, in Judaeo-Christian perspective, the meaning, substance, and consummation of life are found in human *relationships*, and the qualities of justice, respect, concern, compassion, and support that surround them.[88]

The loving and graced relationship or covenant between God and humanity is a metaphor for the human person's social and relational nature.[89] In this relationship, God gives God's love freely and waits for a response. McCormick argues that: "Our radical acceptance of God is tied to the love of neighbor—a love that secures rights, relieves suffering, promotes growth. God is speaking to us in history and we are not free to be uninvolved."[90] If a human person is devoid of the possibility of experiencing human love, then that life has achieved its potential. Lacking the potential for human relationship does not mean that this particular person is not of incalculable worth. McCormick states:

> One can and I believe should say that the *person* is always of incalculable value, but that at some point continuance in physical life offers the person no benefit. Indeed, to keep "life" going can easily be an assault on the person and his or her dignity.[91]

Human reason informed by the Christian story prevents the absolutization of life; human life is not preserved just for biologic processes. To preserve life in this manner is a form of medical vitalism that is rejected by the Judaeo-Christian tradition.[92] What the Christian context prepares us for both intellectually and psychologically is to say at some point, "Enough."[93] For McCormick, it is the quality of a person's life that makes its preservation worthwhile to the person. If the quality of a patient's life would entail an excessive hardship for the patient, then one may be permitted to forgo or withdraw medical treatment. To continue treatment or to initiate treatment in this case would not be acting in the patient's best interests.[94] This is a quality-of-life judgment and, for McCormick, it is based on the potential for relationality, not on any arbitrary judgment about the value of a person's life.[95]

This guideline of the potential for human relationships has been criticized for being too general and open to possible abuse. McCormick himself stated when he advanced this guideline that it had to be further specified. He argues:

> The guideline is general and rather vague. But this is the way it is with all moral norms. They really root in general assertions that must be fleshed out by experience, modified by discussion and consultation, propped up and strengthened by cautions and qualifications. It is in the process of their application that moral norms take on added concreteness.[96]

Despite being convinced that this guideline is fundamentally sound, McCormick understood that he must further concretize it. Specifically, there are those circumstances when the never-competent patient has the potential for human relationships, but the underlying medical condition is critical and will result in imminent death, or after treatment has been initiated it becomes apparent that the treatment is medically futile. In these two situations it is clear that, besides the potential for human relationships, McCormick must incorporate an additional guideline that can weigh the proportionate and disproportionate benefits of certain treatments.

The second guideline of McCormick's quality-of-life criterion is the benefit/burden calculus. McCormick argues:

> Where medical procedures are in question, it is generally admitted that the criterion to be used is a benefits/ burdens estimate. . . . The question posed is: Will the burden of the treatment outweigh the benefits to the patient?

> The general answer: If the treatment is useless or futile,
> or it imposes burdens that outweigh the benefits, it may
> be omitted.[97]

Like his first guideline, McCormick claims the benefit/burden calculus emerges out of the ordinary/extraordinary means distinction. He will justify this claim by examining the sources of Christian ethics.

For McCormick, "moral-theological argument gathers all the warrants it can from revelation, Christian tradition, human experience, and reasoning in an attempt to lift out what appears to be the more human Christian policy."[98] He begins his analysis of the benefit/burden calculus by examining the Catholic tradition. The Catholic tradition maintains that if a medical intervention was judged to be ordinary it was viewed as morally mandatory. If extraordinary, it was morally optional. It was said to be ordinary if it offered some reasonable hope of benefit for the patient and could be used without excessive inconvenience (risk, pain, expense, etc.). If it offered no reasonable hope or benefit or was excessively burdensome, it was extraordinary.[99] Pope Pius XII further clarified the ordinary/extraordinary means distinction when he declared that "we are morally obliged to use only ordinary means to preserve life and health—according to circumstances of persons, places, times, and culture—that is to say means that do not involve any grave burden for oneself or another."[100] Pius XII bases the distinction between ordinary and extraordinary means on the idea that human life is a basic good, but a good to be preserved precisely as a condition of other values. One must examine the particular situation's circumstances, because these circumstances dictate the balance to be considered between life and these other values. McCormick also cites ethicist Gerald Kelly, S.J., and his classic interpretation of ordinary/extraordinary means distinction in the Catholic tradition. Kelly explains that

> *ordinary* means of preserving life are all medicines,
> treatments, and operations, which offer a reasonable
> hope of benefit for the patient and which can be obtained
> and used without excessive expense, pain, or other in-
> convenience. *Extraordinary* means are all medicines,
> treatments, and operations, which cannot be obtained or
> used without excessive expense, pain, or other incon-
> venience, or which, if used, would not offer a reasonable
> hope of benefit.[101]

The theological measure of ordinary and extraordinary means clearly focuses on the patient's best interests.[102] Only the patient or the patient's proxy can weigh adequately the factors of "excessive expense" or "pain."

This is the basis for McCormick's claim that his quality-of-life approach is patient-centered.

McCormick believes that his notion of benefit/burden calculus within his quality-of-life criterion is a logical development of the ordinary/extraordinary means distinction, or what he refers to as an extension of the tradition into new problem areas.[103] McCormick believes that the ordinary/extraordinary means distinction has an honorable history and an enduring validity. However, he argues that these terms "summarize and promulgate judgments drawn on other grounds. It is these 'other grounds' that cry out for explication."[104] McCormick writes:

> We must admit that the terms "ordinary" and "extraordi-
> nary" are but code words. That is, they summarize and
> are vehicles for other judgments. They do not solve
> problems automatically. Rather they are emotional and
> mental preparations for very personal and circumstantial
> judgments that must take into account the patient's atti-
> tudes and value perspectives, or "what the patient would
> have wanted." "Ordinary" and "extraordinary" merely
> summarize other underlying judgments. They say very
> little in and of themselves.[105]

To further explain these "other grounds," McCormick reformulates the ordinary/extraordinary means distinction by advancing his benefit/burden calculus. An extraordinary means is one that offers the patient no real benefit, or offers it at a disproportionate cost. For McCormick, one is called to make a moral judgment: Does the benefit of a proposed medical intervention really outweigh the harm it will inevitably concurrently produce? This is a quality-of-life judgment. McCormick argues: "I see no way out of *some* quality-of-life judgments short of imposing survival on all newborns regardless of their condition and prognosis."[106] For McCormick, this is not a departure from the Catholic tradition. It is a reformulation of the tradition in order to deal with contemporary bioethical problem areas.[107]

The reason for this reformulation of the tradition is that over the centuries the ordinary/extraordinary means distinction has become less objective and more relative because medicine and technology have become more sophisticated. The medical profession is committed to curing disease and preserving life. Today, we have the medical technology to make this commitment a reality. However, McCormick argues that "this commitment must be implemented within a healthy and realistic acknowledgment that we are mortal."[108] Therefore, McCormick believes that we must reformulate the basic value of human life under new circumstances. For many contemporary ethicists the traditional terminology of ordinary/extraordinary means has outlived its usefulness. McCormick argues there are two reasons for this:

> First, the terminology too easily hides the nature of the judgment being made. The major reference point in factoring out what is "reasonable" (benefit) and "excessive" (burden) is the patient—his or her condition, biography, prognosis, and values. The terminology, however, suggests that attention should fall on the means in an all too mechanical way. Second, many people misinterpret the terms to refer to "what physicians ordinarily do, what is customary." This is not what the term means. In their ethical sense, they encompass many more dimensions of the situation.[109]

As a result of being misinterpreted, these terms have led to excessive abuses.[110]

Focusing on the value of human life, McCormick sought to reformulate the ordinary/extraordinary means distinction without abandoning the tradition. For him,

> the theologian's perspective when dealing with the sacredness of life is to question traditional concepts in order to maintain continuity, to express value insights under new circumstances, and to reword judgmental criteria in a way which preserves the tradition and our adhesion to the basic value.[111]

The ordinary/extraordinary means distinction, McCormick realized, could take us only so far. Contemporary medical problems no longer only concern those patients for whom biological death is imminent. Modern medicine and technology have the ability to keep almost anyone biologically alive. This has tended gradually to shift the problem from the means to reverse the dying process to the quality of life sustained and preserved as the result of the application of medical technology.[112] Today, because of the advancements in medicine and technology, it is the kind and quality of life thus saved that establishes a means as extraordinary.

To address this shift in the problem from means to quality of life preserved, McCormick has reformulated the ordinary/extraordinary means distinction to indicate the benefit/burden calculus.[113] In this way, McCormick is still trying to maintain the Catholic tradition by walking a middle course between medical vitalism and medical pessimism. For

McCormick, "it is clear that the judgments of burden and benefit are value judgments, moral choices. They are judgments in which, all things considered, the continuance of life is either called for or not worthwhile to the patient."[114] In making these moral judgments one can see how the principle of proportionate reason is used as a tool for determining whether a particular life-sustaining treatment is a benefit or a burden, that is, whether or not it is in the best interests of the never-competent patient and those involved in the decision-making process.[115]

The benefit/burden calculus was also proposed by the Sacred Congregation for the Doctrine of the Faith in its *Declaration on Euthanasia*, and by the President's Commission for the Study of Ethical Problems in Medicine and Biomedical and Behavioral Research in its *Deciding to Forego Life-Sustaining Treatment.*[116] The issuance of the *Declaration on Euthanasia* in 1980 by the Magisterium gave McCormick further justification for incorporating the benefit/burden calculus into his quality-of-life criterion. The Congregation concludes that:

> It will be possible to make a correct judgment as to the means by studying the type of treatment being used, its degree of complexity or risk, its cost and possibilities of using it, and comparing these elements with the result that can be expected, taking into account the state of the sick person and his or her physical and moral resources.[117]

This statement gave McCormick further proof to anchor his guideline and thus his criterion for treatment decisions in the benefit/burden calculus. Medical treatments are not morally mandatory if they are either gravely burdensome or useless for the patient.[118] The benefit/burden calculus now becomes the basis for McCormick's quality-of-life criterion when a never-competent patient has the potential for human relationships. This entails making a value judgment, and the evaluation of whether a treatment is a benefit or a burden can be open to personal interpretation.[119] That means these evaluations can be "borderline and controversial."[120]

Both guidelines for McCormick's quality-of-life criterion, even though he argued they were reformulations of the ordinary/extraordinary means distinction, came under criticism for being too relative, subjective, and consequential in nature. To address this criticism, McCormick, along with John Paris, S.J., proposed the following norms that would further specify the capacity for human relationships as a summary of the benefit/burden evaluation:

(1) Life-saving intervention ought not to be omitted for institutional or managerial reasons. Included in this specification is the ability of this particular family to cope with a badly disabled baby.

(2) Life-sustaining interventions may not be omitted simply because the baby is retarded. There may be further complications associated with retardation that justify withholding life-sustaining treatment.

(3) Life-sustaining intervention may be omitted or withdrawn when there is excessive hardship on the patient, especially when this combines with poor prognosis (e.g., repeated cardiac surgery, low prognosis transplants, increasingly iatrogenic oxygenization for low birthweight babies).

(4) Life-sustaining interventions may be omitted or withdrawn at a point when it becomes clear that expected life can be had only for a relatively brief time and only with continued use of artificial feeding (e.g., some cases of necrotizing enterocolitis).[121]

These norms or rules do not mandate certain decisions. McCormick argues that concrete rules such as these "do not replace prudence and eliminate conflicts and decisions. They are simply attempts to provide outlines of the areas in which prudence should operate."[122]

McCormick further specified his quality-of-life criterion to shed light on medical situations for the appropriate decision-makers. These rules are "an attempt to make concrete the relations of coalescent values and burdens, even if expressed in nonabsolute form."[123] However, guidelines, even specified by concrete norms and moral principles, cannot cover all circumstances and every possible situation. McCormick's quality-of-life criterion assists the appropriate decision-makers by giving them a range of choices. As rational persons, it is up to the decision-makers to examine each situation using proportionate reason, and the guidelines advanced by McCormick in his quality-of-life criterion, to determine what is in the "best interests" of the never-competent patient and those involved in the decision-making process.[124] McCormick makes clear that no criterion can cover every instance where human discretion must intervene to decide. There is always the possibility of human error because we are finite and sinful people.[125] The margin of error, however, should reflect not only the utter finality of the decision (which tends to narrow it), but also the unavoidable uncertainty and doubt (which tends to

broaden it).[126] With the assistance of these guidelines, McCormick believes that the appropriate decision-makers will be given the necessary
guidance to act responsibly.

In conclusion, McCormick's quality-of-life criterion, as applied to
never-competent patients, is based on a normative understanding of the
"best interests" of the patient. This criterion has been concretized by his
fundamental guidelines of relational potential associated with the infant's
condition and the benefit/burden calculus. However, these are only
guidelines; they do not determine decisions. The quality-of-life criterion
sets parameters and from within these parameters the appropriate decision-makers must use their reason to decide what is in the "best interests"
of the patient.

McCormick understands that these guidelines are open to the possibility of being misinterpreted. However, because there is the potential for
abuse does not mean they should be discarded. McCormick argues:

> Such a threat is inseparable from human living. We must
> reduce such threats by every human and Christian re-
> source available to us; but the existence of threats and
> risks should not lead to the rejection of all exception-
> making, to a type of moral absolutism rejected by Chris-
> tian tradition.[127]

McCormick is attempting to examine new medical situations from within
the value-perceptions and commitments of the Catholic tradition. The
guidelines he proposes for his quality-of-life criterion are an attempt to
help in the decision-making process in regard to never-competent patients. McCormick argues that these guidelines are substantially accurate,
but he is aware that it is only through human experience that they will
become more concrete and meaningful.[128] With this in mind, he places
his guidelines, norms, and moral principles before a broad community
that encompasses not only ethicists but also health care professionals so
that they can be critically scrutinized. McCormick understands that unless his quality-of-life criterion is given the opportunity to be analyzed
and criticized by various disciplines, its usefulness and appropriateness
as a criterion for never-competent patients will always be questioned.
Since McCormick encourages this type of broad, interdisciplinary analysis of his position, the next section will examine criticism, in the hope
that it will lead to further specification and concretization of his moral
criterion.

CRITICISM

Several ethicists have criticized McCormick's patient-centered, quality-of-life criterion over the years. Some of this criticism has been addressed by McCormick in subsequent articles, such as: whether or not he has misinterpreted the ordinary/extraordinary means distinction,[129] whether he has departed from the Catholic tradition on the ordinary/extraordinary means distinction in substance or in formulation,[130] or whether a quality-of-life ethic is completely separate from a sanctity-of-life ethic.[131] Since these criticisms have been addressed by McCormick, there is no need to analyze them in this section. The criticisms that will be addressed focus on ambiguity in regard to language, McCormick's narrow interpretation of social factors, and the relative and subjective nature of his quality-of-life criterion. This section will articulate, evaluate, and analyze these criticisms as they impact McCormick's moral criteriology.

First, several ethicists have criticized McCormick for his lack of precision when it comes to his use of language. This lack of precision has led to a sense of ambiguity in regard to how McCormick understands various terms and to an inconsistency in how he applies various terms. James Walter believes "there is much ambiguity about what 'quality of life' means, and consequently there is little agreement about the definition of this criterion."[132] In particular, Walter believes the word "quality" can refer to several different realities. It can refer to the idea of excellence, or it can be understood as an attribute or property of either biological or personal life. He argues that McCormick, in his first guideline, has isolated one quality or attribute to be considered as the minimum of personal life: the potential for human relationships.[133] Walter suggests that the word "quality" should not primarily refer to a property or attribute. "Rather, the quality that is at issue is the quality of relationship that exists between the medical condition of the patient, on the one hand, and the patient's ability to pursue human purposes, on the other."[134] The ethical concern surrounding those who define quality of life as a property or an attribute is that they do not attribute intrinsic value to physical life.[135]

McCormick's first guideline of the potential for human relationships associated with the patient's condition does appear to be an attribute or property of human life. Relational potential will determine for McCormick, in certain situations, whether a never-competent patient ought to be medically treated. However, in 1986, in an article entitled "The Best Interests of the Baby," McCormick implicitly presents his understanding of "quality" as the quality of relationship that exists between a person's condition and the ability to pursue life's goals. In 1992, McCormick published an article in *America* entitled "'Moral Considerations' Ill Considered," in which he explicitly changed his position. McCormick writes:

> Brodeur correctly rejects a notion of quality of life that
> states that a certain arbitrarily defined level of function-
> ing is required before a person's life is to be valued. But
> if it refers to *the relationship between a person's bio-
> logical condition and the ability to pursue life's goals*, it
> is critical to good decision-making.[136]

Is the potential for human relationships a property of life in his quality-
of-life criterion or does he now view it as the quality of the relationship
that exists between "a person's biological condition and the ability to
pursue life's goals?"[137] It appears that either McCormick has changed his
mind or he was in the process of clarifying his first position. In either
case, McCormick never gave an explanation and justification for his last
position. As a result, one is left wondering how exactly he interpreted the
word "quality."[138]

It is possible to point out additional examples of ambiguities in regard to language and terms. One major example centers on his moral
criterion for decision-making. Based on analysis of McCormick's moral
criteriology, it is clear that he abandoned his notion of the "reasonable
person standard." However, he never explicitly states this nor does he
give a justification for doing so. In addition, it is not at all clear where
McCormick stands in regard to his moral criterion of proportionate reason and his moral criterion of the person "integrally and adequately considered." In the early 1970s, McCormick accepted proportionate reason
as a formal moral criterion and began applying it to ethical issues.
Gradually, however, proportionate reason developed into a "tool" for
determining what actions would promote the good of the whole human
person in particular situations. The result was a new moral criterion, that
is, the person "integrally and adequately considered." Finally, it appears
that McCormick synthesized both criteria into his quality-of-life criterion. How this synthesis occurred and why has never been explained by
McCormick. It is apparent from his writings that he continued to utilize
both proportionate reason and the criterion of the person "integrally and
adequately considered," but again he never explained this evolution, nor
did he ever give justification for it. This lack of clarity regarding the
roles proportionate reason and the person "integrally and adequately considered" play in his quality-of-life criterion leaves this moral criterion
open to serious criticism. McCormick argues that the most important
facet of dealing with treatment decisions for never-competent patients is
the proper approach, not the conclusions. He argues that "with a precisely analyzed and carefully articulated approach, we have our best
chance of keeping the best interests of the baby in clear focus and of
avoiding the traps of sentimentality, ideology, and subjectivism."[139] If

this is true, then it was necessary for him to clarify his moral criterion so that he could eliminate any ambiguity and confusion surrounding it. This is critical because McCormick's moral criteriology is an integral element in his ethical methodological approach.

The last example concerns the role of prudence in McCormick's moral criteriology. McCormick attempts to specify further the two guidelines in his quality-of-life criterion by formulating four norms or rules that provide some guidance for decision-making. However, he argues that prudence plays a major role in the application of his quality-of-life criterion. McCormick writes:

> Concrete rules do not make decisions. They do not re-place prudence and eliminate conflicts and doubt. They are simply attempts to provide outlines of the areas in which prudence should operate.[140]

He refers to the integral role prudence plays in his moral criteriology, but he never defines prudence nor does he explain how he uses it. This is the same criticism that was directed at McCormick in regard to how prudence operates in his moral epistemology.[141] Because McCormick is a "revised" natural law ethicist in the Catholic tradition, one can speculate that he agrees with Aquinas' interpretation of prudence. However, this is speculation at best.[142]

These examples show ambiguities in how McCormick uses language and terminology in his moral criteriology. As a result, this moral criterion has been criticized for being subjective, relative, and consequential by ethicists such as Ramsey, Connery, Reich, and Weber, to name a few. Much of this criticism has been addressed by McCormick directly. However, the point is that if he had carefully articulated his positions in a systematic manner and precisely analyzed them in regard to language and terminology, then much of the confusion surrounding his quality-of-life criterion could have been eliminated. A comprehensive explanation of how his quality-of-life criterion evolved over the years, and an admission that the author, at certain times, had in fact changed his mind, would have benefitted not only McCormick's moral criteriology, but his whole ethical methodology.

Second, as Roman Catholic ethicists Richard Sparks and James McCartney have noted, McCormick may be criticized for having a narrow interpretation of how social factors impact his quality-of-life criterion. This criticism was discussed in chapter two in reference to how it relates to the "essentially social" nature of the human person that McCormick grounds in his doctrine of creation.[143] McCormick argues that when making treatment decisions for handicapped neonates, one ought to take into consideration the effects these decisions have on both the family and society at large. McCormick grounds his position in the Catholic tradition, quoting both Pius XII[144] and moralist Gerald Kelly, S.J.,[145] to show how the Catholic tradition has always included social factors in determining medical decisions. The problem, according to Sparks and McCartney, is that McCormick has not been consistent in how he views and applies these social factors in the area of treatment decisions for handicapped neonates.

Sparks argues that "the ultimate decision as to whether treatment is in a given patient's total best interests ought to incorporate not only medical or individual (i.e., experiential) burden factors, but also broader social factors, viewed from the patient's existentially-contexted vantage point."[146] Therefore, one must allow the never-competent patient's social nature not only to make an impact on the calculation of benefits (e.g., the benefit to the never-competent patient derived from his or her ability to relate to others) but also to allow that same social nature to frame the calculation of burdens (e.g., psychic strain to the family or cost to society).[147] McCartney agrees with Sparks's position and lists the various social factors that should be considered.[148] The major point of the Sparks and McCartney criticism is that McCormick's narrow interpretation of social factors is inconsistent with what he means by "best interests," normatively understood. In a number of articles pertaining to non-competent patients in non-therapeutic medical experimentation situations, McCormick argues that social and familial factors ought to be considered in the benefit/burden calculus.[149] He argues that under certain circumstances, infants and children ought to participate in experimentation situations because, as members of the Christian community, there is a sense of solidarity and Christian concern for others. Infants and children are in some sense volunteer-able to help the common good of society, provided that the individual's well-being is not placed under appreciable burdens.[150] However, when dealing with treatment decisions for never-competent patients, it appears McCormick has a rather narrow interpretation of familial and social factors. In fact, Sparks argues that McCormick "seems to exclude similar social solidarity and familial concerns from the calculus of the patient's best interests in treatment decisions related to non-competents."[151]

Having a narrow interpretation of social and familial factors in the benefit/burden calculus does not mean that McCormick totally excludes these social factors. It appears that he is trying to avoid a "socially-weighted" benefit/burden calculus. Sparks explains a "socially-weighted" benefit/burden calculus:

> The qualitative benefit and burden of treatment for a
> given patient is placed on the ethical scale *over against*

the benefit (utility) and burden of said treatment and patient for the community of affected persons. If the latter social concerns coalesce with the former patient-centered claims, then the patient wins, either receiving the beneficial treatment or else being spared the agony of excessively burdensome, even futile efforts. However, if life-prolonging, even qualitatively beneficial therapy, will inordinately tax that patient's family or society, it is in *their* best interests, and thus morally justified, to withhold or withdraw treatment.[152]

Sparks also rejects a "socially-weighted" calculus in determining the best interests of the patient. However, Sparks believes one can reject a "socially-weighted" calculus without maintaining a restrictive interpretation of social factors.[153] Once again, McCormick is trying to walk a middle course between two extremes. On one side, there are those who categorically exclude social and familial factors in regard to treatment decisions for never-competent patients.[154] On the other side, there are the broad interpreters of social factors in decision-making who have a utilitarian perspective that can lead to the "slippery slope."[155] McCormick, conscious of the criticism that has been directed at his quality-of-life criterion, tends toward a more narrow interpretation of social factors. He is well aware that a broad interpretation of social factors could lead to active infanticide, because it would be more humane, efficient, and the least costly next step. The problem is that McCormick is not in fact walking a middle course. His interpretation of social and familial factors, regarding treatment decisions for handicapped neonates, is not only more restrictive than the Catholic tradition, it also seems to deviate from his normative understanding of "best interests."[156]

For McCormick, in determining what is in the patient's "best interests" he must consider not only familial and social factors, but also the associated medical condition, the capacity for relational potential, and the proportion of the burden of treatment to the benefits derived for the patient. Social and familial factors play a role in determining the benefit/burden calculus, but they must always play a proportionate role. Sparks and McCartney would certainly agree. The problem appears to be that McCormick views the burden to the never-competent patient and the burden to the affected others as being in competition with one another when making treatment decisions. Sparks contends that viewing social burden factors from the patient's perspective can avoid the competition that is constitutive of the socially-weighted position. According to James Walter:

> Sparks seems to be claiming that the child would not,
> and perhaps should not, want to be treated in circum-
> stances of excessive social burden because it would not
> be in the child's best interests to place these burdens on
> those who must care for its existence.[157]

If McCormick has a normative understanding of "best interests," then he should examine the social burden factors from the never-competent patient's perspective. What the handicapped neonate "ought" to want should encompass the needs of those who will care for this child. If the circumstances of treatment will be a grave burden for the family of the never-competent neonate and society as a whole, then this is not in the "best interests" of the never-competent patient.

This criticism by Sparks and McCartney is one of the most substantive critiques of McCormick's quality-of-life criterion. It is substantive because it clearly shows how McCormick's position deviates not only from the Catholic tradition, but also deviates from his own normative understanding of "best interests." This author agrees with the criticism of Sparks and McCartney. However, one can also understand why McCormick has taken this position. First, he fears that a broad interpretation of social factors can easily lead to the slippery slope of social utilitarianism. This, he understands, can lead to infanticide. Second, McCormick is well aware of the finite and sinful nature of humanity. How does one determine if a family is taking the never-competent patient's perspective or their own self-interested perspective?[158] Both of these concerns are legitimate and need to be addressed. This can be accomplished by establishing a middle course between the extremes that follows the Catholic tradition on social burden factors as clarified by Pius XII. The possibility of abuse is always present, but there are safeguards built into McCormick's quality-of-life criterion—guidelines, norms, and moral principles. Being faithful to the Catholic tradition and to his own normative criterion can help alleviate potential abuse.

Third, Richard Sparks criticizes McCormick's relational potential guideline as being limited in its usefulness in many neonatal cases. Sparks writes that McCormick's guideline is

> only minimally helpful in deciding what cases might
> constitute excruciating pain or excessive burdens. He
> leaves the physician the task of providing "more con-
> crete categories or presumptive biological symptoms" to
> enflesh what constitutes a totally non-relational and/or
> an intractably pained mental state.[159]

Sparks commends McCormick for plotting the two extreme cases on the spectrum, but criticizes him for giving physicians the responsibility for filling in the conflictual middle.[160] This criticism seems quite unjustified. It does not appear from McCormick's writings that the sole authority for filling in "the conflictual middle" is left to physicians alone. Clearly, McCormick is convinced that his quality-of-life criterion is "correct as far as it goes."[161] However, he believes that diagnostic categories could assist decision-makers in regard to treatment decisions. He understands that physicians will be at the forefront of determining these diagnostic categories, but he does not believe they are the only ones who can perform this task. He states that, "the most successful recent attempt to concretize in clinical categories the potential for human relationships is that of Robert Weir."[162] Weir is not a physician but an ethicist.

McCormick is well aware that establishing a full set of diagnostic categories is not the cure-all for determining treatment decisions for never-competent patients. He knows that not all medical conditions can be placed in specific categories; there is a marked difference in the severity of conditions within each category. He is also aware that not all physicians or even bioethicists could or would agree to the specific diagnostic categories proposed. However, for McCormick:

> The important point, however, is that we ought to attempt, as far as possible, to approach neonatal disabilities through diagnostic categories, always realizing that such categories cannot deflate important individual differences and that there will always remain gray areas.[163]

How these categories are developed must depend on medical expertise, which is why McCormick relies on physicians and other health care professionals. However, in the final analysis, it is not diagnostic categories that will determine treatment decisions for never-competent patients. Ultimately, these decisions are made by the appropriate decision-makers who will apply the quality-of-life criterion to a particular situation and determine what is in the "best interests" of the never-competent patient.

Finally, Leonard Weber questions whether McCormick's quality-of-life criterion does not, in the long run, negate his position that every human life is of equal value regardless of condition. For Weber, the questions that have to be asked are:

> Once McCormick has made the claim that we must decide to treat or not on the basis of the child's condition, will people really be able to pay much attention to his insistence that every life is valuable regardless of condition? How valuable is a life anyway if it is only a condi-

tion for something else and need not be preserved if that something else cannot be achieved? And though he wants to base his decision on symptoms which physicians can relate to potential for human relationships, is it nevertheless likely that this use of quality of life language will lead others to move away from objective indications to value judgments on the worth of mentally retarded life?[164]

These are justifiable concerns that must be addressed on a continual basis. However, after reviewing McCormick's writings, one can see that he has built-in safeguards that help him ensure that every human life is of equal value regardless of condition. The impetus for Weber's comments comes from the fact that he sees a direct contrast between a sanctity-of-life ethic and a quality-of-life ethic. This is why Weber argues that the extraordinary means approach better provides "for some protection against an arbitrary decision being made on the basis of a judgment about the worth of a particular type of life."[165] Comparing sanctity of life and quality of life allows the focus of attention to be on our obligation to preserve life and avoids degrees of discrimination in the quality-of-life criterion.[166] McCormick understands these two approaches to be correlated, not categorically opposed to one another.[167] There is really only one ethic that holds life to be an intrinsic value with limits on the patient's moral obligation to pursue this value. McCormick writes:

> Quality-of-life assessments ought to be made within an over-all reverence for life, as an extension of one's respect for the sanctity of life. However, there are times when preserving the life of one with no capacity for those aspects of life that we regard as *human* is a violation of the sanctity of life itself. Thus to separate the two approaches and call one *sanctity* of life, the other *quality* of life, is a false conceptual split that can easily suggest that the term "sanctity of life" is being used in an exhortatory way.[168]

In addition to understanding quality of life to be an extension of sanctity of life, McCormick also uses the moral principle of justice to ensure the equal value of every human life regardless of condition. For McCormick, the principle of justice is rooted in charity which emphasizes the dignity of every human person. McCormick's notion of justice is grounded in his theological anthropology. Created in the image and likeness of God, the human person "is a member of God's family and the temple of the spirit."[169] Therefore, God confers on humanity a sense of dignity, which makes everyone equally valuable. Both the principle of justice and the interrelatedness of the quality-of-life and sanctity-of-life criteria allow McCormick to differentiate between every person being of equal value and every life being of equal value. For McCormick, what the "equal value" language is attempting to say is legitimate:

> We must *avoid unjust* discrimination in the provision of
> health care and life supports. But not all discrimination
> (inequality of treatment) is unjust. *Unjust* discrimination
> is avoided if decision-making centers on the benefit to
> the patient, even if the benefit is described largely in
> terms of quality-of-life criteria.[170]

This does not eliminate the possibility that McCormick's quality-of-life criterion could be subject to abuse. Abuse is always possible. However, McCormick believes that the moral principle of justice and the correlation of sanctity of life and quality of life will serve as safeguards against these possibilities of abuse.

In conclusion, in making treatment decisions for never-competent patients, McCormick emphasizes the need for a proper moral criterion that is precisely analyzed and carefully articulated in order to keep the focus on the "best interests" of the never-competent patient. The criticism directed at McCormick's quality-of-life criterion not only highlights the need for McCormick to have been more precise with language and terminology, but also shows the need for a more systematic analysis of his moral criterion. His failure to address these concerns directly opens his moral criterion to ambiguity and misinterpretation, and the real possibility of misapplication and abuse. For McCormick's quality-of-life criterion to be considered beneficial and appropriate for decision-makers, it must stand up to both medical and ethical scrutiny. Unless it does, it will be added to the long list of criteria for moral decision-making found wanting. To avoid this from happening, others who have studied the writings of McCormick must assume the task of clarification and analysis.

CONCLUSION

McCormick's quality-of-life criterion is not a wooden formula that one can apply to any situation and come to a concrete decision. He views his quality-of-life criterion as a "light in a room, a light that allows the individual objects to be seen in the fullness of their context."[171] The two guidelines McCormick proposes as the heart of his quality-of-life criterion serve as a guide to assist the appropriate decision-makers in making treatment decisions for never-competent patients. McCormick believes his quality-of-life criterion is beneficial and appropriate for Christian decision-makers because it is grounded in the Judaeo-Christian tradition and it is reasonable. The quality-of-life criterion proposed for never-competent patients attempts to walk a middle course between extreme positions. To those who believe his criterion is too liberal, McCormick gives two reasons for why he believes it is a "moderate" position. He writes:

> First, there are a good number of people who would like simply to put these children to sleep. This is not my proposal at all. I'm proposing that we shouldn't intervene with artificial medical support or surgery if the child will benefit nothing from them. Second, my position comes out of and is continuous with a conservative tradition— the Judaeo-Christian tradition that life is a basic value, but not an absolute one, and therefore suggests limits with regard to its support.[172]

McCormick constructs his quality-of-life criterion on the foundation of his theological anthropology and his moral epistemology. With the use of discursive reason, informed by the Christian story, people can determine the objective moral rightness and wrongness of an action by determining what constitutes the good of the person "integrally and adequately considered." From this foundation emerges the final element of his ethical methodology.

McCormick has an underlying ethical system; the problem is that he never articulated it in a systematic manner. Being an acknowledged non-system builder does not mean that the structure of a system is not in place.[173] The structure is secure; the problem is that he never articulated it clearly and the particulars are open to ambiguity and misinterpretation. However, demonstrating that McCormick has an ethical methodology and building a case for it is only half the battle. To verify that McCormick's ethical methodology is operable and of value, it will have to be applied to specific ethical situations. The next chapter will take McCormick's ethical methodology and apply it to five specific diagnostic treatment categories of handicapped neonates. These diagnostic treatment categories will attempt to encompass, as far as possible, the entire spectrum of handicapped neonates. McCormick's quality-of-life criterion will be applied to each category to determine if it is a practical and beneficial criterion that can be utilized by the appropriate decision-makers in regard to treatment decisions for handicapped neonates. Before this can be accomplished, one must determine who exactly are the appropriate decision-makers in regard to never-competent patients. Therefore, this next chapter will also examine the procedural issues that focus on the four potential candidates for decision-makers for never-competent patients.

NOTES

[1]Celestine Bittle, *Reality and the Mind* (Milwaukee, WI: Bruce Publishing Company, 1936), 291.

[2]Criteriology comes from the Greek κρίνω meaning to distinguish or judge, which implies the testing of knowledge to distinguish the right from the wrong.

[3]Aaron L. Mackler, "Neonatal Intensive Care," *Scope Note 11*, 1.

[4]James Castelli, "Richard A. McCormick, S.J. and Life/Death Decisions," *St. Anthony Messenger* 83 (August 1975): 34. McCormick, as interviewed by Castelli.

[5]See Lisa Sowle Cahill, "On Richard McCormick," 91.

[6]For a more detailed analysis of McCormick's position on a normative understanding of his patient-centered approach, see McCormick, "The Rights of the Voiceless," *How Brave a New World?*, 99-113.

[7]Allsopp, 105.

[8]McCormick explains Aquinas' reasoning as follows: "That which ordains an act to its end gives it its form. But charity is the virtue which ordains to its end all virtuous acts, either acts or omissions. Therefore, charity gives form to all virtuous acts." McCormick, "The Primacy of Charity," 21; see also Aquinas, *Summa Theologica* IIa-IIae, 23, 8.

[9]McCormick, *Health and Medicine in the Catholic Tradition*, 34. For McCormick, as for Aquinas, "charity does not destroy or replace the other virtues; but the virtues are rooted in and depend on charity, and in such a way that there is no true virtue in the fullest sense without charity. Thus the virtues, while retaining their identity, are participants in charity so that they and their acts are in some sense emanations of and acts of charity." Ibid., 35. The same can be said for the relationship of charity to the moral principles of autonomy, justice, beneficence, and nonmaleficence.

[10]McCormick, "The Moral Right to Privacy," *How Brave a New World?*, 369.

[11]McCormick, *The Critical Calling*, 365. Emphasis in the original.

[12]McCormick, *Health and Medicine in the Catholic Tradition*, 36.

[13]For a more detailed theological analysis, refer to Chapter Two, McCormick's Theological Anthropology section above.

[14]McCormick uses as an example the traditional Christian obligation to preserve life. He argues that the Christian tradition "has always strived to maintain a middle course between two extremes: medical-moral utopianism, i.e., sustaining life at all costs and with all means because when life is over everything is over and death is an absolute end; and its opposite, medical-moral pessimism, i.e., there is no point in sustaining life if it is accompanied by suffering, lack of function, etc. Both of these extremes are basic devaluations of human life because they remove life from the context which gives it its ultimate significance. The middle path is a recognition of the facts that human life is a basic value, the most basic value, because it is the foundation for all other values and achievements, but that life is not the absolute good and death the ultimate and absolute evil." McCormick, "A Proposal for 'Quality of Life' Criteria for Sustaining Life," 76.

[15]McCormick, "To Save or Let Die," *How Brave a New World?*, 342.

[16]Ibid., 342-343.

[17]For a more detailed analysis of Veatch's interpretation of the "reasonable person standard," see Robert Veatch, *Death, Dying and the Biological Revolution* (New Haven, CT: Yale University Press, 1976).

[18]In tort law, the whole theory of negligence presupposes some uniform standard of behavior. The standard of conduct which the community demands must be an external and objective one, rather than the individual judgment, good or bad, of the particular actor; and it must be, so far as possible, the same for all persons, since the law can have no favorites. At the same time, it must make proper allowance for the risk apparent to the actor, for his or her capacity to meet it, and for the circumstances under which he or she must act. The courts have dealt with this very difficult problem by citing a fictitious person, who never has existed on land or sea: the "reasonable man of ordinary prudence." Sometimes he is described as a reasonable man, or a prudent man, or a man of average prudence, or a man of ordinary sense using ordinary care and skill. The actor is required to do what such an ideal individual would do in his place. A model of all proper qualities, with only those shortcomings and weaknesses which the community will tolerate on the occasion, "this excellent but odious character stands like a monument in our Courts of Justice, vainly appealing to his fellow-citizens to order their lives after his own example." For a more detailed analysis of the "reasonable man standard" in tort law, see W. Page Keeton *et al.*, *Prosser and Keeton on the Law of Torts*, 5th ed. (St. Paul, MN: West Publishers, 1984), 149-180.

[19]James J. Walter, "A Public Policy Opinion on the Treatment of Severely Handicapped Newborns," 243; see also McCormick, "The Rights of the Voiceless," *How Brave a New World?*, 109.

[20]McCormick, "The Rights of the Voiceless," *How Brave a New World?*, 109.

[21]McCormick writes: "I believe the broad lines of what is in our best interests is available to human insight and reasoning—that is, there are certain actions objectively destructive or promotive of us as persons. Furthermore, I believe that such perceptions should form the basis on which we build our judgments about what is in the best interests of incompetent persons." Ibid., 108.

[22]For a more detailed analysis of the "ideal observer theory," see Robert Veatch, *A Theory of Medical Ethics* (New York: Basic Books, Inc., 1981), 116-118; see also Roderick Firth, "Ethical Absolutism and the Ideal Observer," *Philosophy and Phenomenological Research* 12 (March 1952): 326. Roderick Firth was the first to originate the "ideal observer theory." Firth defines the statement "X is right" and "X would be approved by an ideal observer who is omniscient, omnipercipient, disinterested, dispassionate, and otherwise normal." Here Firth is taking the view that knowledge that is mediated by our perceptions of reality is something that we obtain under certain kinds of conditions. Stating the conditions under which we obtain particular perceptions will define what we mean by a particular word that we use to identify some part of the real world. For a more detailed analysis, see Arthur J. Dyck, *On Human Care: An Introduction to Ethics* (Nashville, TN: Abingdon, 1977), 141-155.

[23]McCormick, "The Quality of Life, The Sanctity of Life," *How Brave a New World?*, 409.

[24]Walter, "A Public Policy Opinion," 243.

[25]McCormick, *Notes on Moral Theology: 1981 through 1984*, 35. Emphasis in the original.

[26]For a more detailed analysis of this theological grounding, refer to Chapter Two, McCormick's Theological Anthropology section above.

[27]Walter, "A Public Policy Opinion," 243.

[28]Hypothetical substituted judgments are defined as those which judge what would be chosen or decided by a person who for some reason lacks the capacity *de facto* to make a decision in a given case. On the other hand, guardian substituted judgments objectively assess what constitutes a person's best interests all things considered. For a more detailed analysis, see Edmund N. Santurri and William Werpehowski, "Substituted Judgment and the Terminally-Ill Incompetent," *Thought* 57 (December 1982): 484-501; see also Walter, "A Public Policy Opinion," note 19, 244.

[29]McCormick, "The Quality of Life, The Sanctity of Life," *How Brave a New World?*, 409. Emphasis in the original.

[30]Ibid., 410. Emphasis in the original.

[31]After reviewing his "Notes on Moral Theology" in *Theological Studies*, one becomes accustomed to the fact that McCormick becomes attached to a particular notion that he has read about, takes it into consideration for a brief period of time, and then abandons it without explanation or justification. There are numerous examples, such as: the association of basic good, the reasonable person standard, etc.

[32]For an example of how McCormick continues to emphasize the "reasonableness" of the human person, see McCormick, "Life and Preservation," *Theological Studies* 42 (1981): 100-110.

[33]McCormick, *Doing Evil to Achieve Good*, 232-233.

[34]Walter, "Proportionate Reason and Its Three Levels of Inquiry," 32.

[35]For a more detailed analysis, see McCormick, *Doing Evil to Achieve Good*, 193-267; see also Gula, *Reason Informed by Faith*, 273-275.

[36]McCormick, "The New Medicine and Morality," 315-316. Emphasis in the original.

[37]McCormick, *The Critical Calling*, 134.

[38]For a detailed historical analysis of the proportionalism debate and McCormick's involvement, refer to Chapter Three, McCormick's Dual Moral Epistemology section above. It should be noted that the theory of proportionalism for McCormick is the result of a conscious effort to provide a more realistic and rationally satisfying approach to resolving moral conflicts. Allsopp, 105.

[39]For a more detailed analysis of what brought about this shift, refer to Chapter Two, McCormick's Theological Anthropology section above.

[40]McCormick, *The Critical Calling*, 156.

[41]Ibid.

[42]For a more detailed analysis of how the source of McCormick's criterion of the person "integrally and adequately considered" can be found both in the Vatican II document "The Pastoral Constitution on the Church in the Modern World," and in the writings of Thomas Aquinas, refer to Chapter Two, McCormick's Theological Anthropology section above.

[43]Janssens lists eight essential aspects of the human person. For a more detailed analysis, refer to Chapter Two, McCormick's Theological Anthropology section above.

[44]To understand what McCormick means by the person "integrally and adequately considered" it is helpful to examine the American Fertil-

ity Society's "Ethical Considerations of the New Reproductive Technologies." McCormick states that he takes full responsibility for its use in this document. The document states: "'Integrally and adequately' refers to the sum of dimensions of the person that constitute human well-being: bodily health; intellectual and spiritual well-being, which includes the freedom to form one's own convictions on important moral and religious questions; and social well-being in all its forms: familial, economic, political, international and religious." McCormick, "Surrogacy: A Catholic Perspective," *Corrective Vision*, 202; see also American Fertility Society, "Fertility and Sterility," *Supplement 2* 53, no. 6 (1990): 1 S.

[45]McCormick, *Corrective Vision*, 202.

[46]Robert Weir disagrees with McCormick. Weir believes that the quality-of-life criterion and best interests criterion are distinct and separate. McCormick responds to Weir by stating: "I believe Weir is wrong when he asserts that for those who use quality-of-life assessments, 'it is not necessary to consider the best interests of the neonate.' It is precisely because one is focused on best interests that qualitative considerations cannot be ignored but indeed are central. Weir is clearly afraid that quality-of-life considerations will be unfair. But they need not be. It all depends on where the line is drawn. I am all the more convinced of the inseparable unity and general overlap of best interests and quality-of-life considerations when I study Weir's clinical applications of his ethical criteria." McCormick, review of *Selective Nontreatment of Handicapped Newborns*, by Robert Weir, in *Perspectives in Biology and Medicine* 29 (Winter 1986): 328.

[47]McCormick, "The Rights of the Voiceless," *How Brave a New World?*, 112.

[48]Ibid., 101. McCormick argues: "That is one reason why, for instance, a long Christian (in this case Catholic) tradition has held it to be morally acceptable for an individual to forego expensive life-saving medical treatment if such treatment would exhaust family savings, plunge the family into poverty, and deprive other members of the family of, for example, educational opportunity. In such an instance, it would be in the best interests of the ill individual because his best interests include his family." Ibid. For a more detailed analysis on the Catholic tradition on the duty to preserve life, see McCormick and John Paris, "The Catholic Tradition on the Use of Nutrition and Fluids," *America* 156 (May 2, 1987): 356-361.

[49]Walter, "A Public Policy Opinion," 245.

[50]McCormick, "Life and Its Preservation," *Theological Studies* 42 (1981): 108. Emphasis in the original.

[51]Walter writes: "Thus, this test must necessarily exclude all eccentric wants and preferences as well as all sinful desires. Only those desires

that incline us to the fundamental goods and conform to the objective hierarchy of values are included in and interpreted by the reasonable person standard. What McCormick means when he says that most people are or desire to be reasonable is that most people seek what is in their best interests." Walter, "A Public Policy Opinion," 245-246; see also McCormick, "The Rights of the Voiceless," *How Brave a New World?*, 105 and 110.

[52]Ramsey was one of McCormick's major critics in regard to using the "reasonable person standard" as the basis for "best interests." In contrast, Ramsey argues that his "medical indications policy" is more objective. See Paul Ramsey, "Euthanasia and Dying Well," *Linacre Quarterly* 44 (1977); Idem, "Prolonged Dying: Not Medically Indicated," *Hastings Center Report* 6 (February 1976).

[53]For a more detailed analysis of this moral epistemology, refer to Chapter Three, McCormick's Dual Moral Epistemology section, Second Moral Epistemology—After 1983 subsection above.

[54]McCormick, "The Best Interests of the Baby," 20.

[55]Ibid.

[56]On October 2, 1979, Brother Fox, an eighty-three year-old member of the Society of Mary religious order, underwent hernia surgery. During the surgery he suffered severe cardiorespiratory arrest, which resulted in diffuse cerebral and brain-stem anoxia. Brother Fox lost spontaneous respiration and had to be maintained on a respirator. His physicians concluded he was in a "persistent vegetative state." Rev. Philip K. Eichner, religious superior for Brother Fox, after consulting his only surviving relatives (ten nieces and nephews), requested removal of the respirator. For a more detailed analysis of this case, see McCormick, "The Preservation of Life and Self-Determination," *How Brave a New World?*, 381.

[57]For a detailed analysis of the *Quinlan* case, see McCormick, "The Moral Right to Privacy," *How Brave a New World?*, 362-371. For a detailed analysis of the *Saikewicz* case, see Idem, "The Case of Joseph Saikewicz," *How Brave a New World?*, 372-380.

[58]Ibid., 383. Emphasis in the original.

[59]Ibid., 384. Emphasis in the original.

[60]Ibid.

[61]McCormick writes: "If the means could be characterized as 'extraordinary,' there is no obligation *per se* for the patient to use them, or for those with proxy rights (such as parents) to decide to use them for incompetents. If, all things considered, they were to be characterized as 'ordinary,' they were seen as obligatory." McCormick, "The Quality of Life, The Sanctity of Life," *How Brave a New World?*, 394.

[62]McCormick, "To Save or Let Die," *How Brave a New World?*, 347. Emphasis in the original.

[63]McCormick, "A Proposal for 'Quality of Life' Criteria for Sustaining Life," 78.

[64]For a more detailed analysis of these three aspects, see McCormick, "The Best Interests of the Baby," 21-22. Emphasis in the original.

[65]For a more detailed analysis, see Edmund D. Pellegrino, M.D., "Moral Choice, the Good of the Patient and the Patient's Good," in *Ethics and Critical Care Medicine*, ed. J. C. Moskop and L. Kopelman (Dordrecht, Netherlands: D. Reidel, 1985), 117-138.

[66]McCormick, *Health and Medicine in the Catholic Tradition*, 115-116. Emphasis in the original. It should be noted that for both Pellegrino and McCormick there is a hierarchy to these four components. When dealing with situations of conflict the good of last resort takes precedence over the good of the human as human, the good of the human as human takes precedence over patient precedence, and patient preference takes preference over medical good. See Edmund D. Pellegrino, "Moral Choice, the Good of the Patient, and the Patient's Good," in *Ethics and Critical Care Medicine*, 117-138.

[67]McCormick, "The Best Interests of the Baby," 23. McCormick gives two examples how belief systems play a role in decision-making. He writes: "For example, the Orthodox Jew may regard every moment of life as precious, as absolute. For the Catholic, physical existence is relativized by the death-resurrection motif. The accumulation of minutes is not the Catholic criterion of dying well. Therefore, I might be willing to say 'enough' somewhat sooner than others when dealing with problems of life-prolongation. Second, with the always incompetent patient, it will be this good that will undergird the judgment of 'best interests.' Therefore judgments of best interests may differ. Reasonable persons may have differing theologies. For instance, with my beliefs, I could easily conclude that chemotherapy was not in Saikewicz's best interests. Some one else could disagree, and with plausibility, because of a different good of last resort." Ibid.; and McCormick, *Health and Medicine in the Catholic Tradition*, 116.

[68]McCormick, "The Best Interests of the Baby," 23.

[69]Cahill, "On Richard McCormick," 94.

[70]For example, quality of life can mean a clean environment, free of industrial pollution; moderate temperatures and humidity; the absence of excessive noise; or efficient traffic patterns. McCormick, "A Proposal for 'Quality of Life' Criteria for Sustaining Life," 77.

[71]Ibid., 77-78.

[72]Ibid., 77.

[73]McCormick, "To Save or Let Die," *How Brave a New World?*, 343-344.

[74]A guideline for McCormick is a general and fundamental "standard" that serves to specify his normative criterion. A norm is more specific to contexts and more restricted in scope. A norm seeks to specify in content what the guideline requires.

[75]Lisa Sowle Cahill, "On Richard McCormick," 91.

[76]It should be noted that the quality-of-life criterion has various interpretations. McCormick bases his interpretation of quality-of-life on relational potential. Joseph Fletcher uses neocortical function. Earl E. Shelp proposes "minimal independence" as the central property of his quality-of-life position. Jonathan Glover bases his quality-of-life criterion on whether the patient is said to have a life worth living and will this life or death produce beneficial or harmful side effects on other persons. For a more detailed analysis on these positions, see Robert Weir, *Selective Nontreatment of Handicapped Newborns*, 164-170; James J. Walter, "Quality of Life in Clinical Decisions," in *Encyclopedia of Bioethics*, rev. ed., 1354; Joseph Fletcher, "Four Indicators of Humanhood—The Enquiry Matures," *Hastings Center Report* 4 (December 1974): 6-7; Earl E. Shelp, *Born to Die?: Deciding the Fate of Critically Ill Newborns* (New York: Free Press, 1986); and Jonathan Glover, *Causing Death and Saving Lives* (New York: Penguin Books, 1977), 113-114.

[77]McCormick, "To Save or Let Die," *How Brave a New World?*, 351.

[78]McCormick, "The Best Interests of the Baby," 23.

[79]It should be noted here that the basis of these decisions are found in McCormick's theological anthropology, i.e., the meaning of life in love. For a more detailed analysis, refer to Chapter Two, McCormick's Theological Anthropology section above.

[80]McCormick quotes Pius XII as saying that an obligation to use any means possible "would be too burdensome for most men and would render the attainment of the higher, more important good too difficult." Pius XII, "The Prolongation of Life," *Acta Apostolicae Sedis* 49 (1957): 1,031-1,032. McCormick understands Pius XII to say that certain treatments may be refused because they would lead to a life that lacks the proper quality. Weber, *Who Shall Live?*, 69.

[81]McCormick, "To Save or Let Die," *How Brave a New World?*, 349.

[82]For a more detailed analysis, see Ibid., 349-350.

[83]Cahill, "On Richard McCormick," 91.

[84]McCormick, *The Critical Calling*, 202.

[85]McCormick, *Health and Medicine in the Catholic Tradition*, 54.

[86]McCormick, "To Save or Let Die," *How Brave a New World?*, 345.

[87]This is what McCormick means by the principle of charity. It is charity that underlines McCormick's first guideline in his quality-of-life criterion. The good that is higher than human life is the capacity for relationships of love.

[88]McCormick, "To Save or Let Die," *How Brave a New World?*, 346. Emphasis in the original. The religious commitment that the love of God is accomplished through the love of neighbor can be further specified by Josef Fuchs and Karl Rahner. See Josef Fuchs, "Christians Existence and Love of Neighbor," *Personal Responsibility and Christian Morality* (Washington, DC: Georgetown University Press, 1983): 28-31; see also Karl Rahner, "Reflections on the Unity of the Love of Neighbor and the Love of God," *Theological Investigations* vol 6, 231-249.

[89]For a more detailed analysis of the social and relational nature of the human person, refer to Chapter Two, McCormick's Theological Anthropology section, Doctrine of Creation subsection above.

[90]McCormick, *The Critical Calling*, 12.

[91]McCormick, "Quality of Life, Sanctity of Life," *How Brave a New World?*, 406. Emphasis in the original.

[92]This does not mean that once a decision has been made to forgo treatment that the dying person is not treated with dignity and respect. For McCormick, even though a person has reached his or her potential and no treatment is recommended, as members of society we still have a moral obligation to care for the person while he or she is in the dying process. McCormick's position on the dignity of human life is grounded in the Christian context and his position on respect for the treatment of pre-embryos. McCormick's position on the pre-embryo is pertinent because it shows that his respect for human life is consistent from conception to death. If McCormick believes we have a moral obligation to treat the pre-embryo, which has the *potential* for personhood, with dignity and respect, then this should support his belief in the moral obligation to care for the dying *person* when the decision to forgo treatment has been made. See McCormick, "Who Or What Is The Pre-embryo?," *Kennedy Institute of Ethics Journal* 1 (March 1991): 1-5; Idem, "The Pre-embryo As Potential: A Reply To John A. Robertson," *Kennedy Institute of Ethics Journal* 4 (December 1991): 303-305. Emphasis mine.

[93]McCormick, "The Best Interests of the Baby," 20.

[94]Physical life, the condition of other values, would become itself the ultimate value. When this occurs, the value of human life has been distorted out of context. When the condition of human life makes it impossible to realize or attain other values, there is no reason to preserve such

a life. See McCormick, "To Save or Let Die," *How Brave a New World?*, 348.

[95]Weber, *Who Shall Live?*, 71.

[96]McCormick, "To Save Or Let Die: State of the Questions," *America* 131 (October 5, 1974): 171.

[97]Richard A. McCormick, S.J., "Technology and Morality: The Example of Medicine," *New Theology Review* 2 (November 1989): 26.

[98]McCormick continues by stating: "Where values are concerned, especially basic values, we are dealing with something quite original, like color. One can assemble and order a convergence of probabilities to persuade to a point of view, but ultimately we can only be pointed in the direction and asked to see if it is so or not." McCormick, "To Save or Let Die: State of the Questions," 171.

[99]McCormick, *Health and Medicine in the Catholic Tradition*, 145.

[100]Pius XII, "The Prolongation of Life," *Acta Apostolicae Sedis*, 1,032. Pius XII continues stating: "A more strict obligation would be too burdensome for most men and would render the attainment of the higher, more important good too difficult. Life, health, all temporal activities are in fact subordinated to spiritual ends. On the other hand, one is not forbidden to take more than the strictly necessary steps to preserve life and health, as long as he does not fail in some more serious duty." Ibid.

[101]Gerald Kelly, S.J., *Medico-Moral Problems* (St. Louis, MO: The Catholic Health Association of the United States and Canada, 1958), 129. Emphasis in the original.

[102]For a more detailed view of the Catholic tradition's position on the ordinary/extraordinary means distinction, see McCormick & Paris, "The Catholic Tradition on the Use of Nutrition and Fluids," 358-360.

[103]McCormick writes: "A basic human value is challenged by new circumstances, and these circumstances demand that imagination and creativity be employed to devise new formulations, a new understanding of this value in light of these new circumstances while retaining a basic grasp upon the value. For example, in-vitro fertilization poses questions about the meaning of sexuality, parenthood, and the family because it challenges their very biological roots." McCormick, "A Proposal for 'Quality of Life' Criteria for Sustaining Life," 76.

[104]McCormick, "The Best Interests of the Baby," 19.

[105]McCormick, "A Proposal for 'Quality of Life' Criteria for Sustaining Life," 77.

[106]McCormick, "Life and Its Preservation," 105. Emphasis in the original.

[107]McCormick further states that: "It must be remembered that the abiding substance of the Church's teaching, its rock bottom so to speak,

is not found in the ordinary means-extraordinary means terminology. It is found in a basic value judgment about the meaning of life and death, one that refuses to absolutize either. It is *that judgment* that we must carry with us as we face the medical decisions that technology casts upon us." McCormick, "Technology and Morality," 29. Emphasis in the original.

[108]McCormick, *The Critical Calling*, 365.

[109]McCormick, *Health and Medicine in the Catholic Tradition*, 145.

[110]McCormick writes: "Thus, these terms have been badly used in our recent history, especially as vehicles for involuntary homicide, and, at the other end, as mandates for the fruitless and aimless prolongation of dying." Ibid.

[111]To accomplish this McCormick suggests four elements are essential: "first, openness to face new facts; second, the freedom to make an honest and sincere mistake; third, the honesty to admit an error; and, finally, the humility and courage to try again because try we must." McCormick, "A Proposal for 'Quality of Life' Criteria for Sustaining Life," 79.

[112]McCormick, "To Save Or Let Die," *How Brave a New World?*, 344.

[113]Besides McCormick's benefit/burden calculus, other ethicists have suggested various terms to reformulate the ordinary/extraordinary means distinction. Paul Ramsey suggests that the morally significant meaning of ordinary and extraordinary medical means can be reduced almost without remainder to two components—a comparison of treatments to determine if they are "medically indicated" and a patient's right to refuse treatment. See Paul Ramsey, *Ethics on the Edges of Life*, 153-160. Robert Veatch maintains that the terms "ordinary" and "extraordinary" are "extremely vague and are used inconsistently in the literature." Beneath this confusion he finds three overlapping but fundamentally different uses of the terms: usual versus unusual, useful versus useless, imperative versus elective. See Robert Veatch, *Death, Dying and the Biological Revolution*, 110-112. For further examples, see McCormick, "The Quality of Life, The Sanctity of Life," *How Brave a New World?*, 393-405.

[114]McCormick and Paris, "Saving Defective Infants," *How Brave a New World?*, 360.

[115]In making these moral judgments, McCormick will use the principle of justice rooted in charity. As social beings who are interrelated and interdependent, we must realize that decisions we make or that are made for us have a profound impact on family and society. McCormick writes: "Our shared humanity makes us members of a family with ties to each other. Up to a point, we are our sisters' and brothers' keepers. We owe each other. The Christian should sense this even more sharply." Therefore, when making treatment decisions for never-competent patients,

justice, rooted in charity, demands that the patient's "best interests" incorporate not only medical or personal factors but also familial and societal factors. This is based not only on the social nature of persons but also on the goods of creation. Because medical resources are finite, they must be allocated fairly for the good of the whole. It is the principle of justice, rooted in charity, that will help frame parameters within which the right questions about medical treatments can be asked and the right decisions made for the best interests of the patient and all concerned. See McCormick, "Henry the Unknown," *Ethics and Behavior* 1 (1991): 68.

[116]See President's Commission for the Study of Ethical Problems in Medicine and Biomedical and Behavioral Research, "Deciding to Forego Life-Sustaining Treatment: Ethical, Medical and Legal Issues in Treatment Decisions," (Washington, DC, U.S. Printing Office, March 1983): 218-219.

[117]Congregation for the Doctrine of the Faith, "Declaration On Euthanasia," *Origins* 10 (August 1980): 263.

[118]Warren Reich, John Connery, S.J., Leonard Weber, and Donald McCarthy disagree with McCormick's interpretation of the tradition on the benefit/burden distinction. For them, "the burden-to-benefit proportionalism of the ordinary/ extraordinary means tradition admits that quality of life elements impact on the *prima facie* presumption for treatment. It would be historically inaccurate to suggest that the extraordinary means concept referred to means *qua* means, whereas contemporary quality of life ethics speak more to the extraordinary condition or quality of the patient's life." For Reich, Connery, Weber and McCarthy, "the burden must be the burden of a medical treatment, not the burden of handicapped existence." Richard Sparks, *To Treat or Not To Treat?* 110; see also Donald G. McCarthy, "Treating Defective Newborns: Who Judges Extraordinary Means?" *Hospital Progress* 62 (December 1981): 45-50; John Connery, S.J., "Prolonging Life," 151-165; Leonard Weber, *Who Shall Live?*, 88-98; and Warren Reich, "Quality of Life and Defective Newborn Children: An Ethical Analysis," in *Decision-Making and the Defective Newborn*, ed. Chester A. Swinyard (Springfield, IL: Thomas, 1978), 488-511.

[119]To help clarify whether a treatment is a benefit or a burden, McCormick uses the principles of beneficence and nonmaleficence. For McCormick, quality-of-life judgments must avoid doing harm to the patient. Neither physicians nor parents are obliged to initiate or continue medical treatments which do harm to the well-being of the never-competent patient. That well-being consists generally in a life prolonged beyond infancy, without excruciating pain, and with the potential for participating, to at least a minimal degree, in human experience. Pro-

moting the good of another person, seeking the well-being or benefit of a
patient, preventing harm and removing harm from patients, all are rooted
in charity and play an integral role in treatment decisions for never-
competent patients. See McCormick, "A Proposal for 'Quality of Life'
Criteria for Sustaining Life," 79.

[120]McCormick and Paris, "Saving Defective Infants," *How Brave a
New World?*, 358.

[121]Ibid., 358-359. It should be noted that McCormick uses the moral
principles of charity, autonomy, justice, beneficence, and nonmaleficence to help "enflesh" these four norms.

[122]Ibid., 359.

[123]Cahill, "On Richard McCormick," 93.

[124]To further specify how decisions are made for the never-
competent patient by the appropriate decision-makers, McCormick uses
the principle of autonomy rooted in charity. McCormick believes that
autonomy rooted in charity is the middle path between paternalism and
the absolutization of autonomy. McCormick defines paternalism as a
system in which treatment decisions are made against the patient's preferences or without the patient's knowledge and consent. He calls this
"failures of dimension." When autonomy becomes absolutized, then
medicine has been secularized to the point that physicians are simply
technological instruments to carry out the wishes of the patient. Both of
these extremes spell isolation of the person and that can lead to the abandonment of the patient. When autonomy is rooted in charity, the value of
the person "integrally and adequately considered" becomes the focus.
For McCormick, "unless we confront the features that make choices
good or bad, autonomy usurps that role. It trumps every other consideration." When autonomy is rooted in the Christian story, the best interests
of the patient are served. For a more detailed analysis of McCormick's
position on autonomy, see Richard A. McCormick, S.J., "Behind the
Scenes: Some Underlying Issues in Bioethics," *Catholic Library World*
63 (January-June 1992): 158; Idem, "Value Variables in the Health-Care
Reform Debate," *America* 168 (May 29, 1993): 10; Idem, *The Critical
Calling*, 365; and Idem, *Corrective Vision*, 170.

[125]Human error based on our finite and sinful nature is rooted in
McCormick's theological anthropology. For a more detailed analysis,
refer to Chapter Two, McCormick's Theological Anthropology section,
Doctrine of Creation and Doctrine of the Fall subsections above.

[126]McCormick and Paris, "Saving Defective Infants," *How Brave a
New World?*, 360.

[127]McCormick, "To Save Or Let Die: The State of the Question,"
172.

[128]McCormick equates this with the case of the ordinary/extraordinary means distinction where terminal patients are concerned. He explains that: "The first uses of such a distinction were hesitant and terribly anguishing. But as time went along, the distinction meant more to the medical profession and settled into a more helpful policy, precisely through increasing usage. The neonatal problems I was discussing are relatively new. If the guidelines I proposed are substantially accurate, it will be through experience alone that it will become more helpful." Ibid., 173.

[129] Ethicist John Connery, S.J. argues that McCormick has misinterpreted the Catholic tradition regarding the ordinary/extraordinary means distinction. Connery argues that burden and benefit are different issues and that, according to the tradition, it was always the burden that was decisive in constituting a means to be extraordinary. McCormick believes that one cannot separate burden and benefit that sharply. McCormick argues: "It is impossible in some cases to determine what will benefit a patient without presupposing a standard of life. If the standard is bad enough (as in Connery's example of quadruple amputation), the benefit and burden coalesce. Or again, what is a burden to the patient presupposes judgments about the patient's condition, and among the objective conditions to be considered one of the most decisive is the *kind of life* that will be preserved as a result of the interventions. In cases like this, therefore, burden and benefit do not, as Connery thinks, 'deal with different issues . . . and usually apply to different types of cases.'" For a more detailed analysis, see John Connery, S.J., "Prolonging Life: The Duty and Its Limits," 151-165; see also McCormick, "Life and Its Preservation," 104-105. Emphasis in the original.

[130]John Connery, S.J. argues: "McCormick has shifted the emphasis from the nature of means to the quality of life itself. To this extent he departs from the tradition. Failure to employ ordinary means that were useful to prolong life would have been classified in the tradition as suicide." Connery, "Prolonging Life," note 15, 165. McCormick responds to Connery with two points. First, "the quality-of-life ingredient was always present in the very definition of burdensome means. Second, it is one thing to depart from a tradition, and in substance, not merely in formulation; it is another to extend this tradition into new problem areas. If such an extension is true to the substantial value judgments of the tradition, it is a departure only in formulation. This distinction between substance and formulation is clearly proposed by John XXIII and Vatican II." McCormick, "Life and Its Preservation," note 75, 105. For a more detailed analysis of Vatican II and John XXIII on the distinction between formulation and substance, see McCormick, *The Critical Calling*, 16-19;

see also "The Pastoral Constitution on the Church in the Modern World," *Documents of Vatican II*, no. 62, 268-269.

[131]For a more detailed analysis, see Weber, *Who Shall Live?*; McCormick, "The Quality of Life, The Sanctity of Life," *How Brave a New World?*, 393-411; and Idem, "A Proposal for 'Quality of Life' Criteria for Sustaining Life," 76-79.

[132]James J. Walter, "Quality of Life in Clinical Decisions," in *Encyclopedia of Bioethics*, rev. ed., vol. 3, 1353.

[133]Ibid., 1354. For Walter, McCormick is at one end of the quality of life spectrum because he understands "quality" as a property or an attribute. At the other end is Joseph Fletcher, who originally defined the indicators of "personhood" by reference to fifteen positive qualities. In the middle of this spectrum is Earl E. Shelp, who proposes minimal independence as the central attribute of his quality-of-life criterion. Ibid. See also Joseph Fletcher, "Indicators of Humanhood: A Tentative Profile of Man," *Hastings Center Report* 2 (1972): 1-4; and Earl E. Shelp, *Born to Die?: Deciding the Fate of Critically Ill Newborns*. For a more detailed analysis of this "quality of life" spectrum, refer to Chapter One, General Ethical Approaches To Treatment Decisions For Handicapped Neonates section above.

[134]For Walter, "these purposes are understood as the material, social, moral, and spiritual values that transcend physical, biological life. The quality referred to is the quality of a relation and not a property or attribute of life." Walter, "Quality of Life In Clinical Decisions," 1354; Idem, "The Meaning and Validity of Quality of Life Judgments in Contemporary Roman Catholic Medical Ethics," *Louvain Studies* 13 (Fall 1988): 195-208.

[135]Walter uses McCormick as an example. Walter argues: "In some of his writings McCormick has suggested that physical life does not possess inherent value but is a good to be preserved precisely as a condition of other values. Based on his theological convictions that physical life is a created, limited good and that the ability to relate to others is the mediation of one's love of the divine, McCormick resists attributing to physical life the status of an absolute value." Walter, "Quality of Life In Clinical Decisions," 1354.

[136]McCormick, "'Moral Considerations' Ill Considered," *Corrective Vision*, 228. Emphasis mine.

[137]By "quality of the relationship" I am referring to the quality of the relationship that exists between the medical condition of the neonate, on the one hand, and the neonate's ability to pursue human purposes, on the other. For a more detailed analysis, see Walter, "Quality of Life In Clinical Decisions," 1354.

[138]It should be noted that Walter in a footnote states: "It is probably the case that McCormick intended "potential for human relationships" to mean a property or attribute of *life* in his quality of life criterion. Whereas this may be true, I think that the basic thrust of McCormick's position is to assess the quality of *the relation* between the patient's medical condition and the pursuit of life's purposes. For McCormick, the fact that a patient does not possess any capacity for relationality means that the patient will not have any qualitative relation between his/her medical condition and the pursuit of life's values. Indications of my interpretation can be found throughout his more recent writings." Walter, "The Meaning and Validity of Quality of Life Judgments in Contemporary Roman Catholic Ethics," note 23, 207. Emphasis in the original.

[139]McCormick, "The Best Interests of the Baby," 25.

[140]McCormick & Paris, "Saving Defective Infants," *How Brave a New World?*, 316.

[141]For a more detailed analysis, refer to Chapter Three, Criticism section above.

[142]For a detailed explanation on the virtue of prudence in Aquinas, see Aquinas, *Summa Theologica* Ia-IIae, 61.

[143]For a more detailed analysis, refer to Chapter Two, Criticism section above.

[144]For a more detailed analysis, see Pius XII, "The Prolongation of Life," *The Pope Speaks*, 394.

[145]For a more detailed analysis, see Gerald Kelly, S.J., *Medico-Moral Problems*, 132.

[146]Sparks, *To Treat or Not To Treat?*, 198.

[147]James Walter, "Termination of Medical Treatment: The Setting of Moral Limits from Infancy to Old Age," 305.

[148]See Chapter Two, Criticism section above. It should be noted that there are others, especially in the medical profession, who believe that a "broader interpretation" of social factors should be included in the decision-making process for never-competent patients. See Raymond S. Duff and A. G. M. Campbell, "Moral Ethical Dilemmas in the Special Care Nursery," 890-893; Idem, "On Deciding the Care for Severely Handicapped or Dying Persons: With Particular Reference to Infants," *Pediatrics* 57 (April 1976): 487-493; Duff, "On Deciding the Use of Family Commons," in *Developmental Disabilities: Psychological and Social Implications*, eds. Daniel Bergsma and Ann E. Pulver (New York: Alan R. Liss, 1976), 73-84; Anthony Shaw, "The Ethics of Proxy Consent," in *Decision-Making and the Defective Newborn*, 593-600; John Lorber, "Spina Bifida: To Treat or Not To Treat?," *Nursing Mirror* 47 (Septem-

ber 14, 1978): 13-19; and Idem, "Selective Treatment of Myelomeningo-cele: To Treat or Not To Treat?," *Pediatrics* 53 (1974): 307-310.

[149]See McCormick, "Proxy Consent in the Experimentation Situation," *How Brave a New World?*, 51-71; and Idem, "Sharing in Sociality: Children and Experimentation," *How Brave a New World?*, 87-98.

[150]Sparks, *To Treat or Not To Treat?*, 199.

[151]Ibid.

[152]Ibid., 268-269. Emphasis in the original.

[153]Sparks writes: "While preserving unmitigated respect for the inherent dignity and right to life of every human patient, and related *prima facie* prescriptions, it still allows one to incorporate functional potential and social burden into decisions regarding the morality of forgoing treatment. Viewing each handicapped newborn as a multi-faceted rights-bearing person, parents and physicians can factor familial burden and societal limitation into a benefit/burden calculus from the patient's perspective. Such a patient bias or a weighing of the calculus on the side of the individual serves as a prudential wall against the potential abuse and selfishness on the part of burdened others that might take hold if a socially-weighted benefit/burden calculus, particularly with a functional anthropology, were allowed free reign." Ibid., 278.

[154]See Robert Veatch, *Death, Dying and the Biological Revolution: Our Last Quest for Responsibility*, 130-135; see also John Arras, "Toward an Ethic of Ambiguity," *Hastings Center Report* 14 (April 1984): 26-28.

[155]See H. Tristam Engelhardt, Jr., "Ethical Issues in Aiding the Death of Young Children," in *Beneficent Euthanasia*, 180-192; see also Joseph Fletcher, "The 'Right' to Live and the 'Right' to Die," *The Humanist* 34 (July/August 1974): 4-7.

[156] For a more detailed analysis of the Catholic tradition's understanding of social and familial factors, see Pius XII, "The Prolongation of Life," *Acta Apostolicae Sedis*, 1,032.

[157]James J. Walter, "Termination of Medical Treatment: The Setting of Moral Limits from Infancy to Old Age," 305; see also Richard Sparks, *To Treat or Not To Treat?*, 293-326.

[158]James Walter, "Termination of Medical Treatment: The Setting of Moral Limits from Infancy to Old Age," 305.

[159]Sparks, *To Treat or Not To Treat?*, 172.

[160]Sparks shows how McCormick at one extreme uses the anencephalic infant, "whose lack of neocortical function obviously indicates a life wholly without relational potential. Life-saving treatments are therefore optional, even contraindicated. At the opposite extreme of the handicap spectrum is a 'mongoloid' infant or child with Down Syndrome. While retarded mental capacities inhibit these Trisomy 21 victims

from higher education and advanced academic achievements, these infants are still 'aware,' 'conscious,' and capable of interrelating with their environment and with others. If anything, their capacity for uninhibited 'love' is enhanced by the limitation of mental complexity and nuance." Ibid. 172-173.

[161]McCormick, "The Best Interests of the Baby," 23-24.

[162]For a detailed analysis of Weir's clinical categories, see Weir, *Selective Nontreatment of Handicapped Newborns*, 234-243; see also McCormick, "The Best Interests of the Baby," 24.

[163]McCormick, "The Best Interests of the Baby," 24.

[164]Weber, *Who Shall Live?*, 82.

[165]Ibid., 85.

[166]McCormick, "The Quality of Life, The Sanctity of Life," *How Brave a New World?*, 406-407. Those who hold to this position would be Weber, Reich, and Connery. See Weber, *Who Shall Live?*, 78-87; see also Eugene F. Diamond, "'Quality' vs. 'Sanctity' of Life in the Nursery," *America* 135 (1976): 396-398.

[167]Robert Weir maintains that McCormick is moving against the stream of ethical consensus when he makes this claim. Weir writes: "Most ethicists accept the distinction between a sanctity-of-life principle and a quality-of-life principle." Weir, *Selective Nontreatment of Handicapped Newborns*," 165.

[168]McCormick, "The Quality of Life, The Sanctity of Life," *How Brave a New World?*, 407. Emphasis in the original.

[169]McCormick, "Who Or What Is The Pre-embryo?," 12.

[170]McCormick, "The Quality of Life, The Sanctity of Life," *How Brave a New World?*, 407. Emphasis in the original.

[171]Castelli, "Richard A. McCormick and Life/Death Decisions," 34. McCormick, as interviewed by Castelli.

[172]Ibid.

[173]See Odozor, *Richard A. McCormick and the Renewal of Moral Theology*, 23.

5

McCormick's Ethical Methodology
As Applied to Treatment Decisions
for Handicapped Neonates

INTRODUCTION

Dramatic advances in neonatal medical information and technology increase daily, and these advances are being implemented almost immediately. One thing that is clear to serious observers in the field is that the implementation of medical advances and technology for some neonates is a mixed blessing at best. As a result, the appropriate decision-makers are having to decide whether handicapped neonates, such as those with serious congenital anomalies, low-birth-weights, and genetic defects, should be treated aggressively or not at all. McCormick writes: "Here we are dealing with tiny patients who have no history, have had no chance at life, and have no say in the momentous decision about their treatment."[1] Despite proposed federal regulations (1984 Child Abuse Law) and medical guidelines (American Academy of Pediatrics) that have helped to clarify treatment issues, there is still no consensus among responsible decision-makers on substantive and procedural issues surrounding handicapped neonates.[2] There is general agreement within the medical, legal, and ethical professions that there are some handicapped neonates, in particular situations, whose lives need not be saved. Consensus ends, however, when an attempt is made to determine which specific neonates should receive or not receive medical treatment. There is also some general agreement, in certain situations, on the appropriate decision-makers for never-competent patients. Consensus ends, however, when a conflict arises between parents or between parents and health care professionals. This diversity of opinions has brought to the forefront the urgent need for an acceptable set of guidelines on both substantive and procedural issues. McCormick has proposed an ethical methodology, in which a patient-centered, quality-of-life criterion is an integral part, as a public policy option that can be used by the appropriate decision-makers in determining treatment decisions for handicapped neonates.[3] To determine if McCormick's ethical methodology is recommendable to the appropriate decision-makers as a public policy option for the treatment of handicapped neonates, it will be applied to five diagnostic treatment categories of neonatal anomalies.

This chapter will first articulate, analyze, and examine the procedural issues. This entails focusing on a number of questions. Who decides whether a handicapped neonate should be treated or denied treatment? What criterion is used for determining the appropriate decision-makers? How does the criterion apply to these individuals? Finally, on what basis are these treatment decisions made? Second, this chapter will present five diagnostic treatment categories established by this author. These five diagnostic treatment categories span the spectrum of neonatal handicaps so that most congenital anomalies can be placed in one of the five categories. The five diagnostic treatment categories of handicapped neonates include: (1) The handicapped neonate whose potential for human relationships is completely nonexistent. (2) The handicapped neonate who has a potential for human relationships but whose potential is utterly submerged in the mere struggle for survival. (3) The handicapped neonate who has a potential for human relationships but the underlying medical condition will result in imminent death. (4) The handicapped neonate who has the potential for human relationships but after medical treatment has been initiated, it becomes apparent that the treatment may be medically futile. (5) The handicapped neonate who has a potential for human relationships and has a correctable or treatable medical condition. A congenital anomaly has been selected to represent each particular diagnostic category.[4] McCormick's ethical methodology will be applied to each diagnostic treatment category to determine how his approach would guide the appropriate decision-makers in treating the handicapped neonate representative of the particular diagnostic category.

PROCEDURAL ISSUES

Treatment decisions for never-competent patients focus on two distinct but interrelated procedural issues—who are the appropriate decision-makers, and how are these treatment decisions made? This section will first examine who are the appropriate decisions-makers and why McCormick believes these individuals are the appropriate decision-makers. Secondly, this section will examine how McCormick makes these treatment decisions and by which criteria.

Treatment decisions concerning handicapped neonates are difficult under the best of circumstances. They become even more difficult and complex when there is a conflict situation regarding what is in the "best interests" of the handicapped neonate. The factors that add to the complexity of treatment decisions include:

> The high stakes involved in the decisions, the uncertainty of making proxy decisions for incompetent patients who have never been competent, serious time constraints, maximum emotional stress on parents, occasional disagreements between parents about the morally correct course of action, conflicts of interest (between parents and child, physicians and child, parents and physicians), the difficulty of accurately predicting neurological impairment and other future handicaps, inadequate communication of information between responsible parties in cases, and the logistical problems in using hospital committees or courts of law.[5]

The complexity of these issues and the fact that the handicapped neonate must always be represented by a proxy underscore the importance of determining the appropriate decision-maker who will be entrusted to promote the "best interests" of the never-competent patient. To make this determination, ethicist Robert Weir proposes four criteria for determining an appropriate decision-maker. The four criteria are:

> (1) The proxy should have relevant knowledge and information. This means the proxy should be knowledgeable regarding medical facts in particular cases. The proxy should be knowledgeable regarding the family setting into which particular anomalous neonates have been born. The proxy should have knowledge regarding possible alternatives to home care by biological parents.

> (2) The proxy should be impartial. The requirement of impartiality means that such persons should determine, as objectively as possible, whether life-prolonging treatment would be in the best interests of the individual neonate in question.

> (3) The proxy should be emotionally well-equipped to make such treatment decisions. Too often, treatment decisions are made by persons under severe emotional distress.

(4) There should be consistency in moral decision-making from case to case. The proxy, all things being equal, should be consistent in handling cases with the same diagnostic condition. In addition, it is necessary that proxies be consistent in applying the obligatory/nonobligatory distinction to cases.[6]

Weir is well aware that not every proxy can meet all of these conditions. However, he believes that the appropriate decision-maker should meet as many as possible. A review of McCormick's writings regarding procedural issues clearly shows that he would agree with Weir's analysis.[7]

There are four potential candidates for appropriate decision-makers regarding never-competent patients. The potential candidates include: parents, health care professionals, ethics or infant care review committees, and the courts. Parents of the handicapped neonate have their own intrinsic authority because of the nature of their relationship to the neonate. However, there are circumstances in which this intrinsic authority can be and must be limited. Based on Weir's criteria for proxy decision-making, each potential candidate has both positive and negative factors affecting his or her role as an appropriate decision-maker. The potential candidates, along with the positive and negative factors affecting their role as a proxy, will be discussed briefly to give a comprehensive overview of the role of the appropriate decision-maker.

The majority of bioethicists and health care professionals believe that treatment decisions regarding handicapped neonates ought to fall under the jurisdiction of parental authority.[8] The Judicial Council of the American Medical Association adds its support to parents as the appropriate decision-makers by stating: "In desperate situations involving newborns, the advice and judgment of the physicians should be readily available, but the decisions whether to exert maximal efforts to sustain life should be the choice of parents."[9] The President's Commission for the Study of Ethical Problems in Medicine also recommends that parents should be the primary decision-makers, especially in borderline cases.[10] Parents are given this authority as part of the discretionary decision-making power that society grants them in other matters concerning their children. Weir writes that

> society gives parents considerable latitude in providing moral education for their children, in deciding whether their children will attend public or private schools, and in most of the decisions that have to be made about their children's medical care.[11]

Second, parents have anticipated the birth of a child and have made certain commitments to the child prior to birth, therefore, they are the most likely to be most committed to the continuing welfare of the child.

While parents are the most knowledgeable about the family situation into which the neonate is born—emotional, financial, social factors, etc.—they are hampered as decision-makers by several other factors. Given the medical complexity of the situation, the emotional stress parents are under at the time when treatment decisions are being made, and their lack of knowledge concerning alternatives to keeping custody and providing long-term care for the child, some bioethicists and health care professionals believe that parents are not the appropriate decision-makers for never-competent patients. These factors may hinder the parents' decision-making capabilities and have the potential of causing harm to the neonate.[12]

Health care professionals are the second potential candidates for appropriate decision-makers regarding handicapped neonates. Several bioethicists and health care professionals believe that neonatologists are the best decision-makers because they serve as the neonate's advocate and thus are more likely to promote the neonate's best interests.[13] In addition, physicians possess the specialized medical knowledge regarding genetic disorders and congenital anomalies and they understand their long-term effects. They are more impartial and clear-sighted than parents because they are not under emotional stress. Finally, given their professional involvement with daily treatment of handicapped neonates, they have the opportunity to compare neonates with similar anomalous conditions, can assess the effectiveness of various treatment possibilities, and can make comparative judgments about the long-term handicaps associated with various medical conditions.[14]

Despite their medical knowledge, however, neonatologists are not always able to make accurate diagnoses and prognoses. Second, neonatologists are not always impartial and objective. Many have a bias in favor of normal and healthy neonates. Some have a bias toward research and experimentation. Rather than trying to assess treatment options in terms of the best interests of the neonate, neonatologists may tend to view neonates, especially those with serious, possibly exotic conditions, as relatively rare opportunities to advance the cause of neonatal medicine as a science. Finally, there are external pressures that influence neonatologist's opinions. The two dominant external pressures are the law and assertive parents.[15]

The third potential candidate is the Neonatal Infant Review Committee.[16] A number of bioethicists, health care professionals, and attorneys believe that neonates are better served by these review committees because individual decision-makers need advice from an informed group representing different professional disciplines.[17] The reasons advanced for advocating Neonatal Infant Review Committees as the best decision-makers are they ensure emotional stability, impartiality, and consistency. In addition, because of the multi-disciplinary representation on the committee, the members possess the relevant knowledge of medical facts, family setting, and alternatives to home-care that is necessary in making borderline decisions regarding treatment. The Neonatal Infant Review Committee is also able to adjudicate conflicts regarding treatment decisions that often arise between neonatologists and parents. The committee also serves to safeguard the "best interests" of the neonate when both the parents and the neonatologists agree on a course of medical action that is contrary to the "best interests" of the neonate.[18]

The negative aspects surrounding Neonatal Infant Review Committees focus on the fact that neonatal decisions are often made rapidly, in response to a crisis situation. Because of the nature of the committee, logistics and timing are problematic. In addition, committees are often cumbersome ways to make decisions because they can be frustratingly indecisive and occasionally inept. Assertive and outspoken individuals can sometimes dominate committee meetings. Finally, no matter how the committee is composed and how efficient it is, any committee placed in an advisory or decision-making role necessarily means a reduction in parental autonomy and physician discretion in neonatal cases.[19] Realistically, few parents are ever made aware of the fact that such committees exist, and many neonatologists resent having their decisions placed before such committees for review. Even though Weir believes these committees come close to meeting his criteria for proxies in neonatal cases, under these circumstances the practical utilization of such committees as appropriate decision-makers for handicapped neonates is questionable.

The final potential candidate for appropriate decision-maker in regard to treatment decisions for handicapped neonates is the court system.[20] Few parents or health care professionals favor turning treatment decisions over to the courts. Weir writes:

> For parents, the use of the courts as a proxy means the likelihood of court-mandated treatment contrary to parental desires. For physicians, the prospect of judicial involvement in neonatal cases means unnecessary legal intrusion into medical matters.[21]

Despite these objections, the strength of the court system would be that it provides an opportunity for disinterested, dispassionate, and consistent reasoning from case to case. The court system also has the means to ensure that relevant knowledge, information, and opposing points of view are presented for consideration in a public forum. Judges also have the ability to appoint a guardian *ad litem* to be an advocate for the never-competent patient.[22]

On the other hand, the weakness of the court system would be that judges are more remote than other proxies because they are not on the scene in the NICU and often have no personal contact with the case under consideration. This can be viewed as leading to more objectivity, but at the same time it can lead to less sensitivity for the persons involved.[23] In addition, the functioning of judges as proxies depends on the personal views of the judges.[24]

After examining the four potential candidates for decision-makers for handicapped neonates, Weir concludes that, because each is limited in important ways, it is preferable not to regard any of them as the best proxy. Instead, he advocates a serial or sequential ordering of decision-makers for never-competent patients. Weir writes:

> By incorporating each of the possible proxies into a sequential decision-making process, and by restricting the circumstances in which these possible proxies can actually function as decision makers for incompetent patients, the best interests of the defective neonate are more adequately served and protected than if any of the alternative decision makers is permitted to make unilateral decisions about life prolonging treatment in all neonatal cases.[25]

Based on Weir's criteria for proxy decision-makers, McCormick argues that parents in consultation with health care professionals are the appropriate decision-makers for never-competent patients.[26] Like Weir, McCormick believes that when loving and responsible parents are adequately informed about the diagnosis and prognosis of their child, under most circumstances they will make well-informed decisions that all parties concerned can accept as both medically and morally right. To ensure that parents are well-informed and that the neonate's "best interests" are protected, McCormick advocates that parents should seek consultation from health care professionals. McCormick grounds this position both legally and morally.

McCormick maintains that there is a long legal, social, and moral tradition that parents have the right to make their own decisions regarding medical treatments. The legal tradition is based on the principle of self-determination.[27] This tradition also maintains that when the patient is incompetent or never-competent, these decisions are to be made by those who have the "best interests" of the incompetent and never-competent at heart. Since the principle of self-determination is not directly applicable to handicapped neonates, McCormick proposes the principle of familial self-determination to ensure the "best interests" of the neonate are being considered.[28] Someone has to make these treatment decisions for the never-competent patient and McCormick argues that "someone" ought to be the parents.[29] There are two reasons why McCormick proposes that parents have the right to make decisions for handicapped neonates:

> First, the family is normally in the best position to judge the real interests of the incompetent patient. They know his or her life-style, preferences, and values. Second, however—and we think this is the more important reason—our society places great value on the family. The family is a basic moral community affirmed to have not only rights, but also responsibilities in determining how best to serve the interests of its incompetent members. . . . Family members are given enormous responsibility for moral nurture, theological and secular education, and decisions about the best interests of their incompetent members throughout the lifetime of the family unit. It should be no different in the case when the incompetent family member is seriously or terminally ill. Occasionally this may lead a family to decide that the incompetent one's interests can best be served by declining medical intervention.[30]

McCormick argues that familial self-determination has firm support both socially and legally, but he also argues that there are sound theological warrants for supporting familial self-determination. He writes:

> In Christian tradition the family is seen as a tightly bound unit with a sacramental ministry to the world. It is to mirror forth, by its own cohesiveness and solidarity, the love of Christ for his people. It is the school of love and caring, of nourishing and growth. It shares and deepens its values and spiritual life together as a unit. It determines what is to be its Christian life-style. It is the Church in miniature, and therefore like the Church has its own inner dynamics, priorities, and ideals. Since it lives and grows as a unit, its decisions in many important matters are, or ought to be, corporate matters, directions taken as a result of its own familial self-determination.[31]

Firmly grounded by secular and theological warrants, McCormick believes that the parents of never-competent patients have the legal and moral right to act as proxies for their children. However, this does not mean that parents cannot make mistakes or that their authority should go unchecked. McCormick argues:

> The hidden assumption is that responsible and loving families (that is, parents) will make morally right decisions. This is a fair rule of thumb, but only that. Even loving, responsible people can make mistakes, and the assumptions ordinarily warranted in their regard become somewhat more questionable in the bewildering, anguishing, life-death setting of the emergent situation.[32]

Because parents are under emotional stress when treatment decisions have to be made, and because they do not have all the medical knowledge required to make well-informed decisions, McCormick proposes that parents should always consult with the health care professionals involved in the situation. Parents need as much medical information, support, and advice as possible. McCormick argues: "The physician should attempt to lay out, in a sympathetic way, what the future is, what the doubts are, and to elicit from the parents a responsible reaction to the situation."[33] McCormick proposes consultation with health care professionals because they have a tendency to be more objective, have the medical expertise regarding congenital anomalies, can best explain the diagnosis and prognosis based on similar cases, and they have the ability to compare neonates with the same anomalies and know the effectiveness of various treatments.[34] In most situations, health care professionals act as advocates for the neonate and as safeguards against potential abuses. McCormick believes that parents will make reasonable decisions for their children. However, there can be exceptions. McCormick writes:

> As long as those judgments do not deviate too far from what is reasonably in the patient's best interests, the family's wishes should be controlling. If they do deviate so far that the principle of patient benefit is unacceptably compromised, then others involved—medical professionals, friends of the patient, or any others significantly associated with the patient—must seek review to determine the limits of familial autonomy.[35]

If the health care professionals believe that parents do not have the "best interests" of the neonate at heart, then they have the moral and legal responsibility to intervene.

McCormick argues that society also has a responsibility to assure the "best interests" of never-competent patients. Societal intervention should take place "only when the familial judgment so exceeds the limits of reason that the compromise with what is objectively in the incompetent one's best interests cannot be tolerated."[36] If it is suspected that the parents in consultation with health care professionals are acting irresponsibly and not in the "best interests" of the neonate, then society has a *duty* to intervene.[37] McCormick writes:

> That intervention can take many forms, like legislation, criminal prosecution or a child-neglect hearing. The purpose of such proceedings is to guarantee that the primary decision-maker acts in a responsible way, one that should be able to sustain public scrutiny. We believe that public accountability and review, a review that guarantees that the values of the society are respected and adhered to, can be invoked short of judicial intervention.[38]

In this way, McCormick has an additional safeguard in place in the event that parents in consultation with health care professionals fail to keep the "best interests" of the neonate as their primary focus.[39]

McCormick believes his position that parents, in consultation with health care professionals, have the moral responsibility to make treatment decisions for handicapped neonates is firmly rooted in the Catholic tradition, in the social and legal structure of society, and in his own theological anthropology. Decisions by parents in consultation with health care professionals ought to be made in the "best interests" of the handicapped neonate based on the family's beliefs and values. In this way, the "best interests" of the handicapped neonate, normatively understood, are protected.

McCormick determines how treatment decisions are made for handicapped neonates by proposing his category of "best interests," understood normatively.[40] This is a patient-centered, teleological assessment of what is considered to be in the "best interests" of the neonate. Parents should decide what the handicapped neonate ought to want, that is, what is in the "best interests" of the neonate, and all others concerned in the decision-making process. McCormick has a normative understanding of "best interests" because, "as social beings, our good, our flourishing (therefore, our best interests) is inextricably bound up with the well-being of others."[41] McCormick's "best interests" category is a composite category that involves quality-of-life considerations, benefit-burden considerations, and the use of proportionate reason as a tool for establishing what is promotive or destructive for the good of the person "integrally and adequately considered."[42] McCormick's understanding of "best interests" is grounded in his "revised" natural law position. McCormick writes:

> I believe we do have reasons for assuming we know in many cases what an incompetent would want. We may assume that most people are reasonable, and that being such they would choose what is in their best interest. At least this is a safe and protective guideline to follow in structuring our conduct toward them when they cannot speak. The assumption may be factually and *per accidens* incorrect. But I am convinced that it will not often be. . . . I believe most of us want to act reasonably within parameters that are objective in character, even though we do not always do so. Or at least I think it good protective policy to assume this.[43]

The function of parents as the proxy for their children is viewed as protective. Parents protect their children in that they know what their child *ought* to want, that is, what is in their "best interests," normatively understood. McCormick stresses the fact that all reasonable people, not just Christians, can determine what is in the "best interests" of the neonate. He writes:

> The value of human life leading to the traditional evaluation was seen in God's special and costing love for each individual—for fetal life, infant life, senescent life, disabled life, captive life, yes, and most of all unwanted life. These evaluations can be and have been shared by others than Christians, of course. But Christians have particular warrants for resisting any cultural callousing of them.[44]

As social beings who are interrelated, parents in consultation with health care professionals can best determine whether certain treatments will cause excessive social and familial burdens on those who will care for the neonate's existence.[45] Therefore, if McCormick has a normative understanding of "best interests," then it is parents, in consultation with health care professionals, who can best determine what the handicapped neonate ought to want, which should include the needs of those who will

care for the neonate. To help parents determine what is in the "best interests" of the neonate normatively understood, McCormick proposes the
establishment of diagnostic treatment categories. The next section will
propose such diagnostic categories in an attempt to assist parents in the
decision-making process.

APPLICATION OF MCCORMICK'S ETHICAL METHODOLOGY TO FIVE
DIAGNOSTIC TREATMENT CATEGORIES OF HANDICAPPED NEONATES.

This section will address the application of McCormick's ethical methodology to five specific diagnostic treatment categories of handicapped
neonates. These categories attempt to encompass, as far as possible, the
entire spectrum of handicapped neonates. They are based on McCormick's moral criterion of the potential for human relationships.[46] One
example of a congenital anomaly has been selected that is representative
of each particular diagnostic category.

   McCormick has plotted the two extreme positions on this spectrum
of handicapped neonates, but has left the "conflictual middle," to be
filled in by health care professionals and bioethicsts. McCormick writes:

> It is the task of physicians to provide some more con-
> crete categories or presumptive biological symptoms for
> this human judgment. For instance, nearly all would
> likely agree that the anencephalic infant is without rela-
> tional potential. On the other hand, the same cannot be
> said for the mongoloid infant. The task ahead is to attach
> relational potential to presumptive biological symptoms
> for the gray areas between such extremes.[47]

This section will attempt to complete the "conflictual middle." The "conflictual middle" pertains to those neonatal anomalies that fall into the
"gray area" of treatment decisions.[48] These diagnostic treatment categories have been arranged in a way that demonstrates the application of
McCormick's "best interests" criterion. McCormick has established the
two extremes on the spectrum based on his "best interests" criterion. The
middle categories have been arranged in accordance with the two extreme categories by applying McCormick's "best interests" criterion.
There is a logical progression on the spectrum from the neonate who
does not warrant medical treatment to the neonate who does warrant
medical treatment. This author believes that McCormick would agree
with the arrangement of these diagnostic treatment categories.[49] McCormick is well aware that establishing a full set of diagnostic treatment

categories is not a panacea for determining treatment decisions for handicapped neonates. Not all medical conditions can be placed in specific categories; there is a marked difference in the severity of conditions within each category. Not all health care professionals or even bioethicists could or would agree to these specific categories. Nevertheless, McCormick argues:

> The important point, however, is that we ought to attempt, as far as possible, to approach neonatal disabilities through diagnostic categories, always realizing that such categories cannot deflate important individual differences and that there will always remain gray areas.[50]

The establishment of these five diagnostic treatment categories is an attempt to meet the challenge McCormick set before health care professionals and bioethicists to assist parents and health care professionals in making treatment decisions for handicapped neonates.

Before applying McCormick's ethical methodology, and in particular his moral criterion of quality-of-life, it is important to note that, for McCormick, the neonate's life lacks any personal perspectives and thus life-sustaining decisions cannot be individualized.[51] This implies two general stipulations that will impact McCormick's ethical methodology:

> First, the criteria used in determining to save or let die where an infant is concerned are generalizable to all infants. Secondly, and as a consequence, the criteria used must be the strictest possible. That is, the very minimum potential for human experiencing or relationships must be seen as sufficient warrant for attempting to save. Any other view would be racism of the adult world, and would unjustly deprive not simply one but (by logical generalizability) many infants of their chance at life.[52]

This author will add a third stipulation, which is McCormick's position on infanticide. In making treatment decisions for handicapped neonates McCormick argues that "there is no proportionate reason for directly dispatching a terminal or dying patient."[53] McCormick makes a clear distinction between allowing to die and direct termination.[54] Drawing on the doctrine of creation and the lordship of God over all creation, McCormick writes:

> If all persons are equally the creatures of the one God, then none of these creatures is authorized to play God

toward any other. And if all persons are cherished by
God, regardless of merit, we ought to cherish each other
in the same spirit.[55]

This means that even the most handicapped neonates, those who experience extreme pain and suffering, can never be denied dignity and respect by being terminated.[56] These three general stipulations will undergird McCormick's ethical methodology as it is applied to treatment decisions for handicapped neonates.

This section will be structured so that the diagnostic treatment category is presented. The representative anomaly will be examined from a medical point of view by giving a brief description of the anomaly and then the diagnosis and prognosis. McCormick's ethical methodology will be applied to each anomaly to determine whether parents should decide to treat the handicapped neonate representative of the particular diagnostic category. Finally, when applicable, criticisms from the previous three chapters will be addressed.

Category 1: The handicapped neonate whose potential for human relationships is completely nonexistent. An anomaly that would be representative of this category would be anencephaly. Anencephaly is a developmental abnormality of the central nervous system that results in the congenital absence of a major portion of the brain, skull, and scalp. Because anencephalic neonates lack functioning cerebral hemispheres, they never experience any degree of consciousness. They never have thoughts, feelings, sensations, desires, or emotions. There is no purposeful action, social interaction, memory, pain, or suffering. However, anencephalic neonates do have fully or partially functioning brain stem tissue. Consequently, they are able to maintain at least some of the body's autonomic functions (i.e., unconscious activity), including the functions of the heart, lungs, kidneys, and intestinal tract, as well as certain reflex actions. They may be able to breathe, suck, engage in spontaneous movements of the eyes, arms, legs, respond to noxious stimuli with crying or avoidance maneuvers, and exhibit facial expressions typical of healthy infants. While all of this activity gives the appearance that the anencephalic neonate has some degree of consciousness, there is none. Anencephalic neonates are totally unaware of their existence and the environment in which they live.[57]

The cause of anencephaly is usually not known. The data suggests a polygenic or multifactorial etiology. Recognized associations include chromosomal abnormalities and mechanical factors.[58] The appearance of a neonate with anencephaly is unique, and the diagnosis can be made with virtual certainty when the following criteria are met:

(1) A large portion of the skull is absent. (2) The scalp, which extends to the margin of the bone, is absent over the skull defect. (3) Hemorrhagic, fibrotic tissue is exposed because of defects in the skull and scalp. (4) Recognizable cerebral hemispheres are absent.[59]

Some rare neonates fall into a "gray zone" in which it is unclear whether the diagnosis of anencephaly is proper.

The prognosis for an anencephalic neonate is that the life span is very short. Many die within a few hours, less than half survive more than a day, and fewer than 10% survive more than a week.[60] However, because anencephalic neonates do not receive aggressive treatment their potential life span is probably longer than their actual life span.[61]

The first guideline that specifies McCormick's quality-of-life criterion is the potential for human relationships associated with the infant's condition.[62] According to medical authorities, the anencephalic neonate has no potential for human relationships because this neonate lacks functioning cerebral hemispheres, and therefore the neonate will never experience any degree of consciousness. McCormick writes: "I am speaking of an infant with no realistic potential for human relationships, the type of infant whose life will for all practical purposes be vegetative only."[63] Because the anencephalic neonate has no potential for human relationships, parents, in consultation with health care professionals, ought to decide morally to forgo medical treatment for a neonate in this diagnostic category. This is a moral judgment in which, all things considered, the parents decide that further treatment is of no benefit to the neonate.

The decision by parents to forgo medical treatment in this situation is rooted in McCormick's theological anthropology and his moral epistemology. For McCormick, human life is a basic and precious good, but a good to be preserved precisely as a condition for other higher values. According to McCormick, there is a hierarchy of values that is teleological in nature. Each value exists in an interrelationship that consists of a single scale. The ultimate value, the highest value, the End of ends, is God. Therefore, human life is not an absolute good, because there are higher goods for which life can be sacrificed.[64] These other values found the duty to preserve physical life, while they also dictate the limits of this duty. McCormick understands this to mean that physical life is a relative good. The duty to preserve physical life is a limited one. These limits have always been stated in terms of the *means* required to sustain life. Therefore, it is not always morally obligatory to use all means to preserve physical life.[65] For McCormick, when a person no longer has the potential for human relationships—which are the very possibility for growth in love of God and neighbor—then parents are no longer morally required to preserve that life by all human means.[66] To preserve human life in this situation would be to replace the "higher, more important good."[67] "Physical life" would become the ultimate value. When this happens, the value of human life has been distorted. When human life is devoid of the possibility of experiencing human love, that is, no experience or interrelation is possible, then that life has achieved its potential.[68] This is not to say that the anencephalic's life is of no worth. McCormick writes:

> Every human being, regardless of age or condition, is of incalculable worth. The point is not, therefore, whether this or that individual has value. Of course he has, or rather *is* a value. The only point is whether this undoubted value has any potential at all, in continuing physical survival, for attaining a share, even if reduced, in the "higher, more important good." This is not a question about the inherent value of the individual. It is a question about whether this worldly existence will offer such a valued individual any hope of sharing those values for which physical life is the fundamental condition.[69]

After the affections informed by the Christian story discover the basic human values, it is the discursive reason informed by the Christian story that determines if the presence of proportionate reason exists to determine if one value can be sacrificed for another in a conflict situation, for the good of the whole person. In the case of an anencephalic neonate, all things considered, the parents ought to argue that there is a proportionate reason to decide that it is in the "best interests" of the handicapped neonate to allow death to occur naturally. The anencephalic neonate will never experience consciousness and therefore has no potential for human relationships. McCormick argues that there is a point where we judge it to be in the "best interests" of the patient and all concerned to allow death to occur. He writes:

> What we judge to be the good both of the patient and all concerned is rooted in Christian attitudes on the meaning of life and death, attitudes that value life without absolutizing it, and that fear and avoid death without absolutizing it.[70]

The anencephalic neonate has achieved his or her potential. The anencephalic lacks the potential to be oriented toward other, more important and even preferred values. Therefore, medical treatment would not be in the "best interests" of the anencephalic neonate because it would offer no benefit to the neonate.

One criticism directed at McCormick's quality-of-life criterion by Leonard Weber concerns the treatment and value of the handicapped neonate once a decision has been made to withdraw or forgo medical treatment. Weber writes:

> Once McCormick has made the claim that we must de-
> cide to treat or not on the basis of the child's condition,
> will people really be able to pay much attention to his
> insistence that every life is valuable regardless of condi-
> tion?[71]

McCormick argues that even though the anencephalic neonate has reached his or her potential and no treatment is recommended because it is of no benefit to the neonate, as members of society we have a moral obligation to care for the anencephalic neonate while the neonate is in the dying process. McCormick bases this position on the fact that every human life is sacred, is of incalculable worth, and deserves to be treated with dignity and respect, which is rooted in the Christian story. The sacredness of human life and the dignity that is derived from it leads to a particular care for the weakest, most voiceless, voteless, and defenseless members of society.[72] McCormick argues that "sacredness of life demands reverential attitudes and practices."[73] For him, the decision not to treat an anencephalic neonate is a "quality-of-life assessment that is made within an over-all reverence for life, as an extension of one's respect for the sanctity of life."[74] As a result, every life has a value and should be treated with dignity and respect up until the moment of death. McCormick's understanding of the sacredness of human life, his understanding of quality of life as an extension of sanctity of life, and his application of the principles of justice and charity serve to safeguard that anencephalic infants will not be abandoned, but will be treated with dignity and respect while in the dying process.[75] This would include appropriate medical measures, comfort care, and personal psychological and spiritual support to the anencephalic's parents.[76]

In conclusion, when the handicapped neonate's potential for human relationships is completely nonexistent, and further treatment will be of no benefit to the neonate, parents ought to decide, in the neonate's "best interests," not to seek medical treatment. However, once this decision has been made, the anencephalic neonate should be cared for and treated with dignity and respect during the dying process.

Category 2: The handicapped neonate who has a potential for human relationships but whose potential is utterly submerged in the mere struggle for survival. An anomaly that would be representative of this diagnostic treatment category would be a neonate with a Grade IV massive intraventricular hemorrhage (IVH) of the brain[77] and hydrocephalus.[78] Hemorrhage in or around the brain is a major problem in neonates, especially when premature. Hypoxia (lack of oxygen supply), pressures exerted on the neonate's head during labor, and the presence of the germinal matrix (a mass of embryonic cells lying over the caudate nucleus and present only in the fetus) in premature neonates are three major causes of intraventricular hemorrhage. The overall incidence of IVH has decreased in recent years from 40%-60% or less in neonates weighing less than 1500 grams at birth. The incidence and severity are inversely proportional to gestational age.[79] Although there has been a reduction in incidence during the past decade, IVH remains a major concern, principally because of the improved survival rates of very low-birth-weight infants (<1000g), who are at the highest risk for the development of IVH. In the premature neonate, IVH originates from the rupture of fragile vessels in the subependymal germinal matrix. In approximately 80% of patients with intracranial hemorrhage, there is associated IVH, and in approximately 10% to 15%, there is cerebral infarction involving the periventricular tissues. Major IVH occurs in 16% of infants born at $\leq$ 25 weeks and in only 2.1% of infants born at > 25 weeks gestation. The risk period is during the first 3-4 postnatal days: 50% of IVH occurs in the first 6-12 hours of life, 75% by the second day, and 90% by the third day. Ten percent to 65% of newborns with early IVH have progression of the hemorrhage, with maximal extent occurring within 3-5 days of the initial diagnosis.[80]

There are two essential steps in establishing the diagnosis of IVH. First, there is the recognition of the neonate at risk. Second, there is the use of an effective imaging procedure. The neonate at risk would be any premature neonate in a NICU. This is based on the very high incidence of the disorder in this population. Diagnosis of the spectrum of IVH can be done by computed tomography (CT) but cranial ultrasonography is considered the technique of choice because of its portability, high resolution, and lack of ionizing radiation. Nevertheless, CT scanning remains superior for the diagnosis of other varieties of intracranial hemorrhage, including primary subarachnoid, convexity, and posterior fossa subdural and epidural hematomas, and for differentiating hemorrhagic and ischemic parenchymal infarctions.[81] Sonograms are usually obtained via the anterior fontanelle. In the presence of normally sized ventricles, scanning through the posterior fontanelle may increase the rate of detection of IVH.[82] The diagnosis of IVH may be suspected on the basis of clinical signs alone in approximately 50% of neonates. The severity of clinical features range from an asymptomatic state through a saltatory neurologic deterioration over several days to a catastrophic presentation with coma, apnea, tonic extensor posturing, brain stem dysfunction, and flaccid quadriparesis. Associated systemic abnormalities may include hypotension, metabolic acidosis, bradycardia, serum glucose, and electrolyte disturbances. Bloody or xanthochromic cerebrospinal fluid (CSF) supports a diagnosis of intraventricular hemorrhage.[83]

The prognosis for neonates with a Grade IV massive intraventricular hemorrhage is poor, especially if the hemorrhage extends into the parenchyma.[84] The short-term outcome of IVH is related principally to the size of the hemorrhage and may be considered in terms of mortality or hydrocephalus among survivors. Neonates with a Grade IV massive intraventricular hemorrhage and parenchymal involvement have a high mortality rate (60%-80%), and post-hemorrhagic hydrocephalus often develops (65%-100%). The most critical determinant of long-term outcomes is the extent of parenchymal involvement.[85] Major IVH occurs frequently in the context of hypoxic-ischemia cerebral insult, and long-term neurological outcome depends on concomitant or preceding hemorrhagic or nonhemorrhagic hypoxic-ischemic cerebral injury.[86]

A neonate with a Grade IV massive intraventricular hemorrhage and hydrocephalus has the potential for human relationships, but because the intraventricular hemorrhage is so severe and there is the associated complication of progressive hydrocephalus, the potential for human relationships is utterly submerged in the mere struggle for survival.[87] Applying McCormick's ethical methodology and in particular his quality-of-life criterion to this neonate with a Grade IV massive intraventricular hemorrhage, one can see that McCormick would base his decision to withdraw or forgo medical treatment on the Christian tradition that human life is a basic good but a good to be preserved as the condition of other values. Since these other values cluster around and are rooted in human relationships, it follows that when the relational potential is utterly submerged in the mere struggle for survival, that life can be said to have achieved its potential.[88] For McCormick, if the meaning and consummation of life is to be found in love of neighbor, then clearly such meaning is inseparable from human relationships.[89] Therefore, when the potential to love one's neighbor is no longer possible, one does not have a moral responsibility to continue medical treatment. McCormick writes:

> One who must support his life with disproportionate effort focuses the time, attention, energy, and resources of himself and others not precisely on relationships, but on maintaining the condition of relationships. Such con-

centration easily becomes over concentration and dis-
torts one's view of and weakens one's pursuit of the very
relational goods that define our human growth and
flourishing. The importance of relationships gets lost in
the struggle for survival. The very Judaeo-Christian
meaning of life is seriously jeopardized when undue and
unending effort must go into its maintenance.[90]

McCormick grounds his position in the traditional ordinary/extraordinary
means distinction. If the means used to preserve the neonate's life will
bring about a grave hardship for the neonate and those responsible for his
or her care, then this means to preserve life is considered extraordinary
and nonobligatory, that is to say, not beneficial to the neonate.[91]

The moral epistemological basis for this decision is reason informed
by the Christian story. The affections, informed by the Christian story,
assist the parents in determining the value of this neonate's life. However, it is at the level of normative moral judgment that parents must now
rely on discursive reason, informed by the Christian story, to determine if
there is proportionate reason to initiate medical treatment for the "best
interests" of this particular neonate.[92] For McCormick, to continue treatment for a neonate with a Grade IV massive intraventricular hemorrhage
would be "tantamount to elevating a subordinate good in a way that
would prejudice a higher good, eventually making it unrecognizable as a
good."[93] This would be a form of medical vitalism which McCormick
refers to as "idolatry of life." McCormick argues that the Judaeo-
Christian tradition has always sought a middle path between medical vitalism and medical pessimism. Excessive concern for the temporal is at
some point neglect of the eternal.[94] To continue treatment on the neonate
with a Grade IV massive intraventricular hemorrhage and hydrocephalus
would not be in the "best interests" of the neonate because it would cause
a grave hardship and be of little or no benefit for the neonate and those
responsible for his or her care. The medical facts presented confirm that
there is no proportionate reason for prolonging the life of a neonate with
a Grade IV massive intraventricular hemorrhage and progressive hydrocephalus. This neonate has irreversible damage to the brain and other
major organs and the neonate's prognosis is extremely poor with a high
mortality rate. This neonate's ability to relate to others is completely or
almost nearly lost in the mere struggle for physical survival. Human relationships would no longer function as the heart and meaning of this
neonate's life as they should.[95] According to McCormick's ethical methodology, to continue treatment on a neonate in this diagnostic category
would devalue the life of the neonate. This is because it would remove

the neonate's life from the Christian context and story that is the source of its ultimate value.[96]

In support of McCormick's position regarding not treating a neonate with a Grade IV massive intraventricular hemorrhage and hydrocephalus, one can also apply the third norm of his quality-of-life criterion and the moral principles of beneficence and nonmaleficence rooted in charity. The third norm that McCormick uses to specify the capacity for human relationships states: "Life-sustaining interventions may be omitted or withdrawn when there is excessive hardship, especially when this combines with poor prognosis."[97] The prognosis for a neonate with a Grade IV massive intraventricular hemorrhage and hydrocephalus is very poor. The mortality rate is between 60% to 80%. According to neonatologists, to initiate or continue medical treatment would do harm to the well-being of this neonate. For McCormick, quality-of-life judgments must avoid doing harm to all patients.[98] To treat a neonate in this situation would violate a basic principle of bioethics: "*non nocere*" (do no harm). However, McCormick argues that even though a decision has been made to forgo or withdraw medical treatment, neonates in this category should continue to receive humane and necessary palliative care that will relieve pain and suffering, because every human life is sacred, is of incalculable worth, and deserves to be treated with dignity and respect.[99]

In conclusion, when the handicapped neonate has the potential for human relationships but this potential is utterly submerged in the mere struggle for survival, parents can decide in the neonate's "best interests" not to seek medical treatment. The Christian story provides the framework by which the parents can reasonably determine that treatment is not in the "best interests" of this neonate, because it offers no benefit to this neonate "integrally and adequately considered." McCormick believes this moral judgment is not only reasonable but is firmly grounded in the Catholic theological tradition.

Category 3: The handicapped neonate who has the potential for human relationships but the underlying medical condition will result in imminent death. An anomaly that is representative of the neonate who has a potential for human relationships but the underlying medical condition will result in imminent death is a neonate with hypoplastic left heart syndrome. Hypoplastic left heart syndrome encompasses a variety of specific cardiovascular malformations producing similar hemodynamic and clinical manifestations, including aortic atresia, mitral atresia, permanent closure of the foramen ovale, and aortic stenosis. The left heart chamber is usually very small, and endocardial fibroelastosis is common.[100] Hypoplastic left heart syndrome occurs in 10.2% of infants with severe heart disease and is one of the most common lesions presenting in the first week of life. It is less common in very premature neonates (<1.85kg). It is usually an isolated lesion, although it has been described in association with autosomal trisomy syndromes and in infants of diabetic mothers (10.9%). Familial cases occur.[101] The etiology is unknown. However, it is postulated that the cause is premature closure of foramen ovale, abnormally large ductus arteriosus, and autosomal recessive.[102]

The diagnosis can be made with echocardiography by demonstrating a very small or unrecognizable left ventricle.[103] The ascending aorta is small with retrograde flow in cases of aortic atresia, and there is frequently a discrete juxtaductal coarctation. Neonates become symptomatic within the first week of life. It is estimated that 40% are diagnosed in the second day of life, 75% in the sixth day of life and 86% in the thirteenth day of life. The clinical picture of hypoplastic left heart syndrome may be simulated by respiratory distress syndrome, interrupted aortic arch, severe complex coarctation, early neonatal myocarditis, isolated critical valvar aortic stenosis, sepsis, or some inherited metabolic disorders. Within the first few days of life the neonate will develop congestive heart failure and a shocklike picture may develop precipitously. The neonate becomes ashen gray with poor peripheral perfusion, and all pulses are weak. Ductal constriction may be intermittent, with femoral pulses intermittently palpable. Symptoms and signs of congestive heart failure are associated with hypotension and, terminally, with bradycardia.[104] The chest radiograph shows cardiac enlargement and pulmonary plethora, and the electrocardiogram (ECG) usually demonstrates right axis deviation, right atrial hypertrophy, right ventricular hypertrophy, and markedly diminished or absent left ventricular forces.[105]

The prognosis for a neonate with hypoplastic left heart syndrome is very poor. Without surgery, the mortality rate is 98% by one year of age. The mean age of survival is four to twenty-three days. There are few survivors with mitral atresia or hypoplastic left ventricle with severe aortic and mitral stenosis. Therefore, three options are given. The first option is surgical correction, which is done in two or three stages. This technique has variable results; survival is only fair after both procedures.[106] Neonatal cardiac transplantation is a second option with good results at some centers, but the shortage of donors is a serious problem.[107] Palliative care (keeping the neonate comfortable until death) is the third option. Most neonatologists believe that neither reconstructive surgery leading to a Fontan procedure or cardiac transplantation can be viewed as curative. Both methods of treatment have high fiscal and emotional costs.[108]

In this third diagnostic treatment category, since the potential for human relationships is present, McCormick will use the second guideline of his quality-of-life criterion—the benefit/burden calculus—to determine whether neonates ought to be treated. What is to be determined is whether the burden of the treatment will outweigh the benefit to the neo-nate. For McCormick: "If the treatment is useless or futile, or it imposes burdens that outweigh the benefits, it may be omitted."[109] McCormick argues that his notion of benefit/burden calculus is a logical development of the ordinary/extraordinary means distinction, or what he refers to as an extension of the tradition into new problem areas.[110] As is the case in the previous two diagnostic treatment categories, McCormick's second guideline of his quality-of-life criterion—the benefit/burden calculus—is firmly grounded in the Catholic tradition and his theological anthropol-ogy. Human life is a relative good. The duty to preserve physical life is a limited one. These limits have been stated in terms of the means required to sustain life. Therefore, it is not always morally obligatory to use all means to preserve human life.[111]

For McCormick, "it is clear that the judgments of burden and benefit are value judgments, moral choices. They are judgments in which, all things considered, the continuance of life is either called for or not worthwhile to the patient."[112] These value judgments on the meaning of life have an epistemological foundation that is based on reason informed by faith.[113] The Christian story influences not only the parents' disposi-tions, but moral judgments in a rather general way. This moral episte-mology establishes a context in which the parents' reason and calculation ought to operate. It is a context that prevents the absolutization of life, and allows the parents to make treatment decisions based on the neo-nate's "best interests" that will include some consideration of future quality of life. Both the proportionate reason criterion and the criterion of the person "integrally and adequately considered" will play a crucial role in determining these quality-of-life judgments. Parents must determine if a particular treatment will benefit the neonate as a whole.

In examining the neonates in this diagnostic category as applied to hypoplastic left heart syndrome, what must remain at the forefront are the "best interests," normatively defined, of the neonate and those in-volved in the decision-making process. In the case of the neonate with hypoplastic left heart syndrome it appears that further medical treatment would not be in the "best interests" of these neonates. Any benefit ob-tained would be outweighed by the burdens. A neonate diagnosed with hypoplastic left heart syndrome has the additional complication of a high incidence of chromosomal disorders. This is a major factor that must be taken into consideration. Without surgery the mortality rate for this neo-nate is 98%. Heart transplantation is a possible medical option, but it must be remembered that there are very few hearts available for trans-plantation and heart transplantation is still considered an experimental procedure in some circles. Even with surgery, which has a high fiscal and emotional cost, the mortality rate remains high.[114] Any possible medical benefits obtained by this type of surgery would be outweighed by the social and familial burdens.[115]

McCormick's notion of a normative understanding of "best interests" considers not only the relevant medical facts but also the relevant social and familial factors. Financial and emotional costs ought to be considered. That means, if the social factors are excessive, then the neonate should not and would not be treated, because it would place excessive burdens on those who must care for the neonate's existence. What the neonate "ought" to want should encompass the needs of those who care for the child. This anomaly entails excessive surgeries, long-term hospitalization, long-term home care, and there are serious genetic disorders associated with hypoplastic left heart syndrome that will entail additional treatment and serious financial and emotional burdens for the family. Both social and familial factors ought to play a proportionate role in determining the benefit/burden calculus.

McCormick's position on social and familial factors has been criticized for being too restrictive and deviating from both the Catholic tradition and from his own normative understanding of "best interests." McCormick claims that his restrictive notion of social and familial factors, as they pertain to treatment decisions for handicapped neonates, is due to the fact that a broader interpretation could lead to social utilitarianism. This caution is certainly relevant because the possibility of potential abuse is always present. However, the safeguards McCormick has built into his quality-of-life criterion—guidelines, norms, and moral principles—should help to alleviate the possibility of such abuse. In addition, health care professionals serve as safeguards in that they can act as the neonate's advocate should they suspect abuse. If McCormick has a normative understanding of "best interests," then he should examine both social and familial factors from the handicapped neonate's perspective. If the circumstances of treatment will be a grave burden for the family of the neonate and society as a whole, then this is not in the "best interests" of the neonate.[116]

In conclusion, when a handicapped newborn has the potential for human relationships but the underlying medical condition will result in imminent death, parents, in consultation with health care professionals, are not morally obliged to initiate treatment or continue medical treatment. It is clear that the burdens outweigh the benefits to the neonate. Therefore, it is in the best interests of the neonate and all concerned, to withdraw or forgo medical treatment for a neonate in these circumstances.

Category 4: The handicapped neonate who has the potential for human relationships but after medical treatment has been initiated, it becomes apparent that the treatment is medically futile. An anomaly that is representative of a neonate who has the potential for human relationships but after initiating treatment, it becomes apparent that the treatment is medically futile,[117] is a neonate with full length small and large bowel Necrotizing Enterocolitis (NEC) with perforation. It is a major cause of mortality and morbidity in neonates with birth weights less than 1,500 gms.[118] NEC is a condition predominantly seen in premature neonates, which is characterized by partial- or full-thickness intestinal ischemia, usually involving the terminal ileum.[119] NEC is probably the most serious gastrointestinal disorder occurring in neonates. Because NEC appears predominantly in sick, low-birth-weight neonates, the incidence has increased in recent years as the mortality rate for very low-birth-weight neonates has decreased. It has been estimated that 90% of cases occur in premature neonates with an incidence of 8% to 12% in newborns < 1.5 kg. Neonates with NEC represent 2% to 5% of NICU admissions.[120] The age of onset of NEC is related to birth weight and gestational age.[121] Thus, the more premature the neonate, the longer the duration of risk. The etiology is not fully known. Multiple factors appear to be involved, including hypoxia, acidosis, and hypotension, which may lead to ischemic damage of the mucosal barrier of the small intestine. Secondary bacterial invasion of the mucosa may be involved in the pathogenesis of pneumatosis intestinalis. Other factors considered to increase the risk of NEC are umbilical artery catheterization, infection with certain types of bacteria, and hypoalbuminemia.[122] Although the cause is uncertain, the histopathology is well established. Initially, the disease begins as mucosal ischemia, with resultant sloughing of this layer. As the disease progresses, gas develops within the muscular layers and may be seen on x-ray films as pneumatosis cystoides intestinalis.[123] If full-thickness necrosis occurs, perforation and peritonitis develop.[124] The rapidity of disease progression differs in each neonate, but those who perforate usually do so within the first days of the disease.[125]

The diagnosis of NEC is based on both clinical assessment and x-ray studies. The onset of NEC occurs most commonly between day three and day ten of life but may occur as early as the first twenty-four hours of life or as late as three months.[126] Clinical presentations vary widely. Abdominal distension is one of the earliest and most consistent clinical signs, along with an intolerance of feeding with vomiting. The vomitus of about one-half of the neonates is bile stained. Other symptoms include bloody stools, apnea, bradycardia, lethargy, shock, and retention of gastric contents due to poor gastric emptying. Hematest-positive stools help confirm the diagnosis, but blood may be absent or a late finding. Abdominal wall erythema and a palpable abdominal mass are commonly late findings and signify more extensive disease. Radiographic findings in early NEC may show only separated loops of distended intestine, suggesting bowel wall thickening. A persistent large loop of intestine seen on a series of x-ray films has been used by some as an indication of surgery, but these neonates may also be treated medically.[127]

The prognosis for NEC depends on the severity of the disease. Initial management of the neonate with NEC without pneumoperitoneum is standardized.[128] The neonate receives nothing orally, the stomach is decompressed with a gastric sump tube, and intravenous antibiotics are begun. Indications for surgery include pneumoperitoneum, persistent acidosis (i.e., pH less than 7.2), rapidly worsening pulmonary status, and unremitting neutropenia or thrombocytopenia.[129] Mortality is higher in neonates who have perforated before surgery, and it is therefore better to operate before perforation has occurred. Surgery in neonates with perforation should be expeditious and conservative. The frankly necrotic or perforated intestine should be removed and ileostomies formed.[130] When massive resection is necessary, the chance for the neonate's survival is limited, but the premature neonate's intestine still has the potential for growth and adaption, and rarely is the entire intestine involved in the disease.[131] The long-term success rate for treatment for NEC has been good, despite long hospitalization for gastrointestinal adaption when massive resection is necessary. The quoted survival rate for neonates with medically treated NEC is now more than 80%, and the survival rate for those requiring surgery is approximately 20% to 40%.[132]

In this fourth diagnostic treatment category, since the potential for human relationships is present, McCormick will use the second guideline of his quality-of-life criterion—the benefit/burden calculus—to determine whether neonates ought to be treated. What is to be determined is whether the burden of the treatment will outweigh the benefit to the neonate. If the parents, in consultation with the health care professionals, determine that further medical treatment would not improve the neonate's prognosis, or benefit the overall well-being of the neonate, then, all things considered, parents should decide that further treatment would not be in the "best interests" of the neonate. As is the case in the previous diagnostic treatment category, McCormick's second guideline of his quality-of-life criterion—the benefit/burden calculus—is firmly grounded in the Catholic tradition and his theological anthropology. Human life is a relative good. The duty to preserve physical life is a limited one. These limits have been stated in terms of the means required to sustain life. Therefore, it is not always morally obligatory to use all means to preserve human life.[133]

The determination of whether or not further medical treatment for a neonate in this category will be continued entails a value judgment in which all things considered, the parents must decide if this treatment is beneficial or burdensome for the neonate. These value judgments on the meaning and purpose of human life have an epistemological foundation that is based on reason informed by faith. As in the previous categories, the Christian story influences not only the parent's dispositions, but how they will make a moral judgment in this situation. McCormick's moral epistemology serves as a context in which the parents' reason and calculation ought to operate.[134] It is a context that will prevent the absolutization of life, and will allow the parents to make treatment decisions based on the neonate's "best interests" that will include some consideration of future quality of life. Both the proportionate reason criterion and the person "integrally and adequately considered" criterion will be utilized by the parents in determining these quality-of-life judgments. Parents must determine if a medical treatment will benefit the neonate both physiologically and qualitatively. McCormick believes that there is a *prima facie* duty to preserve life. He writes:

> In other words, physicians approach desperately ill patients with a general bias in favor of life. But there are times when this general bias is overwhelmed by the facts, when the attempts to preserve life are not an *actual duty*. That point is reached when attempts at life-preservation are no longer in the child's best interests.[135]

Health care professionals can determine, to the best of their ability, whether further medical treatment would improve the neonate's prognosis, or benefit the overall well-being of the neonate. However, it is the parents who must decide whether further treatment would be beneficial or too burdensome for the neonate as a whole.[136]

In examining neonates in this category with their respective anomalies, what must remain at the forefront are the "best interests," normatively defined, of the neonate and those involved in the decision-making process. A neonate diagnosed as having full-length small and large bowel NEC with perforation has a high mortality rate and, according to medical authorities, further medical treatment is qualitatively futile, that is, any possible medical effect is of no benefit to the neonate.[137] Therefore, it appears that further treatment for neonates in this diagnostic category is not morally obligatory.

In support of McCormick's position regarding not treating a neonate with full length small and large bowel NEC with perforation, one can also apply the fourth norm of his quality-of-life criterion and the moral principles of beneficence, nonmaleficence, and justice rooted in charity. The fourth norm states: "Life-sustaining interventions may be omitted or withdrawn at a point when it becomes clear that expected life can be had for a relatively brief time and only with continued use of artificial feeding (e.g., some cases of NEC)." NEC with perforation has a mortality rate as high as 40% when massive resection is necessary. When a neonate has perforation, and sepsis and peritonitis are present, many neonatologists argue that to continue medical treatment other than palliative care would do harm to the well-being of the neonate.[138] Further aggressive medical treatment would only prolong the dying process. To treat an neonate in this situation would violate a basic principle of bioethics: "*non nocere*" (do no harm). Continuing a medical treatment that is medically futile also violates the principle of justice rooted in charity. For McCormick, as social beings who are interrelated and interdependent, we must realize that decisions we make or that are made for us have a profound impact on family and society. Therefore, justice as the mediation of charity, ought to incorporate both familial and social factors when determining the "best interests" of a handicapped neonate. Our medical resources are limited and must be conserved. Proper stewardship of these resources entails not exhausting them on medical treatments that are futile and inappropriate. Instead, these resources must be rationally allocated. Continuing to use medical resources on a neonate in this diagnostic category when they are in short supply is ethically irresponsible and morally objectionable.[139]

It should be noted that in this category of anomalies, the medical facts regarding diagnosis and prognosis are extremely pertinent. There are less severe cases of NEC that can be treated successfully. Each medical anomaly contains individual differences, and "gray areas" are always a reality. This is an example of why McCormick argues that consultation with health care professionals is essential for parents in making these treatment decisions. Neonatologists have the medical knowledge and the expertise of comparative judgments of neonates with similar anomalous conditions that can assist parents in the decision-making process. They will be able to assist the parents in determining the effectiveness of specific medical treatments and the burdens of such treatments. Health care professionals can also serve as a check and balance to ensure the "best interests" of the neonate are being protected. To serve as an advocate for these neonates, time should be allowed for the clinical picture to emerge, consultation and confirmation with other colleagues must be sought, there should be frequent assessment of the neonate's prognosis, and neonatologists should not categorize neonates too early or change their categories too late. Determining if the burdens outweigh the benefits in this category will depend on the expertise of the health care professionals. Together parents and health care professionals must examine the benefits and the burdens of medical treatments for neonates in this category carefully, because medical futility is not a clinical concept that can be easily determined.

Some critics of McCormick's quality-of-life criterion argue that there is a tendency by some decision-makers to overlook the theological importance of suffering for the neonate and others. These critics believe that a great value in handicapped neonates is the compassion evoked in those who must serve these unfortunates. Some believe that the deprivations and sufferings of others "do often bring out the best in us—affection, tenderness, compassion, selflessness."[140] McCormick responds to these critics by stating:

> Keeping a child alive simply to elicit these responses when he can derive no benefit from continuance in physical life, is getting close to a use of children for adult purposes. . . . I would argue that just as we are "able to give," where the elderly terminal patient is involved, still we judge what form this giving should take exclusively in terms of the benefit to the patient, not in terms of our own opportunity to experience compassionate responses. Any other point of view would get the purpose of treatment mixed up. Is not the same true of the infant?[141]

McCormick follows the Catholic theological tradition and argues that pain and suffering have a special place in God's saving plan. Grave illness is to be seen as an intensifying conformity with Christ. As the human body weakens and is devastated by disease and illness, the strength of Jesus Christ is shared by those who have been baptized into his death and resurrection.[142] However, submitting a neonate to survival for the sake of others is both inhumane and violative of the Christian tradition and the prime rule in medical practice—"*non nocere*" (do no harm). If medical treatment will bring no benefit to the neonate, then there is no moral obligation to treat. Neonates should not be victimized for the good of others.

In conclusion, when a handicapped neonate has the potential for human relationships but after initiating treatment, it becomes apparent that the treatment is medically futile, parents, in consultation with health care professionals, are not morally obliged to continue medical treatment. This is a value judgment that is based on McCormick's guidelines of relational potential and benefit/burden calculus. McCormick's quality-of-life criterion sets basic parameters and enlightens the particular medical situation. Ultimately, the parents will use prudence to examine the medical facts and to weigh, all things considered, whether the burdens of treatment outweigh the benefits to the neonate. In this diagnostic treatment category, the burdens and benefits need to be weighed carefully.

With the severity of this particular medical anomaly, the burdens frequently outweigh the benefits to the neonate. Therefore, in the "best interests" of the neonate and all concerned, parents, in consultation with health care professionals, have the moral obligation to forgo or withdraw treatment for a neonate in these circumstances. However, in certain circumstances, depending on the severity of the medical condition and the parents' view of the child's potential quality of life, the benefits may outweigh the burdens. The notion of medical futility requires a close evaluation of the neonate's best interests from the perspective of both health care professionals and parents. If there is any suspicion about whether parents in consultation with health care professionals are acting responsibly, it is in this type of situation that McCormick's safeguards—Neonatal Infant Review Committees and the courts—can be employed to further protect the best interests of the neonate.

Category 5: The handicapped neonate who has the potential for human relationships and has a correctable or treatable condition. An anomaly that is representative of this diagnostic treatment category is a neonate with trisomy 21 (Down syndrome) and the complication of esophageal atresia with tracheoesophageal fistula. Trisomy 21 or Down syndrome is caused by a faulty chromosome distribution. In about 95% of cases of Down syndrome, there is an extra chromosome 21. The overall incidence is about 1/700 live births, but there is a marked variability depending on maternal age.[143] The extra chromosome 21 comes from the father in one-fourth to one-third of the cases.

Esophageal atresia occurs in approximately 1 of 3000 to 4500 births. In the most common form of esophageal anomaly (86% of neonates), the blind-ending upper esophageal segment usually extends into the upper portion of the thorax, and the lower portion of the esophagus is connected to the trachea at or just above the tracheal carina. This connection is usually 3-5 mm in diameter and easily admits air or, in a retrograde fashion, acidic gastric secretions.[144]

The clinical diagnosis of a neonate with Down syndrome would be a neonate who tends to be placid, rarely cries, and demonstrates muscular hypotonicity. Nuchal lymphedema, similar to that seen in Turner's syndrome, also occurs in Down syndrome and is being detected with increasing frequency prenatally by fetal ultrasonography.[145] Physical and mental development are retarded; the mean IQ is about 50. Microcephaly, brachycephaly, and a flattened occiput are characteristic. The eyes are slanted, and epicanthal folds are present. Brushfield's spots (gray to white spots resembling grains of salt around the periphery of the iris) usually are visible in the neonatal period and disappear during the first twelve months of life. The bridge of the nose is flattened, the mouth is often held open because of a large, protruding tongue that is furrowed and lacks the central fissure, and the ears are small with down-folded helixes. The hands are short and broad, with single palmar crease (simian crease); the fingers are short, with clinodactyly (incurvature) of the fifth finger, which often has two phalanges. The feet have a wide gap between the first and the second toes, and a plantar furrow extends backward. Hands and feet show characteristic dermal prints (dermatoglyphics). Congenital heart disease is found in about 35% of patients; atrioventricular canal defects and ventricular septal defects are most common.[146]

The diagnosis of esophageal atresia may not be obvious on the initial examination of a neonate unless an attempt is made to pass a tube into the stomach. The earliest clinical signs are excessive oral secretions, regurgitation of saliva, and cyanosis. The saliva collects in the blind-ending esophagus and then accumulates until it is apparent around the lips as excessive mucus. The first feeding is followed by choking, coughing, and regurgitation. Abdominal distention is a prominent feature, occurring as inspired air is transmitted through the fistula and distal esophagus into the stomach. Gastric juice may pass upward in the distal esophagus, transversing the tracheoesophageal fistula and spilling into the trachea and lungs, leading to chemical pneumonia. A contrast x-ray film confirms the diagnosis of atresia; a lateral projection with 1 ml of dilute barium or an isoosmolar contrast agent (e.g., metrizamide) shows the length of the upper pouch, defines its precise extension into the chest, and demonstrates the rare upper pouch fistula. Esophageal atresia has become more frequently recognized during maternal ultrasonography. Failure to visualize a fetal stomach in a mother who has polyhydramnios suggests esophageal atresia. Prenatal diagnosis permits a search for associated problems and allows a comprehensive, coordinated approach to the family and neonate in the prenatal period.[147]

The prognosis for a Down syndrome neonate who has esophageal atresia with tracheoesophageal fistula is excellent.[148] The aim of preoperative management is to prevent aspiration pneumonia, which makes surgical correction more hazardous. Oral feedings are withheld. A double lumen suction catheter is inserted into the upper esophageal pouch and attached to continuous suction to prevent aspiration of swallowed saliva. When the neonate is stable, immediate primary repair is undertaken. If unstable, surgery is delayed until the clinical status is stabilized, the impact of associated anomalies is determined, and the neonate can be anesthetized and operated on safely. When the neonate is stable, a thoracotomy can be done to repair the esophageal atresia and close the tracheoesophageal fistula.[149] Occasionally, the gap between the esophageal segments is too great for a primary repair. Gentle stretching of the esophageal segments before later anastomosis may be beneficial, or repair by interposing a segment of colon or forming a gastric tube between the

esophageal segments may be required. The most common acute complications are leakage at the site of anastomosis and stricture formation. If
there is no leakage, feedings are begun and quickly advanced.[150] The
survival rate for neonates who were classified as stable and had primary
repair is 100%. Survival in the unstable group who had staged repair is
57%. The deaths were due to associated anomalies, including congenital
diaphragmatic hernia and hypoplastic left heart syndrome.[151]

To determine whether a Down syndrome neonate who has esophageal atresia with tracheoesophageal fistula ought to be treated, McCormick will apply both guidelines of his quality-of-life criterion. In this
situation, the handicapped neonate has the potential for human relationships. This neonate will, in relative comfort, be able to experience our
caring and love. Thus, both the parents and the neonate will be able to
share in the higher, more important good. Continued physical existence
will offer this neonate hope of sharing those values for which physical
life is a fundamental condition.[152] This position is firmly grounded in
McCormick's theological anthropology. Secondly, the benefits of proper
medical treatment clearly outweigh the burdens. According to the medical authorities, a neonate with Down syndrome associated with esophageal atresia and tracheoesophageal fistula has an excellent chance of living
a productive life with corrective surgery. Therefore, all things considered, there is a proportionate reason to seek corrective surgery in this
situation, because it is in the "best interests" of the neonate and those
involved in the decision-making process.

The decision to treat is also supported by the second norm established by McCormick and John Paris, S.J., as a further specification of
the capacity for human relationships as a summary of the benefit/burden
calculus. The norm states: "Life-sustaining interventions may not be
omitted simply because the baby is retarded. There may be further complications associated with retardation that justify withholding life-
sustaining treatment."[153] In this situation, all things considered, there is a
proportionate reason to treat this Down syndrome neonate because the
complication associated with the retardation can be corrected with a very
high probability of success. As long as the medical condition is treatable
or correctable and the corrected condition will result in improvement of
the neonate's prognosis, comfort, and well-being or general state of
health, then this is looked upon as a beneficial treatment and under the
benefit/burden calculus it ought to be made available to this neonate.[154]
Failure to treat a Down syndrome neonate with a correctable condition
would be allowing a cultural bias to distort the basic value of human life.
For McCormick, it is reason informed by the Christian story that allows
parents to determine what is truly in the "best interests" of the handicapped neonate against such cultural biases.

In conclusion, when a handicapped neonate has the potential for human relationships and an associated medical condition that is treatable or correctable, and thus there is a great benefit to the patient, parents have a moral obligation to treat this neonate. The decision to treat has its basis in McCormick's moral epistemology, which is based on reason informed by the Christian story. The decision to treat is rooted in the sensitivities and emotions of the parents as well as in rational analysis, both of which are enlightened by the Christian story. The guidelines, norms, and moral principles advanced by McCormick's quality-of-life criterion assist parents, in consultation with health care professionals, to examine the range of moral choices and to determine what is in the "best interests" of this neonate, normatively understood.

McCormick's patient-centered, quality-of-life criterion, which is rooted in his theological anthropology and his moral epistemology, provides guidelines, norms, and moral principles that parents can utilize in making treatment decisions for handicapped neonates. However, this criterion is not a mathematical formula that parents can apply to a particular situation and come up with a certain answer. The quality-of-life criterion sets certain parameters for parents in the decision-making process. However, parameters do not replace prudence nor do they eliminate doubts and conflicts. McCormick writes:

> Doubts and agonizing problems will remain. Hence a certain range of choices must be allowed to parents, a certain margin of error, a certain space. Guidelines can be developed which aid us to judge when parents have exceeded the limits of human discretion. They cannot cover every instance where human discretion must intervene to decide. The margin of error tolerable should reflect not only the utter finality of the decision (which tends to narrow it), but also the unavoidable uncertainty and doubt (which tends to broaden it).[155]

It is prudence that will direct parents in making the right moral decision among the range of choices available.

One of the major criticisms that has been directed against McCormick's ethical methodology is that he never defines prudence nor does he explain how he uses it. He refers to the integral role that prudence plays in both his moral epistemology and his moral criteriology. He explains that concrete rules and guidelines cannot replace prudence. Yet, McCormick never gives any guidance on how parents should exercise prudence in moral decision-making. As a "revised" natural law ethicist in the Catholic tradition, McCormick understands that prudence listens to human experience (one's own and others') it seeks counsel, and it looks into the future to anticipate and size-up the consequences. But McCormick is also aware that because of our finite nature and the effects of the Fall, ambiguity has become part of the human condition. Both reason and free will have become more vulnerable and are open to potential abuse.[156] If McCormick had articulated how prudence should operate in situations of conflict and doubt, parents would be given more guidance in moral decision-making that would help safeguard the "best interests" of the neonate.[157] This is a substantive criticism that needs to be addressed and clarified if McCormick's ethical methodology is to become a public policy option concerning treatment decisions for handicapped neonates.

In conclusion, McCormick has always underscored the primacy of method. His ethical methodology has been constructed from his writings and has been applied to treatment decisions for handicapped neonates. Criticisms of his ethical methodology remain due to inconsistencies in terminology and ambiguities in the application of various concepts. These inconsistencies and ambiguities that exist in regard to his ethical methodology could be overcome with a systematic and coherent articulation of his theoretical foundations. This articulation is crucial if McCormick's ethical methodology is being proposed as a public policy option on the treatment of handicapped neonates. When making treatment decisions for handicapped neonates, parents and health care professionals need clarity, not ambiguity, because these decisions affect the life and death of these neonates. Unfortunately, the task of clarifying these inconsistencies in terminology and ambiguities in application will be left to those of us who have studied his writings.

CONCLUSION

McCormick's ethical methodology has been articulated, examined, critically analyzed, and systematically applied to five diagnostic treatment categories that represent the spectrum of neonatal anomalies. In the final chapter, McCormick's ethical methodology will be evaluated as a public policy option for the treatment of handicapped neonates. Two questions will be examined and analyzed. The first: Is McCormick's ethical methodology practical, beneficial, and appropriate for Christian parents and health care professionals in making treatment decisions for handicapped neonates? A brief evaluation will be given of its positive and negative points from the Christian decision-maker's perspective. The second: Can it be recommended to all decision-makers, both Christian and non-Christian, as a public policy option for the treatment of handicapped neonates? This second area concerns the question of the uniqueness of

Christian ethics. McCormick claims that the sources of faith do not originate concrete moral obligations that are impervious to human insight and reasoning. However, they do confirm them. Christian values and norms are open to all reasonable people, but does this mean that McCormick's ethical methodology is sustainable without the religious content? If one strips away the religious content does his ethical methodology hold together as a public policy option that can be employed by all reasonable people? These issues will be examined in depth in the final chapter and a recommendation will be proposed regarding McCormick's ethical methodology as a public policy option for the treatment of handicapped neonates.

NOTES

[1]McCormick, "The Quality of Life, The Sanctity of Life," *How Brave a New World?*, 393-394.

[2]For a more detailed analysis of the 1984 Child Abuse Law and the guidelines of the American Academy of Pediatrics, refer to Chapter One, Neonatology: A United States Perspective section above.

[3]It should be noted that McCormick believes morality and public policy are both related and distinct. He writes: "They are related because law or public policy has an inherently moral character due to its rootage in existential human ends (goods). The common good of all persons cannot be unrelated to what is judged to be promotive or destructive to the individual—in other words, judged to be moral or immoral. Morality and public policy are distinct because it is only when individual acts have ascertainable public consequences on the maintenance and stability of society that they are the proper concerns of society, fit subjects for public policy." McCormick, "Public Policy and Fetal Research," *How Brave a New World?*, 72.

[4]It should be noted that this author verified the five diagnostic treatment categories and the representative anomalies with Dr. Jonathan Muraskas, Associate Professor of Pediatrics and Assistant Clinical Director of Neonatology, at the Loyola Medical Center Chicago, Illinois. The five diagnostic categories and their representative anomalies were also confirmed by Dr. Apollo Maglalang, Professor of Pediatrics and Director of Neonatology, at the Atlantic City Medical Center Atlantic City, New Jersey. These two neonatologists were selected because this author has done a bioethics clinical rotation under each physician's supervision in the past.

[5]Weir, *Selective Nontreatment of Handicapped Newborns*, 254.

[6]Ibid., 255-257. It should be noted that Robert Weir is being quoted because McCormick has been greatly influenced by Weir's writings, especially in the area of treatment decisions for handicapped neonates. See McCormick, "The Best Interests of the Baby," 18-25. It should also be noted that Weir advocates the child's best interests as his fundamental decision-making standard. Weir writes: "As potential persons, neonates have *prima facie* claims to life and the medical treatment necessary to prolong life. Although there are some instances in which these *prima facie* claims are justifiably overridden by other considerations, such considerations should have only one focal point: the best interests of the anomalous child." Ibid., 194-195. Weir understands the "best interests" criterion to be distinct from the "quality-of-life" criterion, however, both McCormick and Richard Sparks disagree that these two criteria are really distinct or separable. McCormick writes: "It is precisely because one is focused on best interests that qualitative considerations cannot be ignored but indeed are central. Weir is clearly afraid that quality-of-life considerations will be unfair. But they need not be. It all depends on where the line is drawn." McCormick, review of *Selective Nontreatment of Handicapped Newborns*, by Robert Weir, in *Perspectives in Biology and Medicine* 29 (Winter 1986): 328; see also Sparks, *To Treat or Not To Treat?*, 189-192. For a more detailed analysis of McCormick's notion of "best interests," refer to Chapter Four, McCormick's Ethical Criteria section above.

[7]See McCormick, "The Best Interests of the Baby," 18-25; Idem, "The Preservation of Life and Self-Determination," *How Brave a New World?*, 381-389; and McCormick and Paris, "Saving Defective Infants," *How Brave a New World?*, 352-361.

[8]Examples of bioethicists who believe parents are the appropriate decision-makers would include: John Fletcher, "Choices of Life or Death in the Care of Defective Newborns," in *Social Responsibility: Journalism, Law, and Medicine*, ed. Louis W. Hodges (Lexington, VA: Washington and Lee University Press, 1973), 60-79; Michael J. Garland, "Care of the Newborn: The Decision Not to Treat," *Perinatology/Neonatology* 1 (September-October 1977): 10-17; and Terence Ackerman, "Meningomyelocele and Parental Commitment: A Policy Proposal Regarding Selection for Treatment," *Man and Medicine* 5 (Fall 1980): 295-300. Examples of health care professionals who believe parents are the appropriate decision-makers include: Raymond S. Duff, M.D., and A. G. M. Campbell, M.D., "Moral and Ethical Dilemmas: Seven Years into the Debate and Human Ambiguity," *Annals of the American Academy of Political and Social Science* 447 (January 1977): 19-28; Anthony Shaw, M.D., "Who Should Die and Who Should Decide?," in *Infanticide and*

the Value of Life, ed. Marvin Kohl (Buffalo, NY: Prometheus Books, 1978), 104-109; and R. B. Zachary, M.D., "Ethical and Social Aspects of Treatment of Spina Bifida," *The Lancet* 2 (1969): 270-276.

[9]The Judicial Council of the American Medical Association, "Current Opinions of the Judicial Council of the American Medical Association," (Chicago, IL: American Medical Association, 1982): 9.

[10]According to the President's Commission: "Parents are usually present, concerned, willing to become informed, and cognizant of the values of the culture in which the child will be raised. They can be expected to try to make decisions that advance the newborn's best interests." For a more detailed analysis, see The President's Commission For the Study of Ethical Problems in Medicine and Biomedical Research, *Deciding to Forego Life-Sustaining Treatment* (Washington, DC: U.S. Government Printing Office, 1983), 6-7; 197-229.

[11]Weir, *Selective Nontreatment of Handicapped Newborns*, 258.

[12]Weir argues that according to his criteria for proxy decision-makers, there are three circumstances in which parents should not have the final word in treatment decisions: "when they simply cannot understand the relevant medical facts of a case, when they are emotionally unstable, and when they appear to put their own interests before those of defective newborns." Ibid., 269.

[13]Examples of bioethicists and health care professionals who believe neonatologists are the best decision-makers for handicapped neonates include: Carson Strong, "Decision Making in the NICU: The Neonatologist as Patient Advocate," *Hastings Center Report* 25 (1984): 17-23; C. Everett Koop, M.D., "The Seriously Ill or Dying Child: Supporting the Patient and the Family," in *Death, Dying, and Euthanasia*, eds. Dennis J. Horan and David Mall (Washington, DC: University Publications of America, 1977), 537-539; John Lorber, M.D., "Spina Bifida Cystica: Results of Treatment of 270 Consecutive Cases with Criteria for Selection for the Future," *Archives of Diseases in Childhood* 47 (1972): 850-871; and John M. Freeman, M.D., Kenneth Schoolman, M.D., and William Reinke, M.D., "Decision Making and the Infant with Spina Bifida," in *Decision Making and the Defective Newborn*, ed. Chester A. Swinyard (Springfield, IL: Charles C. Thomas, 1978), 103-115.

[14]Weir, *Selective Nontreatment of Handicapped Newborns*, 260-261.

[15]Ibid., 261-263.

[16]A Neonatal Infant Review Committee is an advisory committee used to safeguard the best interests of the handicapped neonate. Physicians and parents can refer cases to the committee for treatment recommendations. The committee typically consists of one or more neonatologists, appropriate medical consultants, the senior Neonatal Intensive Care

Unit (NICU) nurse, other NICU nurses, a social service representative, a hospital administrator, one or more pediatricians, the hospital attorney, one or more bioethicists, and one or more members of the clergy. For a more detailed analysis of Neonatal Infant Review Committees, see Ibid., 263-266.

[17]Examples of bioethicists and health care professionals who believe Neonatal Infant Review Committees are the most appropriate decision-makers include: Paul Ramsey, *Ethics at the Edges of Life*, 145-227; John A. Robertson and Norman Fost, M.D., "Passive Euthanasia of Defective Newborn Infants: Legal Considerations," *Journal of Pediatrics* 88 (1976): 887-889; and Paul Bridge and Maryls Bridge, "The Brief Life and Death of Christopher Bridge," *Hastings Center Report* 11 (December 1981): 18-20.

[18]Weir, *Selective Nontreatment of Handicapped Newborns*, 263-265.

[19]Ibid., 264-266.

[20]Examples of those who advocate the courts as the appropriate decision-makers include: Paul A. Freund, "Mongoloids and 'Mercy Killing,'" in *Ethics in Medicine*, eds. Stanley J. Reiser, Arthur J. Dyck, and William J. Curran (Cambridge, MA: The MIT Press, 1982), 530-542. Physicians Fost and Koop advocate a possible appropriate role for the courts. See Norman Fost, M.D., "Ethical Problems in Pediatrics," *Current Problems in Pediatrics* 6 (October 1976): 13-17; and C. Everett Koop, M.D., "The Handicapped Child and His Family," *Linacre Quarterly* 48 (February 1981): 19-24.

[21]Weir, *Selective Nontreatment of Handicapped Newborns*, 266.

[22]A guardian *ad litem* is an adult appointed by the court to represent the interests of a minor or an incompetent/never-competent person.

[23]Weir, *Selective Nontreatment of Handicapped Newborns*, 266-268.

[24]Weir writes: "For instance, in cases involving neonates with Down's syndrome complicated with esophageal or duodenal atresia, some judges in some jurisdictions are reluctant to override parental autonomy—and other judges in other jurisdictions override parental autonomy in such cases simply on the basis of a telephoned request from the attending pediatrician." Ibid., 268.

[25]Ibid. It should be noted that Weir begins with parents then moves to physicians, Neonatal Infant Review Committees and then to the courts. For a more detailed analysis of his serial ordering of decision makers for never-competent patients, see Ibid., 268-270. It should also be noted that Weir agrees with James Childress on this issue of serial ordering. For a more detailed analysis of Childress' position, see James F. Childress, *Who Should Decide?* (New York: Oxford Press, 1982): 172-174.

[26]It can be assumed that when McCormick refers to parents he is referring to parents who abide by the Christian story or are of the Christian faith. In chapter six I will evaluate whether McCormick's ethical methodology is applicable to non-Christian parents.

[27]The principle of self-determination entails that it is the person himself or herself who is best situated to implement treatment decisions. The underlying supposition for self-determination in the acceptance or refusal of treatment is that the over-all good of the patient will best be served if treatment is controlled by the person. For a more detailed analysis, see McCormick, "The Moral Right To Privacy," *How Brave a New World?*, 369. It should be noted that, even though individual self-determination is not applicable with never-competent patients, McCormick believes that "a fuller understanding of the principle of autonomy and benefit to the patient may still provide a basis for making responsible decisions about the care of such patients." Idem, "The Preservation of Life and Self-Determination," *How Brave a New World?*, 386.

[28]McCormick argues that the principle of patient benefit forms the foundation for the principle of familial self-determination. The principle of patient benefit states: "Incompetent patients and formerly competent patients who have not expressed themselves adequately while competent must be accorded full dignity as human beings. We must affirm the moral obligation placed upon others that this implies. Someone must have the responsibility of determining what is the patient's best interest." Ibid.

[29]In the event that no family member or family surrogate is willing to be appointed guardian for an incompetent or never-competent patient, then the principle of familial self-determination no longer has any significance for that specific case. McCormick writes: "The principle of patient benefit remains and becomes the exclusive principle for determining the case. Even then, however, when the only principle is that of choosing the course that will best serve the patient's best interests, someone will have to make the determination. In these most tragic cases often a public official such as a judge may have to be called upon. By this method due process will be provided to protect the interests of a most vulnerable group in our society." Ibid., 388.

[30]Ibid., 387. It should be noted that these two reasons are similar to the criteria for proxy decision-makers that Weir advocates. The parents have the knowledge regarding the family setting into which this particular anomalous neonate has been born. The parents know the emotional, financial, and social factors that will play a major role in determining if this neonate should be treated.

[31]Ibid., 387-388. McCormick's notion of familial self-determination has its roots in the notion of love of God and love of neighbor. For a more detailed analysis of McCormick's position on the love of God and love of neighbor, refer to Chapter Two, McCormick's Theological Anthropology section, Doctrine of Creation subsection above.

[32]McCormick, "The Best Interests of the Baby," 19.

[33]Editorial Staff, "When The Neonate Is Defective," *Contemporary OB/GYN* 7 (June 1976): 103. McCormick, as interviewed by the editorial staff.

[34]It should be noted that McCormick's rationale for having parents consult with health care professionals seems to be based on Weir's criteria for proxy decision-makers.

[35]McCormick, "The Preservation of Life and Self-Determination," *How Brave a New World?*, 389.

[36]Ibid., 388.

[37]When McCormick states that under certain circumstances "society" has a duty to intervene, he is referring to agencies such as the Department of Children and Family Services, etc.

[38]McCormick and Paris, "Saving Defective Infants," *How Brave a New World?*, 360.

[39]It should be noted that McCormick's notion of safeguards corresponds to Weir's use of sequential arrangement of decision-makers. Weir writes: "A sequential arrangement of decision makers also incorporates the possibilities of (a) appeals to a 'higher' proxy and (b) overriding the decision of a 'lower' proxy when circumstances merit." Weir, *Selective Nontreatment of Handicapped Newborns*, 268. McCormick does not have this sequential arrangement, but he does believe that Neonatal Infant Review Committees and the courts can play a role when necessary.

[40]It should be noted that there are other ethical approaches and criteria used by bioethicists in making treatment decisions for handicapped neonates. For a more detailed analysis of these other criteria, refer to Chapter One, General Ethical Approaches to Treatment for Handicapped Neonates section above.

[41]McCormick, "The Rights of the Voiceless," *How Brave a New World?*, 101. The basis for this is in McCormick's theological anthropology. For a more detailed analysis, refer to Chapter Two, McCormick's Theological Anthropology section, Doctrine of Creation subsection above.

[42]For a more detailed analysis of McCormick's category of "best interests," refer to Chapter Four, McCormick's Ethical Criteria section above. It should be noted that when McCormick refers to benefits in his "best interests" category it is not restricted to medical benefits. Benefits

also apply to social and familial benefits. This notion of "benefit" originates in Pellegrino's four components of "best interests" that McCormick
has incorporated into his "best interests" category. For a more detailed
analysis of Pellegrino's position, refer to Chapter Four, McCormick's
Ethical Criteria section above; see also Edmund Pellegrino, M.D.,
"Moral Choice, The Good of the Patient and the Patient's Good," in
Ethics and Critical Care Medicine, 117-138.

[43]McCormick, "The Rights of the Voiceless," *How Brave a New
World?*, 104-105.

[44]McCormick, "Public Policy on Abortion," *How Brave a New
World?*, 197-198.

[45]This is grounded in McCormick's theological anthropology which
states that persons are created in the image and likeness of God; therefore, all persons are social and relational creatures. This sense of sociality and relationality suggests that the well-being of persons is interrelated. Further, the well-being of one person cannot be conceived of or
realistically pursued independently of the good of others since a social
creature is part of human being and becoming. This sense of sociality
and relationality pertains to neonates as much as it does to adults.
McCormick writes: "The good of infants is inseparably interlocked and
interrelated to the good of others, for infants are human beings. Clearly,
they cannot experience this or respond to its implications as claims. But
we may for them—to the extent that it is reasonable to do so, a reasonableness founded on their common share in our human nature. *On this
basis* we conclude to the reasonableness of certain interventions and try
to convey and limit this reasonableness (rooted in the continuity of our
share in the sociality of human nature) by the language of *ought*."
McCormick, "Sharing In Sociality: Children and Experimentation," *How
Brave a New World?*, 90-91. Emphasis in the original. For a more detailed analysis of McCormick's understanding of the social and relational
nature of the human person, refer to Chapter Two, McCormick's Theological Anthropology section, Doctrine of Creation subsection above.

[46]By relational potential McCormick means "the hope that the infant
will, in relative comfort, be able to experience our caring and love."
McCormick, "To Save or Let Die," *How Brave a New World?*, 351. For
a more detailed analysis of McCormick's relational potential, refer to
Chapter Four, McCormick's Ethical Criteria section above.

[47]McCormick, "To Save or Let Die," *How Brave a New World?*,
349-350.

[48]This would include anomalies in which the neonate has the potential for human relationships, but the potential is utterly submerged in the
mere struggle for survival, or the medical condition will result in immi-

nent death, or it has been determined that further treatment is medically futile. Certain anomalies that would fall within this category would be spina bifida, hypoplastic left heart syndrome, trisomy 13, trisomy 18, Lesch-Nyhan syndrome, etc.

[49]I base this opinion on McCormick's evaluation of Weir's attempt to concretize in clinical categories two categories of nontreatment for handicapped neonates. For a more detailed analysis, see McCormick, "The Best Interests of the Baby," 24. I also base this on personal conversations this author had with McCormick after he read the manuscript.

[50]Ibid.

[51]This is in contrast to individuals who are competent or who were once competent. For these individuals, life-sustaining decisions can be individualized to the person. McCormick writes: "That is, the notion of 'benefit to the patient' can be individualized. The adult has a past, perspectives on life and its meaning, aspirations and achievements. All these things can be weighed by the patient making life-sustaining decisions or by those who know the patient best and presumably have his best interests at heart." McCormick, "The Preservation of Life," *Linacre Quarterly* 43 (May 1976): 100.

[52]Ibid.

[53]McCormick, "The New Medicine and Morality," 316.

[54]For a more detailed analysis of McCormick's position on the distinction between allowing to die and direct termination, as well as his position on infanticide, refer to Chapter Three, Practical Implications of McCormick's Moral Epistemology As Applied To Treatment Decisions For Handicapped Neonates section above.

[55]McCormick, "Public Policy on Abortion," *How Brave a New World?*, 197.

[56]This is an important safeguard because there are a number of bioethicists and health care professionals who argue that there is no moral difference between direct termination and allowing to die. See Joseph Fletcher, "Ethics and Euthanasia," *American Journal of Nursing* 73 (1973): 670-765. This article also appears as a chapter in *To Live and To Die*, ed. Robert H. Williams (New York: Springer-Verlag, 1973), 113-124. Paul Ramsey also offers a critique of this view in *Ethics at the Edges of Life*, 212-227.

[57]American Medical Associations's Council of Ethical and Judicial Affairs, "The Use of Anencephalic Neonates As Organ Donors," *Journal of the American Medical Association* 273 (May 24-31, 1995): 1615.

[58]According to the members of the Task Force on Anencephaly: "Mechanical factors that cause disruption of the normal processes of development include amniotic bands and fetal adhesions to the placenta.

For anencephaly to develop, these conditions must occur at or before the induction of cerebral development; if they occur later, they may be associated with preservation of the cerebrum. Poorly understood geographic factors (reflected, for example, in a high incidence along the Eastern seaboard of the United States and the western coastal regions of Europe), and the maternal reproductive history influence the incidence and perhaps the causes of anencephaly. The incidence of anencephaly is increased in twins. Several maternal factors have been associated with anencephaly, including hyperthermia and deficiencies of folate, zinc, and copper." David A. Stumpf, M.D. et al., "The Infant with Anencephaly," *The New England Journal of Medicine* 322 (March 8, 1990): 670.

[59]Ibid.

[60]It should be noted that there is one case where Stephanie Keene, known as "Baby K," lived for two and one half years before dying. Many question if anencephaly was the proper diagnosis in this case. For a more detailed analysis of this case, see Mark A. Bonano, "The Case of Baby K: Exploring the Concept of Medical Futility," *Annals of Health Law* 4 (1995): 151.

[61]For a more detailed analysis of anencephaly, see A.D. Abbattista, F. Vigevano, G. Catena, and F. Parisi, "Anencephalic Neonates and Diagnosis of Death," *Transplant Process* 8 (December 29, 1997): 3634-3635; C. Lantz, "The Anencephalic Infant As Organ Donor, *Health Law Journal* 4 (1996): 179-195; D. A. Shewmon, "Anencephaly: Selected Medical Aspects," *Hastings Center Report* 18 (1988): 11-19; P. A. Baird and A. D. Sadovnick, "Survival in Infants with Anencephaly," *Clinical Pediatrics* 23 (1984): 268-271; Malcolm Levene and David Tudehope, *Essentials of Neonatal Medicine* (Oxford: Blackwell Scientific Publications, 1993), 278-281; and Gordon Avery, Mary Ann Fletcher and Mhairi MacDonald, *Neonatology: Pathophysiology and Management of the Newborn*, 4th ed., 1155-1156.

[62]For a more detailed analysis of this guideline, refer to Chapter Four, McCormick's Ethical Criteria section above.

[63]McCormick, "To Save or Let Die: State of the Question," 172.

[64]For a more detailed analysis of McCormick's position on life as a good but not an absolute good, refer to Chapter Two, McCormick's Theological Anthropology section above.

[65]McCormick, "To Save or Let Die," *How Brave a New World?*, 345.

[66]McCormick, "The Judaeo-Christian Tradition and Bioethical Codes," *How Brave a New World?*, 14. For a more detailed analysis of McCormick's position on how human relationships are the very possibility of growth in love of God and neighbor, refer to Chapter Two,

Practical Implications of McCormick's Theological Anthropology As Applied to Treatment Decisions for Handicapped Neonates section, Life Is a Value To Be Preserved Only Insofar As It Contains Some Potentiality for Human Relationships subsection above.

[67]Lisa Sowle Cahill states: "McCormick identifies the good 'higher' than human life as the capacity for relationships of love." Cahill, "On Richard McCormick," 92.

[68]McCormick, "The Quality of Life, The Sanctity of Life," *How Brave a New World?*, 405.

[69]McCormick, "To Save or Let Die," *How Brave a New World?*, 350. Emphasis in the original. As I have stated prior, McCormick makes a distinction here between every person being of equal value and every life being of equal value. He writes: "What the 'equal value' language is attempting to say is legitimate: We must avoid *unjust* discrimination in the provision of health care and life supports. But not all discrimination (inequality of treatment) is unjust. *Unjust* discrimination is avoided if decision-making centers on the benefit to the patient, even if that benefit is described largely in terms of quality-of-life criteria." Ibid., 407. Emphasis in the original.

[70]McCormick, "The New Medicine and Morality," 317.

[71]Leonard Weber, *Who Shall Live?*, 82.

[72]McCormick, "The Judaeo-Christian Tradition and Bioethical Codes," *How Brave a New World?*, 10-11. For a more detailed analysis of the practical implications of McCormick's notion that human life is sacred, refer to Chapter Two, Practical Implications of McCormick's Theological Anthropology As Applied to Treatment Decisions for Handicapped Neonates section, Human Life As Sacred subsection above.

[73]McCormick, *The Critical Calling*, 268.

[74]McCormick, "The Quality of Life, The Sanctity of Life," *How Brave a New World?*, 407.

[75]For a more detailed analysis of McCormick's understanding of quality of life as an extension of sanctity of life and his understanding of the moral principles of justice and charity, refer to Chapter Four, Criticism section above.

[76]It should be noted that no pain relief is necessary because the anencephalic neonate lacks the ability to feel pain.

[77]There are four grades of severity of Intraventricular Hemorrhage that can be detected by ultrasound scan. Grade I—the germinal matrix hemorrhage with no or minimal intraventricular hemorrhage (<10% of ventricular area on parasagittal view). Grade II—intraventricular hemorrhage (10-50% of ventricular area on parasagittal view). Grade III—intraventricular hemorrhage (>50% of ventricular area on parasagittal

view; usually distends lateral ventricle). Grade IV—intraventricular hemorrhage with parenchymal involvement. For a more detailed analysis of the grading of intraventricular hemorrhages, see Tricia Lacy Gomella, M. Douglas Cunningham, Fabien Eyal and Karin Zent, *Neonatology* 4th Ed. (Stamford, CT: Appleton & Lange, 1999), 462; and Joseph Volpe, M.D., "Intraventricular Hemorrhage and Brain Injury in the Premature Infant: Diagnosis, Prognosis, and Prevention," *Clinics in Perinatology* 16 (June 1989): 388-389.

[78]Hydrocephalus is caused by a pathological obstruction along the pathway of cerebrospinal fluid circulation. This condition is a progressive enlargement of the head from increased amounts of cerebrospinal fluid into the ventricles of the brain. Neonates with IVH usually experience progressive hydrocephalus and show evidence of irreversible damage of the brain or other major organs (i.e., multiple congenital anomalies and cerebral atrophy secondary to meningitis). In this group, prognosis is uniformly poor, and shunting operations have little to offer. For a more detailed analysis, see Avery *et al.*, *Neonatology* 1145.

[79]The incidence of major IVH (large IVH or any intraparenchymal hemorrhage) was 5.2% (versus 13%-28% in earlier studies) in infants of less than 1500 grams who did not receive any prenatal or postnatal pharmacotherapy for the prevention of IVH other than antenatal steroids administered to accelerate pulmonary maturity. Gomella *et al.*, 460-461. See also R.D. Sheth, "Trends in Incidence and Severity of Intraventricular Hemorrhage," *Journal of Child Neurology* 13 (June 1998): 261-264.

[80]Gomella *et al.*, *Neonatology*, 460-461; and Avery *et al.*, *Neonatology*, 1127.

[81]Because of the high risk of IVH, routine cranial ultrasonography is recommended at four days of age for high risk neonates younger than 32 weeks gestation. Ultrasound scanning should be performed sooner if there are clinical concerns. Because there may be progression in the size of the hemorrhage in 20% to 40% of patients with IVH, the ultrasound scans should be repeated after the first week of life to establish the maximal extent of the hemorrhage. For a more detailed analysis of cranial ultrasonography, see Avery *et al.*, *Neonatology*, 1128.

[82]Gomella *et al.*, *Neonatology*, 462. Although CT scanning and magnetic resonance imaging (MRI) are acceptable alternatives they are more expensive and require transport from the intensive care unit to the imaging device. Ibid.; See also A. Hill, "Intraventricular Hemorrhage: Emphasis on Prevention," *Seminar in Pediatric Neurology* 5 (September 1998): 152-160.

[83]Avery *et al.*, *Neonatology*, 1128.

[84]Parenchyma is the distinctive tissue characteristic of an organ and responsible for its functioning.

[85]In a study by F. Guzzetta, M.D. *et al.*, it was determined that the prognosis for neonates with a massive intraventricular hemorrhage and periventricular parenchymal injury, identified on ultrasound scan as intraparenchymal echodensity (IPE) greater than 1cm, was unfavorable. Thus, neonates with extensive IPE (that is, IPE that included fronto-parieto-occipital regions), 30 of 37 (81%) died, and of the seven survivors, all had subsequent motor deficits. For a more detailed analysis, see F. Guzzetta, M.D. *et al.*, "Periventricular Intraparenchymal Echodensities in the Premature Newborn: Critical Determinant of Neurological Outcome," *Pediatrics* 78 (1986): 995.

[86]For a more detailed analysis of IVH, see Avery *et al.*, *Neonatology*, 1132; B. Vohr, W.C. Allan, D.T. Scott *et al.*, "Early-Onset Intraventricular Hemorrhage in Preterm Neonates: Incidence of Neurodevelopmental Handicap," *Perinatology* 23 (June 1999): 212-217; L. Barton, J.E. Hodgman, and Z. Pavlova, "Causes of Death in the Extremely Low Birth Weight Infant," *Pediatrics* 103 (February 1999): 446-451; Joseph J. Volpe, M.D., A. Ernest, M.D., and Jane G. Stein, M.D., "Intraventricular Hemorrhage and Brain Injury in the Premature Infant," *Clinics in Perinatology* 16 (June 1989): 387-411; John J. Paris and Kevin O'Connell, "Withdrawal of Nutrition and Fluids from a Neurologically Devastated Infant: The Case of Baby T," *Journal of Perinatology* 11 (1991): 372-373; Michael Jellinek, Elizabeth Catlin, I. Davis Todres, and Edwin Cassem, "Facing Tragic Decision with Parents in the Neonatal Intensive Care Unit: Clinical Perspectives," *Pediatrics* 89 (January 1992): 119-122.

[87]To clarify what McCormick means by the potential for human relationships being utterly submerged in the mere struggle for survival, he writes: "Something other than the 'higher, more important good' would occupy first place. Life, the condition for other values and achievements, would usurp the place of these and become itself the ultimate value. When that happens, the value of human life has been distorted out of context." McCormick, "To Save or Let Die," *How Brave a New World?*, 347-348.

[88]McCormick, *Health and Medicine in the Catholic Tradition*, 54.

[89]McCormick, "The Best Interests of the Baby," 23. For a more detailed analysis of McCormick's position on how our love of neighbor is in some real way our love of God, refer to Chapter Four, McCormick's Ethical Criteria section above.

[90]McCormick, "To Save or Let Die," *How Brave a New World?*, 346.

[91]It should be noted that McCormick claims his quality-of-life criterion has its foundation in the traditional ordinary/extraordinary means distinction that was later clarified by Pius XII. McCormick quotes Pius XII as saying that an obligation to use any means possible "would be too burdensome for most men and would render the attainment of the higher, more important good too difficult. Life, health, all temporal activities are in fact subordinated to spiritual ends." Pius XII, "The Prolongation of Life," *Acta Apostolicae Sedis*, 1,031-1,032.

[92]For a more detailed analysis of McCormick's moral epistemology after 1983, and specifically, how he determines if one value can be sacrificed for another in a conflict situation, refer to Chapter Three, McCormick's Dual Moral Epistemology section, Second Moral Epistemology—After 1983 subsection above.

[93]McCormick, *Health and Medicine in the Catholic Tradition*, 52

[94]Ibid. For a more detailed analysis of McCormick's argument, refer to Chapter Three, Practical Implications of McCormick's Moral Epistemology As Applied to Treatment Decisions for Handicapped Neonates section, Human Life Is a Good But Not an Absolute Good subsection above.

[95]McCormick, "To Save or Let Die," *How Brave a New World?*, 347.

[96]For a more detailed analysis of the key elements of the Christian story, refer to Chapter Three, McCormick's Dual Moral Epistemology section above.

[97]McCormick and Paris, "Saving Defective Infants," *How Brave a New World?*, 358. For a more complete analysis of this third norm and McCormick's position on the moral principles, refer to Chapter Four, McCormick's Ethical Criteria section above.

[98]For McCormick, the well-being of a patient consists generally in a life prolonged beyond infancy, without excruciating pain, and with the potential for participating, to at least a minimal degree, in human experience. For a more detailed analysis of this position, see McCormick, "A Proposal for 'Quality of Life' Criteria for Sustaining Life," 79; and refer to Chapter Four, McCormick's Ethical Criteria section above.

[99]For a more detailed analysis of McCormick's position on pain and suffering, refer to Chapter Two, Practical Implications of McCormick's Theological Anthropology As Applied to Treatment Decisions for Handicapped Neonates section, Pain and Suffering Can Have Redemptive Meaning subsection above.

[100]Endocardial fibroelastosis is the thickening of endocardium into a fibroelastic layer of tissue which may occur in the left ventricle of the

hypoplastic heart. For a more detailed analysis, see Avery *et al.*, *Neonatology*, 551-552.

[101]Ibid., 551. It should be noted that a study performed by Marvin Natowicz, M.D. *et al.*, found that as in other complex congenital heart lesions, the prevalence of underlying genetic causes of and major extra cardiac anomalies associated with hypoplastic left heart syndrome is substantial—28% in this study. Natowicz writes: "For many of the genetic disorders we identified, the association with hypoplastic left heart syndrome that we observed is not unexpected. Thus, the association of the syndrome with the chromosomal disorders that we found in our series is not surprising because all of these chromosomal syndromes are associated with high incidence of congenital heart disease. An association between hypoplastic left heart syndrome and trisomy 13, trisomy 18, trisomy 21, and Turner syndrome has, in fact, been noted previously, as has an association with duplication 12p, duplication 16q, monosomy 4p, and monosomy 11q syndromes. Similarly, an association between Smith-Lemli-Opitz, Apert, and Holt-Oram syndromes and hypoplastic left heart syndrome is probably not fortuitous in that each is frequently associated with congenital heart disease." Marvin Natowicz, M.D. *et al.*, "Genetic Disorders and Major Extra Cardiac Anomalies Associated with Hypoplastic Left Heart Syndrome," *Pediatrics* 82 (November 1988): 702-704. This is an important point because in addition to the anomaly of hypoplastic left heart syndrome, other serious genetic disorders are usually associated with this anomaly. These associated genetic disorders will play a major role in the decision-making process of whether such neonates should receive medical treatment.

[102]This information was obtained from Dr. Apollo Maglalang, Professor of Pediatrics at the Atlantic City Medical Center Atlantic City, New Jersey, in an interview on December 28, 1995. The foramen ovale is a normal feature of the heart allowing blood to flow between atria. A ductus arteriosus is a normally occurring shunt between the aorta and the pulmonary artery. In utero, the ductus arteriosus allows blood flow to be diverted from the high-resistance pulmonary circulation to the descending aorta and the low-resistance placental bed. Functional closure of the ductus arteriosus occurs soon after birth but can be delayed in premature infants and in certain situations. Finally, autosomal has to do with any of the 22 chromosome pairs not associated with sex determination. For a more detailed analysis, see Avery *et al.*, *Neonatology*, 551-553; see also Denise Kirsten, "Patent Ductus Arteriosus in the Preterm Infant," *Neonatal Network* 15 (March 1996): 19-26.

[103]Echocardiography is examination of the structures and movements of the heart with reflected pulsed ultrasound. As a non-invasive investi-

gation employing non-ionizing energy, it has become established as a useful additional method of evaluating heart disease. For a more detailed analysis, see Avery *et al.*, *Neonatology*, 552-553.

[104]Bradycardia is an abnormally slow rate of heart beat (usually taken as 60 per minute or less). For a more detailed analysis, see Ibid., 1361-1362.

[105]Ibid., 552.

[106]The first is palliation (the Norwood procedure), redirecting the blood flow so that the right ventricle serves as the "systemic ventricle," and is high risk intervention. The second stage (Fontan procedure) directs the systemic venous to return directly to the pulmonary circulation and the atrial septal defect is closed. The Fontan procedure may be done in two stages. See Avery *et al.*, *Neonatology*, 551-553.

[107]It should be noted that cardiac transplantation has been used recently as an alternative approach with good results, but there is limited timely availability of neonatal donors and limited documentation of long-range survival. For a more detailed analysis, see L. L. Bailey, M.D., "Role of Cardiac Transplantation in the Neonate," *Journal of Heart Transplant* 4 (1985): 506.

[108]For a more detailed analysis of hypoplastic left heart syndrome, see Gomella *et al.*, *Neonatology*, 339-340; D.L. Williams, A.C. Gelijns, A.J. Moskowicz *et al.*, "Hypoplastic Left Heart Syndrome: Valuing the Survival," *Journal of Thorascic Cardiovascular Surgery* 19 (April 2000): 720-731; S. Weinstein, G.W. Gaynor, N.D. Bridges *et al.*, "Early Survival of Infants Weighing 2.5 Kilograms Or Less Undergoing First-Stage Reconstruction for Hypoplastic Left Heart Syndrome," *Circulation* 100 (November 9, 1999): Supplement III: 167-170; W. A. Long, *Fetal and Neonatal Cardiology* (Philadelphia, PA: W. B. Sanders, 1990); J. H. Moller and W. A. Neal, *Fetal, Neonatal, and Infant Cardiac Disease* (Norfolk, CT: Appleton and Lange, 1989); S. C. Mitchell, S. B. Korones, and H. W. Berendes, "Congenital Heart Disease In 56,109 Births," *Circulation* 43 (1971): 323-335; and Leonard L. Bailey *et al.*, "Cardiac Allotransplanation in Newborns As Therapy for Hypoplastic Left Heart Syndrome," *The New England Journal of Medicine* 315 (October 9, 1986): 949-951.

[109]McCormick, "Technology and Morality: The Example of Medicine," 26.

[110]For a more detailed analysis of McCormick's reformulation of the ordinary/ extraordinary means distinction into his benefit/burden calculus, refer to Chapter Four, McCormick's Ethical Criteria section above.

[111]McCormick, "To Save or Let Die," *How Brave a New World?*, 345. For a more detailed analysis of McCormick's belief that human life

is a relative good, refer to Chapter Two, McCormick's Theological Anthropology section above.

[112]McCormick and Paris, "Saving Defective Infants," *How Brave a New World?*, 360.

[113]For a more detailed analysis of McCormick's second moral epistemology after 1983, and how prediscursive and discursive reason informed by the Christian story play an essential role in the parent's discernment, refer to Chapter Three, McCormick's Dual Moral Epistemology section, Second Moral Epistemology—After 1983 subsection above.

[114]It should be remembered that Avery *et al.* believe that neither reconstructive surgery leading to the Fontan procedure or cardiac transplantation can be viewed as curative. See Avery *et al.*, *Neonatology*, 552.
For a more detailed analysis of heart transplantation in neonates, see
Leonard L. Bailey *et al.*, Cardiac Allotransplantation in Newborns As
Therapy for Hypoplastic Left Heart Syndrome, " *New England Journal
of Medicine.* 949-951.

[115]In McCormick's notion of "best interests," the benefits are not restricted to medical benefits. Benefits also apply to social and familial
factors. This can be seen in how McCormick has incorporated Pellegrino's four components of "best interests" into his interpretation. For a
more detailed analysis of Pellegrino's four components, see Pellegrino,
"Moral Choice, the Good of the Patient and the Patient's Good," in *Ethics and Critical Care Medicine*, 117-138.

[116]For a more detailed analysis of McCormick's position on social
and familial factors and the criticism of his position by Richard Sparks
and James McCartney, refer to Chapter Four, Criticism section above;
see also Chapter Two, Criticism section above.

[117]It should be noted that the term "futile" is an elusive and ambiguous term. There are four major types of futility. First, physiological futility—an intervention cannot lead to the intended physiological effect.
Second, imminent demise futility—an intervention may be futile if, despite that intervention, the patient will die in the very near future (this is
sometimes expressed as the patient will not survive to discharge, although that is not really equivalent to dying in the very near future).
Third, lethal condition futility—an intervention may be futile if the patient has an underlying lethal condition which the intervention does not
affect and which will result in death in the not too far future (weeks, perhaps months, but not years) even if the intervention is employed. Fourth,
qualitative futility—an intervention may be futile if it fails to lead to an
acceptable quality of life. For a more detailed analysis of futility, see
Baruch A. Brody and Amir Halevy, "Is Futility a Futile Concept?" *Journal of Medicine and Philosophy* 20 (April 1995): 126-129. McCormick

has a normative understanding of futility which does not solely rely on physiological futility. McCormick's normative understanding of futility considers whether the agreed on potential effect is of any value and benefit to the patient, that is, in the patient's "best interests," normatively understood. For McCormick, a medical treatment might be successful in achieving an effect (physiologically effective), but the effect might not be beneficial to the patient (qualitatively effective). Since the goal of medical treatment is to benefit the patient, it follows that nonbeneficial treatment is medically futile. This is determined by the parents, in consultation with the health care professionals, because a determination must be made of the patient's medical status and an evaluation must be made of the medical intervention. The determination of medical futility entails balancing the values of patients, the values of medicine, and the fact that there is much uncertainty in making "predictive medical judgments." McCormick's notion of medical futility is rooted in the principles of beneficence and nonmaleficence—do no harm to the patient. For a more detailed analysis of medical futility, see Peter A. Clark, S.J., and Catherine M. Mikus, "Time for a Formalized Medical Futility Policy," *Health Progress* 81 (July-August, 2000): 24-32; Edmund Pellegrino, "Decisions at the End of Life: The Use and Abuse of the Concept of Futility," in *The Dignity of the Dying Person: Proceedings of the Fifth Assembly of the Pontifical Academy of Life* (Vatican City, Italy: 2000), 219-241; Robert Veatch and Carol Mason Spicer, "Futile Care: Physicians Should Not Be Allowed to Refuse to Treat," *Health Progress* 74 (December 1993): 22-27; James F. Drane and John L. Coulehan, "The Concept of Futility: Parents Do Not Have a Right to Demand Medically Useless Treatment," *Health Progress* 74 (December 1993): 32; Glenn G. Griener, "The Physician's Authority to Withhold Futile Treatment," *Journal of Philosophy and Medicine* 20 (April 1995): 209; Peter A. Clark, S.J., "Medical Futility in Pediatrics: Is It Time for a Public Policy?" *Journal of Public Health Policy* 23 (2002): 66-89; and Peter A. Clark, S.J., "Building a Policy in Pediatrics for Medical Futility," *Pediatric Nursing* 27 (March-April 2001): 180-184.

[118]NEC is the most common surgical emergency in neonates; the mortality exceeds that of all gastrointestinal tract congenital malformations combined. It is the third leading cause of neonatal death, with a 30 to 50 percent mortality rate. For a more detailed analysis, see Leslie A. Parker, "Necrotizing Enterocolitis," *Neonatal Network* 14 (September 1995): 17.

[119]The ileum is the part of the small intestine between the jejunum (the second part of the small intestine extending from the duodenum to the ileum) and the caecum (the first part of the large intestine, situated in

the right lower quadrant of the abdomen, which forms a pouch-like cavity connecting the terminal ileum to the ascending colon and the vermiform appendix). For a more detailed description, see *The Oxford Medical Companion*, eds. John Walton, Jeremiah Barondess, and Stephen Lock (Oxford: Oxford University Press, 1994), 397.

[120]The incidence increases with decreasing gestational age. Sixty percent to 80% of cases occur in high-risk premature newborns, while 10%-25% occur in low-risk and full-term newborns. Gomella *et al.*, *Neonatology*, 452.

[121]It has been noted that smaller, more immature neonates (<26 weeks of gestation) tend to have NEC at an older age than larger, more mature (>31 weeks of age) neonates. For a more detailed analysis, see R. D. Uauy *et al.*, "Necrotizing Enterocolitis in Very Low Birth Weight Infants: Biodemographic and Clinical Correlates," *Journal of Pediatrics* 119 (1991): 630.

[122]It can be noted that NEC has been observed to occur in epidemics in neonatal intensive care units, further supporting the role of microbial agents in pathogenesis. For a more detailed analysis, see Avery *et al.*, *Neonatology*, 614. It should also be noted that another risk factor for NEC that is gaining acceptance is maternal cocaine use. Leslie Parker writes: "Cocaine may cause mesenteric ischemia via two mechanisms: (1) Cocaine causes maternal vasoconstriction, which decreases uterine blood flow and leads to fetal hypoxia. (2) Cocaine crosses the placenta and causes fetal vasoconstriction and subsequent hypoxia. Cocaine exposed neonates with NEC tend to be more critically ill than other infants with NEC. Because the bowel is more necrotic, these infants have an increased need for surgical intervention, and their overall mortality is increased." For a more detailed analysis, see Parker, "Necrotizing Enterocolitis," 20.

[123]Pneumatosis intestinalis appears as submucosal or subserosal cysts filled with a gaseous mixture consisting of hydrogen, methane, and carbon dioxide. On x-ray it appears as linear or bubbly air in the intramural area. For a more detailed analysis, see Ibid., 17.

[124]Peritonitis is an inflammation of the peritoneum, usually resulting from a rupture of a hollow viscus such as the appendix. For a more detailed description, see *The Oxford Medical Companion*, 738.

[125]Avery *et al.*, *Neonatology*, 614-615; 937-938. It should be noted that there are new studies that breast milk has a protective mechanism against NEC. The studies show that very few infants who were fed exclusively breast milk developed NEC, and most of these were fed breast milk that had been either heated or frozen. At birth, neonates have no secretory IgA (Immunoglobulin A) in their intestinal tract. Breast milk

provides this IgA and other immunocompetent cells that are partially protective against gastrointestinal infections. As preventive strategies, oral IgA and corticosteroids have been shown to decrease the incidence of NEC. Oral IgA appears to decrease the incidence of NEC by exerting an immunoprotective effect on the gastrointestinal tract. It provides antibodies against numerous pathogens that may cause gastrointestinal infection. In the near future, all low-birth-weight neonates may receive IgA supplementation to prevent NEC. For a more detailed analysis, see E. Halac *et al.*, "Prenatal and Postnatal Corticosteroid Therapy to Prevent Neonatal Necrotizing Enterocolitis: A Controlled Trial," *Journal of Pediatrics* 117 (1990): 132-138; B. J. Stoll *et al.*, "Epidemiology of Necrotizing Enterocolitis: A Case Control Group," *Journal of Pediatrics* 96 (1980): 447-451; see also Parker, "Necrotizing Enterocolitis," 20.

[126]For a more detailed analysis, see Parker, "Necrotizing Enterocolitis," 17.

[127]Elizabeth H. Thilo, M.D., Raul Lazarte, M.D., and Jacinto Hernandez, M.D., "Necrotizing Enterocolitis in the First Twenty-Four Hours of Life," *Pediatrics* 73 (April 1984): 476-480; and Avery *et al.*, *Neonatology*, 937-938.

[128]Pneumoperitoneum is air in the peritoneal cavity. Artificial pneumoperitoneum is sometimes induced in order to assist radiological diagnosis; it was formally a common procedure in the treatment of pulmonary tuberculosis, to help in immobilization of the lung. For a more detailed analysis, see *The Oxford Medical Companion*, 775.

[129]Thrombocytopenia results from either decreased platelet production or increased peripheral platelet destruction or sequestration. A bone marrow examination is usually required to make this distinction. Normally, bone spicules contain 3-10 megakaryocytes per low-power field. Normal or increased numbers of megakaryocytes imply increased platelet consumption. Decreased numbers suggests decreased platelet production. For a more detailed analysis, see William Claiborne Dunagan, M.D. and Michael L. Ridner, M.D., eds., *Manual of Medical Therapeutics* 26th ed. (Boston, MA: Little, Brown and Company, 1986), 330.

[130]An ileostomy is a surgically created opening of the ileum onto the abdominal surface. For a more detailed description, see *The Oxford Medical Companion*, 397.

[131]If an extensive amount of necrotic bowel is resected, there may be an insufficient amount of bowel remaining for digestion. This could result in short gut syndrome and possibly be incompatible with life. See Parker, "Necrotizing Enterocolitis," 21.

[132]For a more detailed analysis of NEC, see Gomella *et al.*, *Neonatology*, 452-456; Avery *et al.*, *Neonatology*, 614-616; 937-939; M.D.

Kamitsuka, M.K. Horton, and M.A. Williams, "The Incidence of Necrotizing Enterocolitis After Introducing Standardized Feeding Schedules for Infants Between 1250 and 2500 Grams and Less than 35 Weeks of Gestation," *Pediatrics* 105 (February 2000): 379-384; J. Neu and M.D. Weiss, "Necrotizing Enterocolitis: Pathophysiology and Prevention," *Journal of Parenteral Enteral Nutrition* 23 (September-October 1999): Supplement 1-3-7; J. Sontag, M.H. Wagner, J. Waldschmidt *et al.*, "Multisystem Organ Failure and Capillary Leak Syndrome in Severe Necrotizing Enterocolitis of Very Low Birth Weight Infants," *Journal of Pediatric Surgery* 33 (March 1998): 484-494; R.C. Holman, B.J. Stoll, M.J. Clark *et al.*, "The Epidemiology of Necrotizing Enterocolitis Infant Mortality in the United States," *American Journal of Public Health* 87 (December 1997): 2026-2031; C.L. Snyder, G.K. Gittes, J.P. Murphy *et al.*, "Survival After Necrotizing Enterocolitis in Infants Weighing Less than 1,000 Grams: 25 Years' Experience at a Single Institution," *Journal of Pediatric Surgery* 32 (March 1997): 434-437; E. Tallo-Martinez, N. Claure and E. Bancalari, "Necrotizing Enterocolitis in Full-Term and Near-Term Infants: Risk Factors," *Biological Neonate* 71 ((1997): 292-298; W. A. Ballance *et al.*, "Pathology of Neonatal NEC: A Ten Year Experience," *Journal of Pediatric Medicine, Supplement 1, Pt. 2* 117 (1990); D. Anderson, and R. M. Kliegman, "The Relationship of Neonatal Alimentation Practices to the Occurance of Endemic Necrotizing Enterocolitis," *American Journal of Perinatology* 8 (1991); and R. Covert *et al.*, "Factors Associated with Age of Onset of Necrotizing Enterocolitis," *American Journal of Perinatology* 6 (1989).

[133] McCormick, "To Save Or Let Die," *How Brave a New World?*, 345. For a more detailed analysis of McCormick's belief that human life is a relative good, refer to Chapter Two, McCormick's Theological Anthropology section above.

[134] For a more detailed analysis of McCormick's second moral epistemology after 1983, and how prediscursive and discursive reason informed by the Christian story play an essential role in the parent's discernment, refer to Chapter Three, McCormick's Dual Moral Epistemology section, Second Moral Epistemology—After 1983 subsection above.

[135] McCormick, "The Best Interests of the Baby," 21. Emphasis in the original.

[136] It should be noted that physician-bioethicist Edmund Pellegrino has established a combination of subjective and objective criteria which will allow decision-makers in consultation with physicians to make medical decisions about when certain treatments are no longer beneficial. Pellegrino's approach is similar to McCormick's approach. Pelligrino's approach, which is historically based, strikes a balance between three

criteria: *effectiveness, benefits,* and *burdens. Effectiveness* is an estimate of the capacity of the medical treatment to alter the natural history of the disease or symptoms in a positive way. This is an objective determination which is dependent upon outcome studies and within the domain of the physician's expertise. It centers on the medical good and on measurable clinical data about prognoses and therapeutics. *Benefit* refers to that which is valuable to the patient as perceived by the patient or his or her surrogate. This is a subjective determination and not within the physician's domain but in that of the patient or surrogate decision-maker. Benefit centers on the patient's assessment of his or her own good, that is, the values and goals in undergoing treatment. *Burden* refers to the physical, emotional, fiscal, or social costs imposed on the patient by the medical treatment. Burdens are both subjective and objective and within the domain of both the physician, when factual, and patient/surrogate, when subjective and personal. Those burdens imposed on the medical team or society would, in certain rare circumstances, be considered as well as burdens on the patient. To determine if a medical treatment is beneficial or futile will depend on an assessment of these three criteria. If the assessment is favorable and in the patient's best interest, all things being equal, then the treatment is morally justifiable. When the assessment is unfavorable and not good for the patient, then the treatment in question is not morally justifiable. See, Pellegrino, "Decisions at the End of Life," 227-228.

[137]Qualitative futility claims that although the treatment may be successful in achieving an effect (physiologically effective), the effect is not worth achieving. Effective treatment may not be beneficial for the patient. Since the goal of medical treatment is to benefit the patient, then nonbeneficial treatment is medically futile. For McCormick, this is a value judgment that is made by the parents, in consultation with health care professionals. Once complete information about medical outcomes and about the patient's goals and values are exchanged, then this decision can be made. For a more detailed analysis of qualitative futility, see Glenn G. Griener, "The Physician's Authority to Withhold Futile Treatment," *Journal of Philosophy and Medicine,* 212-215.

[138]For a more detailed analysis of McCormick's position on pain and suffering, refer to Chapter Two, Practical Implications of McCormick's Theological Anthropology As Applied to Treatment Decisions for Handicapped Neonates section, Pain and Suffering Can Have Redemptive Meaning subsection above.

[139]It should be noted that the distributive justice argument does have its critics. The United State's health care system does not have a defined budget and is not centrally regulated. Therefore, money saved in one area

of health care is not necessarily spent in another area of health care, or even on other worthwhile programs such as education and welfare. In fact, several studies argue that termination of treatment at the point that patients reach any plausible definition of futility would save only a modest amount of money. Those who are cynical by nature would say that the savings most likely end up as a positive balance on the corporate earnings sheet of the hospital. See, A. Halevy, R.C. Neal and B.A. Brody, "The Low Frequency of Futility in an Adult Intensive Care Unit Setting," *Archives of Internal Medicine* 156 (1996): 100-104; R.C. Sachdeva *et al.*, "Resource Consumption in a Pediatric Intensive Care Unit Setting," *Journal of Pediatrics* 128 (1996): 742-747; and Robert Truog, "Futility in Pediatrics: From Case to Policy," *The Journal of Clinical Ethics* 11 (Summer 2000): 136-141.

[140]McCormick, "To Save or Let Die: State of the Question," 172.

[141]Ibid.

[142]For a more detailed analysis of McCormick's position on redemptive suffering, refer to Chapter Two, Practical Implications of McCormick's Theological Anthropology as Applied to Treatment Decisions for Handicapped Neonates section, Pain and Suffering Can Have Redemptive Meaning subsection above.

[143]In the early childbearing years, the incidence of Down syndrome is about 1/2000 live births; for mothers over 40 years of age, it rises to about 1/40 live births. Just over 20% of neonates with Down syndrome are born to mothers > 35 years of age, yet these older mothers have only 7% to 8% of the children. However, the number of women having babies after age 35 has been rising rapidly in the last few years. For a more detailed analysis, see Robert Berkow, M.D., *The Merck Manual*, 2299.

[144]Avery *et al.*, *Neonatology*, 923.

[145]Lymphedema is the accumulation of excessive lymph fluid and swelling of subcutaneous tissues due to obstruction, destruction, or hypoplasia of lymph vessels. For a more detailed analysis, see Robert Berkow, M.D., *The Merck Manual*, 593. Turner's syndrome, also known as Gonadal Dygenesis or Bonnevie-Ullrich syndrome, is a complete or partial absence of one of the two X chromosomes in the female. Its incidence is about 1/3000 live female births. For a more detailed analysis, see Ibid., 2305.

[146]Ibid., 2299-2301.

[147]Avery *et al.*, *Neonatology*, 923-924.

[148]It should be noted that the life expectancy of a Down syndrome neonate without major heart defects is about 45-50 years of age. Robert Berkow, M.D., *The Merck Manual*, 2301-2302.

[149]The fistula is identified and carefully divided from the trachea. The tracheal opening is closed with several sutures, with care to avoid narrowing the tracheal lumen. The circumference of the lower esophageal fistula is usually small and is enlarged by trimming and spatulating its open end. The tip of the upper pouch is mobilized extensively and cut across to expose the lumen. For a more detailed analysis, see Avery *et al., Neonatology*, 924-925.

[150]It should be noted that in the early 1900s, virtually all neonates born with esophageal atresia and tracheoesophageal fistula died. In 1941, Haight and Towsley were the first to bring a neonate with esophageal atresia and tracheoesophageal fistula through the rigors of primary transthoracic reconstruction. This landmark accomplishment occurred before antibiotics, respiratory support, or sophisticated intravenous nutrition were available. This surgical approach formed the basis of modern operative and postoperative care of neonates with this anomaly. Fifty years after the first survivor was announced, every neonate born with atresia of the esophagus who is spared coexisting fatal anomalies and is offered appropriate care has an excellent chance of leading a normal life. In a study done at Children's National Medical Center in Washington, DC, 118 patients with blind upper esophageal pouch and a fistula arising from the bifurcation of the trachea were treated between 1966 and 1989. Eighty-eight percent of the patients survived. For a more detailed analysis, see Ibid., 923-926.

[151]Ibid., 923-927; Gomella *et al.*, 533-534; and Berkow, *The Merck Manual*, 2065-2067. For a more detailed analysis of esophageal atresia with tracheoesophageal fistula, see L. Spitz, E. Keily, R. J. Brereton, "Esophageal Atresia: A Five Year Experience with 148 Cases," *Journal of Pediatric Surgery* 22 (1987): 103-106; J. G. Randolph, K. Newman, K. D. Anderson, "Current Results and Repair of Esophageal Atresia with Tracheoesophageal Fistula Using Physiologic Status as a Guide to Therapy," *Annals of Surgery* 209 (1989): 520-526; and E. C. Pohlson, R. Schaller, and D. Trapper, "Improved Survival with Primary Anastomosis in the Low-Birth-Weight Neonate with Esophageal Atresia and Tracheoesophageal Fistula," *Journal of Pediatric Surgery* 24 (1988): 415-420.

[152]McCormick, "To Save or Let Die," *How Brave a New World?*, 351.

[153]McCormick and Paris, "Saving Defective Infants," *How Brave a New World?*, 358.

[154]It should be noted that McCormick uses the moral principles of charity, autonomy, justice, beneficence, and nonmaleficence to help "en-

flesh" his four norms. For a more detailed analysis of these moral principles, refer to Chapter Four, McCormick's Ethical Criteria section above.

[155]McCormick and Paris, "Saving Defective Infants," *How Brave a New World?*, 360.

[156]For a more detailed analysis of the effects of the Fall on humanity, refer to Chapter Two, McCormick's Theological Anthropology section, Doctrine of the Fall subsection above.

[157]One could assume that because McCormick is a natural law ethicist, albeit revised, in the Catholic Thomistic tradition, that he agrees with Aquinas' understanding of prudence. However, this would be speculation at best. For a detailed analysis of Aquinas' view on prudence, see Aquinas, *Summa Theologica* Ia-IIae, 61.

6

Conclusion

INTRODUCTION

Books, like other forms of communication, are never completely finished products. Rather, they are each one conversation in an ongoing dialogue that hopes to advance the overall discussion by producing new insights and developing new directions. Bernard Lonergan, S.J., explains my point this way:

> For concrete situations give rise to insights which issue
> into policies and courses of action. Action transforms the
> existing situation to give rise to further insights, better
> policies, more effective courses of action. It follows that
> if insight occurs, it keeps recurring; and at each recur-
> rence knowledge develops, action increases its scope,
> and situations improve.[1]

This book has systematically analyzed and critiqued McCormick's ethical methodology as applied to treatment decisions for handicapped neonates. In the process, insights have occurred, which may give rise to a public policy option that will result in a more effective course of action in the treatment of handicapped neonates. At the same time, the insights gained have given rise to further questions that will need to be examined in the future. The aim of this book has not been to conclude the debate surrounding treatment decisions for handicapped neonates, but to deepen our understanding of the issues involved principally through an analysis of McCormick's ethical methodology. Neonatal medical knowledge and technology will continue to advance and new ethical dilemmas will continue to confront us. As a result, new courses of action and further public policies will be needed to meet the new challenges.

The scope of this book has been twofold: First, to articulate, exam-ine, and critically analyze McCormick's ethical methodology. Second, to apply it systematically to five diagnostic treatment categories of handicapped neonates, to determine if this ethical methodology is a viable option for parents and health care professionals in determining treatment decisions for these neonates. This critical analysis is necessitated by the fact that parents and health care professionals are often forced to draw lines between neonates who will be treated and those who will not be. These lines are already being drawn and there is a need for an ethical methodology that can be used by decision-makers to assist them in making these decisions because the life and death of a handicapped neonate hangs in the balance. McCormick offers an ethical methodology that he believes could be beneficial and recommendable to decision-makers. Such an assumption has been clinically tested and now waits to be assessed critically to determine if McCormick's ethical methodology can be a public policy option for the treatment of handicapped neonates.

This chapter will consist of two substantive areas of discussion. The first will focus on a critical assessment of McCormick's ethical methodology as applied to the spectrum of handicapped neonates. Two major questions form the basis for this critical assessment. Is McCormick's ethical methodology practical, beneficial, and appropriate for Christian parents and health care professionals in making treatment decisions for handicapped neonates? Can it be recommended to all decision-makers, both Christian and non-Christian, as a public policy option for the treatment of handicapped neonates? Both of these questions will be critically assessed from McCormick's perspective and from my own perspective. Second, this author will conclude with a personal assessment of what has been learned from McCormick's ethical methodology and from this book.

CRITICAL ASSESSMENT OF MCCORMICK'S ETHICAL METHODOLOGY

Complex bioethical dilemmas challenge society to search for answers and to formulate policies regarding issues ranging from the first moments of life to the last moments before death. Contemporary theologians have been challenged to address these issues from a theological perspective, but there has been little clarity about how this should be done and what impact this will have on reasonable people. Alasdair MacIntyre has attempted to make this challenge more clear. MacIntyre writes:

> What ought we to expect from contemporary theologians
> in the area of medical ethics? First—and without this
> everything else is uninteresting—we ought to expect a

> clear statement of what difference it makes to be a Jew
> or a Christian or a Moslem rather than a secular thinker.[2]

McCormick has attempted to answer MacIntyre's challenge from a Christian perspective. He has specified in his ethical methodology what it means to be a Christian and how the Christian story impacts on the decision-making process in bioethics. After applying his ethical methodology to the five diagnostic treatment categories of handicapped neonates, I must now assess whether his ethical methodology is practical, beneficial, and appropriate for Christian decision-makers.

McCormick believes, and I concur, that his ethical methodology is practical, beneficial, and appropriate for Christian decision-makers in making treatment decisions for handicapped neonates, because it is reasonable and is grounded in the Judaeo-Christian tradition. Before making an assessment on this statement it is first necessary to examine what these terms mean. The term "practical" means useful. In this context, it refers to whether McCormick's ethical methodology is capable of being used or put into effect by Christian decision-makers. Specifically, when it is applied to neonatal anomalies, does it assist Christian decision-makers in coming to a well-reasoned conclusion? Does his ethical methodology give Christian decision-makers various choices within given parameters? "Beneficial" refers to promoting the well-being of the handicapped neonate. When applied to neonatal anomalies, does McCormick's ethical methodology promote the "best interests," normatively understood, of the handicapped neonate and all concerned in the decision-making process? "Appropriate" refers to suitability. Is McCormick's ethical methodology fitting for the needs of particular handicapped neonates? That is, does it adequately consider the relevant medical data, the pertinent circumstances of the situation, the religious and cultural values of the family, and other applicable factors that should be considered in the process of decision-making? These questions will have to be addressed in order to give McCormick's ethical methodology a proper assessment.

As a "revised" natural law ethicist, McCormick believes that reason is shaped by faith, and this shaping takes the form of perspectives, themes, and insights associated with the Christian story.[3] For McCormick, reasoning about the Christian story reveals "the deeper dimensions of the universally human."[4] As a result of this "compenetration" of faith and reason, McCormick relies on a more experiential, commonsense basis for his natural law thinking. Reason can discover and know the basic human goods, and the Christian story nourishes the overall perspectives of the person and serves as a "corrective vision" to the secularism of the culture. McCormick argues that, because his ethical methodology is reasonable and objective, it can be applied to any situation by all reasonable people.

Rooted in "revised" natural law, McCormick believes his ethical methodology is practical for decision-makers because it sets certain parameters for parents in the decision-making process. His ethical methodology is not a wooden formula that parents can apply to any situation and come to a concrete decision. Instead, his ethical methodology illuminates a certain situation so that the facts of the situation are made clearer and the decision-makers can see, as much as possible, the full content and context of the situation. The guidelines, norms, and moral principles that make-up McCormick's moral criteria serve to guide and assist parents and health care professionals, not to make decisions for them. They cannot assure moral certitude. Doubts and conflicts will always be part of the decision-making process. What McCormick's ethical methodology does is to allow parents a certain range of choices, a certain margin of error, a certain space, so that within those parameters they can use prudence to come to a well-reasoned moral decision.[5] As long as the decisions reached are reasonable and do not deviate too far from the neonate's "best interests," normatively understood, these decisions should be respected. McCormick believes, and most parents and health care professionals would agree, that his ethical methodology, being reasonable and grounded in a time honored tradition, can assist Christian decision-makers on a practical level in making treatment decisions for handicapped neonates.

I would agree with McCormick's assessment that his ethical methodology is practical for Christian decision-makers. Rooted in right reason informed by faith, McCormick's ethical methodology keeps Christian decision-makers focused on the "best interests" of the handicapped neonate. The Christian story provides a framework that illuminates the situation for Christian decision-makers. It clarifies what it means to be truly human, thus assisting Christian decision-makers to remain focused on the "best interests" of the neonate. McCormick's quality-of-life criterion sets limits and helps to guide Christian decision-makers in their use of right reason in deciding whether certain medical treatments will promote the "best interests" of the handicapped neonate. McCormick's ethical methodology is practical because it sets up a structure with certain parameters in which Christian decision-makers have the flexibility to use their prudence in making well-reasoned decisions.

To determine if certain medical treatments are beneficial for a handicapped neonate, that is, if they will promote the well-being of the neonate, McCormick proposes his category of "best interests," normatively understood. This is a patient-centered, teleological assessment of what is considered to be in the "best interests" of the handicapped neonate and those involved in the decision-making process. McCormick's "best interests" category is a composite category that involves quality-of-life considerations benefit-burden considerations, and the use of proportionate reason as a tool for establishing what is promotive or destructive for the good of the person "integrally and adequately considered." His understanding of "best interests" is grounded in his "revised" natural law position and in the Judaeo-Christian tradition.[6] McCormick assumes that most people are reasonable, and because they are reasonable that they will choose what is in the "best interests" of the handicapped neonate. He believes this is a safe and protective guideline. McCormick argues that most people want to act reasonably within parameters that are objective in character, even though they do not always do so.[7] In the event that decision-makers fail to act reasonably, McCormick proposes several internal and external safeguards that can be used to protect the neonate's "best interests."

The internal safeguards would be the guidelines, norms, and moral principles McCormick proposes in his quality-of-life criterion. These are objective criteria that can be used by parents and health care professionals in discerning treatment decisions.[8] The external safeguards, proposed by McCormick, are in the form of checks and balances that serve and protect the "best interests" of the neonate against the possibility of irresponsible decision-makers. These checks and balances are both individual and societal. Parents are the primary decision-makers. For McCormick, however, health care professionals should always be consulted because they have the medical expertise, can best explain the diagnosis and prognosis based on similar cases, and they have the ability to compare neonates with the same anomalies and know the effectiveness of various treatments. In this capacity, health care professionals serve as a resource for parents and advocates for the handicapped neonate. McCormick also advocates societal intervention should it be suspected that parents, in consultation with health care professionals, are not acting in a morally responsible manner. These safeguards include both Neonatal Infant Review Committees and the court system.[9]

In my judgment, McCormick's ethical methodology is beneficial in determining treatment decisions for the handicapped neonate, because it is reasonable and it is grounded in a tradition that keeps the focus of the decision on what will promote the "best interests," normatively understood, of the neonate. I agree with McCormick's assumption that most people do want to act reasonably within parameters that are objective in character. His ethical methodology sets those objective parameters and, after applying them to the five diagnostic treatment categories of handicapped neonates, McCormick has shown them to be reasonable. His category of "best interests," normatively understood, allows parents and health care professionals a certain discretion in their decision-making, but at the same time, there are built-in safeguards to protect the neonate against irresponsible decision-making.

McCormick argues that his ethical methodology is appropriate for decision-makers because it considers not only the relevant medical facts and the pertinent circumstances of the situation, but also familial and social factors, such as, religious, cultural, emotional, and financial factors. Parents, in consultation with health care professionals, can best determine what the handicapped neonate ought to want and protect his or her "best interests" by using McCormick's quality-of-life moral criterion. Parents are most knowledgeable about the family situation into which the neonate is born. This includes knowing the financial, emotional, and social factors. Parents can also weigh and balance the religious and cultural values that inform their decision-making. Health care professionals have the specialized medical knowledge and clinical expertise that can assist parents in the decision-making process. They also have a level of objectivity that parents may lack because of the overwhelming emotional stress of the situation. Together, parents and health care professionals are able to determine what are the appropriate needs of this neonate, to assess these needs, and to determine whether medical treatment is in the "best interests" of the neonate "integrally and adequately considered."

In my judgment, McCormick's ethical methodology is appropriate for Christian decision-makers because it emphasizes "the reasonable" from within a Christian context. It stresses the need for decision-makers to examine the medical facts, the circumstances of the situation, foreseeable consequences, social and familial factors, and other pertinent data before deciding on an appropriate course of action. McCormick's ethical methodology also stresses that these facts are to be considered always within the context of the Christian story, so that the "best interests" of the handicapped neonate are always promoted and protected. Treatment decisions for handicapped neonates are value judgments that must be based on the appropriate needs of the neonate. These value judgments can possibly become distorted by self-interested perspectives and technological considerations. Christian decision-makers who use McCormick's ethical methodology are not immune from making mistakes. We are a finite and sinful people. However, because the content of this ethical methodology is reasonable, and because these decisions are made within the context of the Christian story, less chance exists that such treatment decisions will be pushed to the extremes.[10] McCormick's ethical methodology is appropriate for Christian decision-makers because it protects the "best interests" of the handicapped neonate by promoting value judgments that are grounded in reason and informed by the Christian story.

In conclusion, having applied McCormick's ethical methodology to the five diagnostic treatment categories of handicapped neonates, and after a careful personal assessment, I believe McCormick has demonstrated the practicality, beneficial nature, and appropriateness of this ethical methodology for Christian decision-makers. His ethical methodology is not only reasonable and coherent, but is grounded in a tradition that promotes the "best interests," normatively understood, of handicapped neonates.

The second area of concern pertains to whether McCormick's ethical methodology can be recommended to all decision-makers, both Christian and non-Christian, as a public policy option for the treatment of handicapped neonates. If Christian values and norms are open to all reasonable people, does this mean that McCormick's ethical methodology is sustainable without the religious content? That is, once the religious content is stripped away, does McCormick's ethical methodology hold together as a public policy option that can be employed by all reasonable people? To determine if McCormick's ethical methodology can be recommended to all decision-makers, an assessment will have to be made of the three components of a methodology. These components are the formal elements of the methodology itself, the material content of the methodology, and the moral content of its conclusions and judgments. Before this can be accomplished, the phrase "public policy option" must be explained. A public policy option in the bioethical field includes public laws, policies, regulations, and guidelines that bear on ethical aspects of medical practice and health care.[11] A public policy becomes a standard way of operating in a clinical situation by all parties involved. Once a public policy has been approved it begins to take on a life of its own which requires all people, Christian and non-Christian alike, to abide by its laws, guidelines, norms, and principles.

The formal elements of McCormick's ethical methodology concern his anthropology, epistemology, and criteriology. At the formal level, McCormick's ethical methodology is not unique because any valid ethical methodology must contain these formal components. His ethical methodology is rooted in an anthropology that critically reflects on the origin, purpose, and destiny of the human person. It considers human persons precisely in terms of their relationships with God, others, self, and the world. His moral epistemology is a systematic and critical study of morality as a body of knowledge. Specifically, McCormick's moral epistemology is concerned with the human ways of knowing values and disvalues and moral obligations. Finally, once the human ways of knowing have been established, McCormick formulates a set of moral criteria that guide moral reasoning in measuring human actions. At the formal level of methodology, then, McCormick's ethical methodology can be shared by those who are not Christian or even not religious. In my

judgment, it can be recommended to both Christians and non-Christians
at the level of formal content.

The material component of McCormick's ethical methodology is
based on reason informed by the Christian story.[12] For McCormick, the
Christian story as religious content shapes moral perspectives, motivation, and processes of reasoning, but only in a general way. McCormick
writes:

> The Christian story nourishes our overall perspectives,
> telling us through Christ the kinds of people we ought to
> be and become, and the type of world we ought to create.
> It does not give us concrete answers to tragic conflict
> cases or relieve us of the messy and arduous work of
> search, deliberation, and discussion.[13]

The Christian story as religious content informs reason so that our concrete moral deliberations can remain truly human and promote our well-
being.[14] The religious content of McCormick's ethical methodology may
be unique in that it is based on the Christian story and is rooted in the
Judaeo-Christian tradition. However, the uniqueness of religious content
does not translate into the moral content being unique.

The moral content of McCormick's ethical methodology concerns
the question of the distinctiveness of Christian ethics. When McCormick
refers to ethics he is referring to essential ethics.[15] He believes that at the
level of essential ethics, in principle, all reasonable people can reach the
same ethical conclusions because the moral content of ethics is the same
for all. What the Christian tradition does is to illuminate human values,
support them, and provide a context for their reading at any given point
in history.[16] McCormick writes:

> Since there is only one destiny possible to all men, there
> is existentially only one *essential* morality common to
> all men, Christians and non-Christians alike. Whatever is
> distinctive about Christian morality is found essentially
> in the style of life, the manner of accomplishing the
> moral tasks common to all persons, not in the tasks
> themselves. Christian morality is, in its concreteness and
> materiality, *human* morality. The theological study of
> morality accepts the human in all its fullness as its start-
> ing point. It is the *human* which is then illumined by the
> person, teaching and achievement of Jesus Christ. The
> experience of Jesus is regarded as normative because he

is believed to have experienced what it is to be human in the fullest way and at the deepest level.[17]

The Christian faith profoundly affects one's perspectives, analyses, and judgments in very important ways, but not to the point that there are concrete moral demands that are in principle unavailable to human insight and reasoning. McCormick's morality is based on a "revised" notion of natural law; therefore, in principle, all reasonable people can reach the moral truth through human insight and reasoning. McCormick writes:

> Since Christian ethics is the objectification in Jesus Christ of every person's experience of subjectivity, "it does not and cannot add to human ethical self-understanding as such any material content that is, in principle 'strange' or 'foreign' to man as he exists and experiences himself in this world."[18]

What reasoning about the Christian story does is to reveal the deeper dimensions of what it means to be truly human. As a result, McCormick argues that his ethical methodology can be a public policy option for Christians and non-Christians because it is based on human reason and experience.

In my judgment, McCormick's ethical methodology can be recommended to Christians and non-Christians at the material moral content level. The foundation of McCormick's ethical methodology is the centrality of the human person, not the Christian story itself. McCormick bases his ethical methodology on the fact that human nature is essentially the same for all. Therefore, by reason reflecting on human experience, every person, in principle, can know the good that ought to be done and the evil that ought to be avoided. The moral law is not logically dependent on faith or the Christian tradition. The Christian story and symbols nourish the faith of the Christian and affect one's perspectives. They sharpen one's focus on those basic human goods that are definitive of our human flourishing. But they do not originate concrete moral obligations such that they would be considered impervious to human reasoning. The Christian story provides a context or a framework in which human reason can operate. The material moral content of McCormick's ethical methodology is Christian but it is not impervious to human reasoning. I agree with McCormick that what the Christian story does is to aid us in "staying human by underlining the truly human against all cultural attempts to distort the human."[19] The Christian story illuminates who we are as human persons, where we come from, where we are destined, and who we ought to be. It is within this framework, that is knowable to all,

that reason determines what will promote the "best interests" of each individual.[20]

The final element of McCormick's ethical methodology that must be
examined to determine if it can be recommended to all decision-makers
as a public policy option is the content of the moral conclusions or judgments that are drawn from his ethical methodology. McCormick argues
that the Christian story or the religious content of his ethical methodology influences not only personal dispositions, but also moral judgments
in a rather general way.[21] At the level of prediscursive reason, the Christian story sinks deep into the person and sensitizes the person to the
meaning of life and to the values that are definitive of human flourishing.
At the level of discursive reason, the Christian story helps to shape the
person's moral vision. The very meaning, purpose, and value of a person
is grounded and ultimately explained by this story.[22] However, McCormick emphasizes that the moral conclusions or judgments a Christian
reaches will not be substantially different from those yielded by objective
and reasonable but nonreligious analysis. For McCormick, "Christian
emphases do not yield moral norms and rules for decision-making, nor
do they conduce to concrete answers unique to that tradition."[23] In other
words, the sources of faith do not originate concrete moral obligations
that are impervious to human insight and reasoning; however, they do
confirm them. McCormick writes:

> It is persons so informed, persons with such "reasons"
> sunk in their being, who face new situations, new
> dilemmas, and reason together as to what is the best
> policy, the best protocol for the service of all the values.
> They do not find concrete answers in their tradition, but
> they bring a worldview that informs their reasoning—
> especially by allowing basic human goods to retain their
> attractiveness and not be tainted by cultural distortions.[24]

For McCormick, if the insights yielded from the Christian story were
impervious to human reason, then any hope of a public policy option
would be paralyzed in the "irreconcilable stand-off of conflicting stories
and worldviews."[25] Human reason, unaided by explicit faith, can come to
the same insights because they are inherently intelligible and recommendable. Christian insights do not automatically yield moral obligations
but they will deeply condition them.[26]

In my opinion, the moral conclusions or judgments that are derived
from McCormick's ethical methodology are not unique to Christians. By
the light of right reason, in principle, all human persons can know which
actions are objectively morally right and which actions are objectively

morally wrong. This entails a complete analysis of the human person and his or her actions before one can give an adequate account of objectivity. The dignity of the person, the social and relational character of personhood, life as a basic but not an absolute good, and love as the crowning human relationship are foundational Christian insights. The Christian story is not the only cognitive source for these insights. The insights and perspectives that are produced by McCormick's ethical methodology and form the basis for moral conclusions are, in principle, inherently intelligible. They are reasonable and, therefore, can be and are shared by non-Christians.

In applying McCormick's ethical methodology to the five diagnostic treatment categories, it is apparent that the reference point for his ethical methodology is the human person "integrally and adequately considered." In reaching a moral conclusion or judgment for each category of handicapped neonate, a comprehensive analysis was made of both the medical and the non-medical facts. This data was interpreted from a rational point of view. And the "best interests," normatively understood, of the neonate were the primary focus. The moral conclusions produced by applying McCormick's ethical methodology to each diagnostic category are not unique to Christians. Each moral conclusion or judgment is inherently intelligible and recommendable to both Christians and non-Christians. The strength of McCormick's ethical methodology is that reasoning about the Christian story reveals the deeper dimensions of what it means to be truly human.[27]

In conclusion, it is my judgment that McCormick's ethical methodology can be recommended to both Christians and non-Christians as a public policy option for the treatment of handicapped neonates. The formal component of his ethical methodology is firmly rooted in anthropology, epistemology, and criteriology. The moral content of McCormick's ethical methodology is based on reason informed by the Christian story. The human person is the central focus and the Christian story illuminates what it means to be truly human. Finally, the moral conclusions or judgments that a Christian reaches by applying McCormick's ethical methodology are not substantially different from those yielded by an objective and reasonable but nonreligious analysis. If the moral content of McCormick's ethical methodology is reasonable and available, in principle, to all persons, then the moral conclusions derived from it must also be reasonable and available, in principle, to all persons. This is not to say that the individual values that generate a norm cannot experience a special grounding and ratification in revelation. The point is that they are also grounded in human reason and experience.[28]

FUTURE CONSIDERATIONS

McCormick's ethical methodology has much to offer both parents and health care professionals in making treatment decisions for handicapped neonates. In the process of this systematic evaluation of McCormick's ethical methodology as applied to treatment decisions for handicapped neonates, a number of other significant issues relevant to this area have arisen that will need to be examined in the future. First, McCormick argues that the sanctity-of-life ethic and the quality-of-life ethic are not categorically opposed to one another, but that these two approaches are correlated. There is only one ethic that holds life to be an intrinsic value with limits on the patient's moral obligation to pursue this value.[29] McCormick is moving against the stream of ethical consensus in making this claim. However, if his ethical methodology, which includes his quality-of-life criterion, is to be implemented as a public policy option, this distinction should be reexamined, and McCormick's notion that the two ethics are correlated should be reconsidered. This aspect of the quality-of-life approach is essential in a public policy option in order to protect the "best interests" of handicapped neonates.

Second, another major element of the quality-of-life approach that must be further examined and analyzed is the ambiguity that surrounds "medical futility." Together, bioethicists and health care professionals must further clarify the distinction between physiological futility and qualitative futility and how both operate within a quality-of-life criterion. As a public policy option, the quality-of-life criterion advocates a normative understanding of medical futility. For McCormick, a medical treatment might be successful in achieving an effect (physiologically effective), but the effect might not be beneficial to the patient (qualitatively effective). Since the goal of medical treatment is to benefit the patient, it follows that nonbeneficial treatment is medically futile. This is a significant distinction that must be clarified within both the bioethical realm as well as within the medical realm. Health care professionals and bioethicists need to examine this issue critically and enter into a constructive dialogue that will add clarity to this ambiguous and elusive term. Once the terms have been clarified, if this is possible, there is a need for the establishment of guidelines that would concretize qualitative futility. Some will say that such guidelines are impossible to establish, and others will say they are not necessary. This issue will become, and many say has already become, a crucial element in the quality-of-life debate. Unless the term "medical futility" is clarified and guidelines are established for qualitative futility, my fear is that some neonates will continue to be treated who should not be, and others who should be treated will be denied treatment. This could be a form of abuse and even torture, because the qualitative aspect of their treatment has not been adequately considered.[30]

Third, if McCormick's ethical methodology is approved as a public policy option for the treatment of handicapped neonates, then a more constructive and open dialogue needs to be initiated between neonatal health care professionals, bioethicists, and legal professionals. A comprehensive public policy concerning treatment decisions for handicappped neonates requires the expertise and mutual understanding of professionals in these three specialities in order to evaluate all pertinent information. Neonatologists and lawyers need to understand the ethical dimensions surrounding treatment decisions; bioethicists and lawyers need to be more knowledgeable about medical procedures and their consequences; and finally, neonatologists and bioethicists need to be more informed about the possible legal ramifications of certain treatment decisions. This dialogue could be advanced by the establishment of more Neonatal Infant Review Committees. These committees would not only foster constructive dialogue on the ethical, legal, and medical levels, but they could assist parents in their decision-making process by adding a sense of consistency, emotional stability, and impartiality to very difficult medical, ethical, and legal issues.

A major stumbling block to fostering this constructive dialogue through the formation of Neonatal Infant Review Committees seems to be that neonatologists feel threatened to bring cases before such interdisciplinary committees for review. A sense of mistrust seems to pervade the relationships between bioethicists, neonatologists, and lawyers. This may be based more on misperceptions than on facts. There is a need for dialogue between these professionals because, even with the assistance of diagnostic treatment categories, there will always be "gray areas" into which some neonatal anomalies will fall. Treatment decisions in the future regarding these particular handicapped neonates will continue to be highly technical, ethically ambiguous, and legally unprecedented. As neonatal technology and medicine continue to advance and become more complex, it is likely so too will the ethical dilemmas. To meet the challenge concerning the discernment of these treatment decisions, parents will need to rely on the expertise of neonatologists, bioethicists, and lawyers. They cannot be in an adversarial position. Individually, each has valuable knowledge and expertise that is crucial in making these treatment decisions. Together, they act as a safeguard to promote the "best interests" of the handicapped neonate in the event that decision-makers fail to act responsibly. Unless this sense of mistrust is rectified, a constructive dialogue cannot begin, and both parents and neonates could suffer. The implementation of Neonatal Infant Review Committees with a well-balanced, inter-disciplinary membership can bring these essential advocates to the table where a well-informed discussion can lead to recommendations that will be in the "best interests" of these voiceless neonates.

PERSONAL ASSESSMENT—CONCLUSION

In conclusion, this book has made explicit McCormick's ethical methodology and has applied it to five diagnostic treatment categories of handicapped neonates. In a critical assessment of McCormick's ethical methodology and its clinical application, I have shown that it is practical, beneficial, and appropriate for Christian parents and health care professionals to use in making treatment decisions for handicapped neonates, because it is reasonable and is rooted in a time honored tradition. I have also demonstrated that it can be a public policy option for both Christian and non-Christian decision-makers, because the formal and material components of his ethical methodology and the moral content of the conclusions or judgments that are derived from it are reasonable and objective. McCormick's ethical methodology is rooted in the Christian tradition. However, I am convinced that the Christian tradition does not originate moral rules or norms for decision-making. Rather, it informs the Christian person's reason and leads the Christian person to moral conclusions that can, in principle, be known by all reasonable people. In conclusion, I recommend McCormick's ethical methodology to all as a public policy option for the treatment of handicappepd neonates.

Following this recommendation, this book concludes having attempted to advance the ethical dialogue and open up the possibility of further ethical discussions. I have invigorated the ethical dialogue by systematically articulating, examining, and assessing McCormick's ethical methodology. Until now McCormick's ethical methodology was only implied in his writings. Being committed to, as he says, "putting out fires," McCormick never systematically articulated his ethical methodology. As a result, ambiguities and inconsistencies have plagued McCormick and his bioethical positions. The systematic articulation, examination, and assessment of McCormick's ethical methodology in this book will not only help to clarify these ambiguities and inconsistencies, but will also provide people with an ethical strategy to assist them in living a good life in the midst of conflicting values. This is particularly true for parents and health care professionals as they discern treatment decisions for handicapped neonates. McCormick's ethical methodology can assist them in understanding various neonatal anomalies by illuminating the situation and it can guide them in making treatment decisions that are promotive of the "best interests" of the handicapped neonate. As neonatal technology and medicine continue to advance, parents and health care professionals will continue to be called upon to draw lines regarding treatments for handicapped neonates. In my judgment, the future of neonates born with congenital anomalies will be more humane, because McCormick's ethical methodology can now be advanced as a public policy option that will result in more effective courses of action in the medical treatment of handicapped neonates.

Hopefully, this book has represented Richard McCormick as a man of vision and courage. His contributions to moral theology and bioethics have been widely recognized and will have a lasting impact into the future. Though not all will agree with McCormick's moral positions, his rigor and intellectual passion to make a concrete difference in the world have provided both leadership and guidance to a whole generation of Catholic and Protestant, and even non-Christian, readers of his work. He has accomplished this by combining humility with courage, dialogue with decisiveness, and support with criticism.[31] Perhaps McCormick's greatest legacy will be his courage in confronting complex ethical dilemmas, his commitment to formulating well-reasoned moral arguments, and his openness to and respect for the wisdom of his Christian and non-Christian colleagues. This will be his greatest legacy because Richard McCormick and his writings have already begun to have a profound impact on the next generation of bioethicists.

NOTES

[1]Bernard Lonergan, S.J., *Insight: A Study of Human Understanding*, xiv.

[2]Alasdair MacIntyre, "Theological Ethics and the Ethics of Medicine and Health Care," *Journal of Medicine and Philosophy* 4 (1979): 435.

[3]For a more detailed analysis of McCormick's "revised" natural law approach, refer to Chapter One, Bioethical Methodologies section above.

[4]McCormick, *The Critical Calling*, 204. McCormick elaborates on this statement by stating: "a person within the Christian community has access to a privileged articulation, in objective form, of this experience of subjectivity. Precisely because the resources of Scripture, dogma and Christian life (the 'storied community') are the fullest available objectifications of the common human experience, 'the articulation of man's image of his moral good that is possible within historical Christian communities remains privileged in its access to enlarged perspectives on man.'" Ibid.

[5]McCormick and Paris, "Saving Defective Infants," *How Brave a New World?*, 360.

[6]This refers to McCormick's claim that his quality-of-life criterion has its foundation in the traditional ordinary/extraordinary means distinction that was later clarified by Pius XII. For a more detailed analysis, see Pius XII, "The Prolongation of Life," *Acta Apostolicae Sedis*, 1,031-1,032; refer also to Chapter Four, McCormick's Ethical Criteria section above.

[7]McCormick, "The Rights of the Voiceless," *How Brave a New World?*, 104-105.

[8]For a more detailed analysis of McCormick's quality-of-life criterion, refer to Chapter Four, McCormick's Ethical Criteria section above.

[9]For a more detailed analysis of these societal safeguards, refer to Chapter Five, Procedural Issues section above.

[10]The two extremes would range from medical vitalism—preserve life at all costs to medical pessimism—abbreviate the dying process by active euthanasia. The Judaeo-Christian tradition has always walked a middle path, that is, human life is a basic and precious good, but a good to be preserved precisely as the condition of other values. For a more detailed analysis of the Judaeo-Christian tradition's view, see McCormick, "To Save or Let Die," *How Brave a New World?*, 345-346.

[11]For a more detailed analysis of public policy and the bioethical field, see Dan W. Block, "Public Policy and Bioethics," *Encyclopedia of Bioethics*, rev. ed., vol. 4, 2181-2188.

[12]For a more detailed analysis of the Christian story, refer to Chapter Two, McCormick's Theological Anthropology section above.

[13]McCormick, *Health and Medicine in the Catholic Tradition*, 48.

[14]Ibid., 51.

[15]There are four levels in which the term "ethics" can be understood where rightness and wrongness of conduct is concerned. First, essential ethics—this refers to those norms that are regarded as applicable to all persons, where one's behavior is but an instance of a general, essential moral norm. Second, existential ethics—this refers to the choice of a good that the individual as individual should realize, the experience of an absolute ethical demand addressed to the individual. Third, essential Christian ethics—this refers to those ethical decisions a Christian must make precisely because he or she belongs to a community to which the non-Christian does not belong. Finally, existential Christian ethics—this refers to those ethical decisions that the Christian as individual must make, e.g., the choice to concentrate on certain political issues not only because these seem best suited to one's talent, but above all because they seem more in accord with the gospel perspectives. For a more detailed analysis of these four levels, see McCormick, "Does Religious Faith Add to Ethical Perception?" in *Readings in Moral Theology No. 2*, 157-158.

[16]Ibid., 169.

[17]Ibid., 168. Emphasis in the original.

[18]McCormick, *Health and Medicine in the Catholic Tradition*, 60; see also James F. Bresnahan, "Rahner's Christian Ethics," 352.

[19]McCormick, "Does Religious Faith Add to Ethical Perception?" in *Readings in Moral Theology No. 2*, 169.

[20]It should be noted that McCormick is developing an "in principle" argument and he realizes *de facto* that not everyone will adhere to its normative conclusions. Not all people will accept an afterlife, the sacredness of human life, etc. For McCormick, an in principle argument is not a *de facto* argument.

[21]McCormick, "Best Interests of the Baby," 20.

[22]For a more detailed analysis of McCormick's moral epistemology, refer to Chapter Three, McCormick's Dual Moral Epistemology section, Second Moral Epistemology—After 1983 subsection above.

[23]McCormick, "Theology and Biomedical Ethics," 329.

[24]McCormick, "The Judaeo-Christian Tradition and Bioethical Codes," *How Brave a New World?*, 16.

[25]Ibid.

[26]McCormick writes: "The Christian story is not the only cognitive source for the radical sociality of persons, for the immorality of infanticide and abortion, etc. even though historically these insights may be strongly attached to the story. In this epistemological sense, these insights are not specific to Christians. They can be and are shared by others." Ibid., 329-330.

[27]McCormick, "Theology and Biomedical Ethics," 331.

[28]McCormick, "Does Religious Faith Add to Ethical Perception?," in *Readings in Moral Theology No. 2*, 163.

[29]For a more detailed analysis of McCormick's position on the correlation of the sanctity-of-life ethic and the quality-of-life ethic, see McCormick, "The Quality of Life, The Sanctity of Life," *How Brave a New World?*, 393-411; refer also to Chapter Four,

[30]Peter A. Clark, S.J., "Medical Futility in Pediatrics: Is it Time for a Public Policy?" 66-89.

[31]Charles E. Curran, "Why This Book?" in *Moral Theology: Challenges for the Future*, 10.

Bibliography

PRIMARY SOURCES

McCormick, S.J., Richard A. "Ghosts in the Wings." *America* 86 (January 5, 1952): 377-379.

_____. "Standards and the Stagirite." *America* 87 (May 3, 1952): 135-137.

_____. *The Removal of a Fetus Probably Dead to Save the Life of the Mother.* Rome: Pontifica Universitas Gregoriana, 1957.

_____. "The Primacy of Charity." *Perspectives* (August-September 1959): 18-27.

_____. "Adolescent Masturbation: A Pastoral Problem." *Homiletic and Pastoral Review* 60 (March 1960): 527-540.

_____. Review of *The Primacy of Charity in Moral Theology*, by Gerald Gilleman. In *The Priest* 16 (July 1960): 346-347.

_____. Review of *Morality and the Homosexual*, by Michael J. Buckley. In *Homiletic and Pastoral Review* 61 (August 1960): 1031-1034.

_____. "Adolescent Affection: Toward a Sound Sexuality." *Homiletic and Pastoral Review* 61 (December 1960): 244-261.

_____. Review of *Counseling the Catholic*, by George Hagmaier. In *Review for Religious* 19 (1960): 391.

_____. Review of *Population, Resources, and the Future*, by William J. Gibbons. In *The Catholic World* 194 (October 1961): 56-59.

_____. "Moral Considerations in Autopsy." *Linacre Quarterly* 28 (November 1961): 161- 169.

_____. Review of *Family Planning and Modern Problems*, by Stanislas de Lestapsis. In *America* 106 (December 9, 1961): 370.

_____. "Anti-Fertility Pills." *Homiletic and Pastoral Review* 62 (May 1962): 692-700.

_____. Review of *Alcoholism and Society*, by Morris E. Chafetz. In *America* 107 (June 9, 1962): 386-387.

_____. Review of *Our Crowded Planet*, by Fairfled Osborn, ed. In *America* 107 (November 3, 1962): 1000-1001.

_____. "Is Professional Boxing Immoral?" *Sports Illustrated* 17 (November 5, 1962): 71- 72, 74, 76, 78-80, 82.

_____. "Heterosexual Relationships in Adolescence." *Review for Religious* 22 (January 1963): 57-92; reprinted as "Heterosexual Relationships in Adolescence: The Ideal and the Problem," In *Adolescence: Special Cases and Special Problems,* by Raymond J. Steimel, ed. Washington, DC: The Catholic University of America Press, 1963, 42-65.

_____. Review of *Birth Control and Catholics,* by George A. Kelly. In *America* 109 (October 19, 1963): 465-466.

_____. "Conjugal Love and Conjugal Morality." *America* 110 (January 11, 1964): 38-42.

_____. Review of *Marriage Questions: Contemporary Moral Theology, Vol. II,* by John C. Ford and Gerald Kelly. In *America* 110 (January 18, 1964): 112.

_____. Review of *Personality and Sexual Problems,* by William C. Bier, ed. In *America* 110 (May 23, 1964): 738.

_____. "Toward a Dialogue." *Commonweal* 80 (June 5, 1964): 313-317.

_____. Review of *Love in Marriage,* by Henri Gilbert. In *America* 111 (June 27, 1964): 870.

_____. "Whither the Pill." *The Catholic World* 199 (July 1964): 207-214.

_____. Review of *Psychiatry and Religious Faith,* by Robert G. Gassert. In *America* 111 (September 19, 1964): 312-313.

_____. "Psychosexual Development in Religious Life." *Review for Religious* 23 (November 1964): 724-741.

_____. Review of *Contraception and Catholics,* by Louis Dupre. In *America* 111 (November 14, 1964): 628-629.

_____. Review of *Contraception and Holiness,* introduction by Archbishop Thomas D. Roberts. In *America* 111 (November 14, 1964): 624-628.

_____. "Family Size, Rhythm, and the Pill." Chap. in *The Problem of Population: Moral and Theological Considerations,* ed. Donald N. Barrett, 58-84. South Bend, IN:University of Notre Dame Press, 1965, 58-84.

_____. "The Priest and Teen-age Sexuality." *The Homiletic and Pastoral Review* 65 (February 1965): 379-387.

_____. Review of *The Authentic Morality,* by Ignace Lepp. In *America* 112 (March 27, 1965): 433-434.

_____. Review of *Christian Renewal in a Changing World,* by Bernard Häring. In *America* 112 (March 27, 1965): 433.

_____. "Abortion." *America* 112 (June 19, 1965): 877-881.

_____. Review of *Contraception and the Natural Law,* by Germain G. Grisez. In *The American Ecclesiastical Review* 153 (August 1965): 119-125.

_____. "Toward a New Sexuality." *The Catholic World* 202 (October 1965): 10-16.

_____. Review of *Sin, Liberty, and Law*, by Louis Monden. In *America* 113 (November 13, 1965): 602-604.

_____. "Notes on Moral Theology." *Theological Studies* 16 (December 1965): 596-662.

_____. "Practical and Theoretical Considerations." Chap. in *The Problem of Population: Vol. III Educational Considerations*, 50-73. South Bend, IN: The University of Notre Dame Press, 1964.

_____. "The Council on Contraception." *America* 114 (January 8, 1966): 47-48.

_____. "The History of a Moral Problem." *America* 114 (January 29, 1966): 174-178.

_____. "Worship in Common." *Catholic Mind* 64 (April 1966): 20-25.

_____. "General Confession." *Catholic Mind* 64 (May 1966): 10-12.

_____. Review of *The Time of Salvation*, by Bernard Häring. In *America* 114 (June 18, 1966): 859-860.

_____. "Modern Morals in a Muddle." *America* 115 (July 30, 1966): 116.

_____. "The Polygraph in Business and Industry." *Theological Studies* 27 (September 1966): 421-433.

_____. "Notes on Moral Theology." *Theological Studies* 17 (December 1966): 607-654.

_____. "Abortion and Moral Principles." Chap. in *The Wrong of Abortion*, 1-13. New York: America Press, 1966.

_____. "Conjugal Morality." Chap. in *Married Love and Children*, 24-32. New York: America Press, 1966.

_____. "Panel Talk on Curriculum: Anti-Semitism and Christian Ethics." Chap. in *Judaism and the Christian Seminary Curriculum*. Edited by J. Bruce Long, 94-98. Chicago, IL: Loyola University Press, 1966.

_____. Review of *Christian Maturity*, by Bernard Häring. In *America* 116 (April 8, 1967): 538.

_____. Review of *The Human Mystery of Sexuality*, by Marc Oraison. In *Homiletic and Pastoral Review* 67 (May 1967): 707-708.

_____. "Conference with Consensus." *America* 117 (September 23, 1967): 320-321.

_____. "Aspects of the Moral Question." *America* 117 (December 9, 1967): 716-719.

_____. "Notes on Moral Theology: January-June, 1967." *Theological Studies* 67 (May 1967): 749-800.

____. Review of *The Celibate Condition and Sex*, by Marc Oraison. In *Homiletic and Pastoral Review* 68 (February 1968): 446-448.

____. "The New Morality." *America* 118 (June 15, 1968): 769-772.

____. "Past Church Teaching on Abortion." *CTSA Proceedings* 23 (June 17-21, 1968): 131-151.

____. "Notes on Moral Theology: January-June, 1968." *Theological Studies* 29 (December 1968): 679-741.

____. "Human Significance and Christian Significance." Chap. in *Norm and Content In Christian Ethics*. Edited by Gene H. Outka and Paul Ramsey, 233-261. New York: Charles Scribner and Sons, 1968.

____. "The Moral Theology of Vatican II." Chap. in *The Future of Ethics and Moral Theology*, 7-18. Chicago, IL: Argus Communications, 1968.

____. "The Theology of Revolution." *Catholic Mind* 67 (April 1969): 23-32.

____. "When Priests Marry." *America* 120 (April 19, 1969): 471-474.

____. Review of *The Catholic Case for Contraception*, by Daniel Callahan. In *America* 120 (May 24, 1969): 239-254.

____. "The Teachings of the Magisterium and Theologians." *CTSA Proceedings* 24 (June 16-19, 1969): 239-254.

____. "Reflections on Sunday Observance." *The American Ecclesiastical Review* 161 (July 1969): 55-61.

____. "Notes on Moral Theology: January-June, 1969." *Theological Studies* 30 (December 1969): 635-692.

____. "Christian Morals." *America* 122 (January 10, 1970): 5-6.

____. "Ethics of Political Protest." *Catholic Mind* 68 (March 1970): 11-12.

____. "What We Expect from a Priest—What He Expects from Us." *Emmanuel* 76 (April 1970): 163-166.

____. Review of *Who Shall Live?*, by Kenneth Vaux. In *America* 122 (April 18, 1970): 424-425.

____. Review of *Contemporary Problems in Moral Theology*, by Charles E. Curran. In *America* 122 (May 16, 1970): 527.

____. Review of *Road to Relevance*, by Bernard Häring. In *America* 122 (May 16, 1970): 527.

____. "Loyalty and Dissent: The Magisterium—A New Model." *America* 122 (June 27, 1970): 674-676.

____. "A Moralist Report." *America* 123 (July 11, 1970): 22-23.

____, George W. MacRae, and Ladislas Örsy. "Brussels Hosts the Theologians." *America* 123 (October 3, 1970): 232, 234.

____. "Notes on Moral Theology: April-September, 1970." *Theological Studies* 23 (March 1971): 66-122.

____. Review of *Abortion: The Myths, the Realities, and the Arguments*, y Germain Grisez. In *America* 124 (April 17, 1971): 412-413.

____. "Presidential Address." *CTSA Proceedings* 26 (June 14-17, 1971): 239-250.

____. Review of *Morality Is for Persons*, by Bernard Häring. In *America* 125 (September 11, 1971): 155-159.

____. "Not What Catholic Hospitals Ordered." *America* 125 (September 11, 1971): 155- 159; reprint, *Linacre Quarterly* 39 (February 1972): 16-20.

____. *"Vom Umgang Mit Dem Lebensraum,"* *Theologie der Gegenwart* 14 (1971): 209- 216.

____. Review of *Christian Ethics and the Community*, by James Gustafson. In *America* 126 (February 26, 1972): 214-215.

____. "Notes on Moral Theology: April-September, 1971." *Theological Studies* 33 (March 1972): 68-119.

____. "Autonomy and Coercion: Moral Values in Medical Practice." *Linacre Quarterly* 39 (May 1972): 101-105; reprint, *Catholic Mind* 71 (March 1973): 8-11.

____. Review of *Catholic Moral Theology in Dialogue*, by Charles E. Curran. In *America* 127 (July 22, 1972): 44-45.

____. "Genetic Medicine: Notes on the Moral Literature." *Theological tudies* 33 (September 1972): 531-552; reprinted in *Moral Theology No. 10*. eds. Martin E. Marty and Dean G. Peerman. New York: The Macmillan Company, 1973.

____, and CTSA Study Committee. "The Problem of Second Marriages: An Interim Pastoral Statement by the Study Committee Commissioned by the Board of Directors of CTSA-Report of August 1972." *CTSA Proceedings* 27 (September 1-4, 1972): 234-240; reprint, *America* 127 (October 27, 1972): 258-260.

____. "The New Directives and Institutional Medico-Moral Responsibility." *Chicago Studies* 11 (Fall 1972): 305-314.

____. "Theologians View the Directives." *Hospital Progress* 53 (December 1972): 51, 53, 54, 68.

____. "Theologians View the Directives." *Hospital Progress* 54 (February 1973): 73-74.

____. "The Abortion Ruling: Analysis and Prognosis Commentary: Fr. McCormick." *Hospital Progress* 54 (March 1973): 85, 96.

____. "Notes on Moral Theology: April-September, 1972." *Theological Studies* 34 (March 1973): 53-102.

____. "The Silence Since *Humanae Vitae*." *America* 129 (July 21, 1973): 30-33; reprint, *Linacre Quarterly* 41 (Fall 1974): 26-32.

____. "What the Silence Means." *America* 129 (October 20, 1973): 287-290.

____. "The New Medicine and Morality." *Theology Digest* 21 (Winter 1973): 308-321.

____. *Ambiguity in Moral Choice*. Milwaukee, WI: Marquette University Press, 1973.

____. "Issue Areas for a Medical Ethics Program." Chap. in *The Teaching of Medical Ethics*, eds. Robert M. Veatch, Willard Gaylin, and Councilman Morgen, 103-114. New York: Hastings Center Publication, 1973.

____. "The Problem of Motivation." Chap. in *The Population Crisis and Moral Responsibility*, ed. J. Philip Wogaman, 320-323. Washington, DC: Public Affairs Press, 1973.

____. "Response to Professor Curran-II." *CTSA Proceedings* 29 (June 10-13, 1974): 161-164.

____. "Notes on Moral Theology: The Abortion Dossier." *Theological Studies* 35 (June 1974): 312-359.

____. "To Save or Let Die." *America* 130 (July 13, 1974): 6-10; simultaneously published in *The Journal of the American Medical Association* 229 (July 1974): 172-176.

____. "The Teaching Role of the Magisterium—And of the Theologians." *The Catholic Leader* (August 11-17, 1974): 7-8.

____. "Fr. Richard McCormick, S.J., On Pope Paul's Encyclical '*Humanae Vitae*' and the Church's Magisterium." *The Catholic Leader* (September 22-28, 1974): 10-16.

____. "To Save or Let Die: State of the Question." *America* 131 (October 5, 1974): 169-173.

____. "Personal Conscience." *Chicago Studies* 13 (Fall 1974): 241-252.

____. "Proxy Consent in the Experimentation Situation." *Perspectives in Biology and Medicine* 18 (Autumn 1974): 2-12; reprinted in *Love and Society: Essays in the Ethics of Paul Ramsey*, eds. James T. Johnson and David H. Smith, 209-227. Missoula, MT: Scholars Press, 1974).

____. "The Concept of Authority." Chap. in *Seminar on Authority: The Proceedings of A Dialogue Between Catholics and Baptists Sponsored by the Ecumenical Institute of Wake Forest University and Belmont Abbey College*, ed. J. William Angel, 9-18. Winston-Salem, NC: The Ecumenical Institute of Wake Forest University, 1974.

____. "H. V. In Perspective." *The Tablet* (February 8, 1975): 126-128.

____. "Notes on Moral Theology: April-September, 1974." *Theological Studies* 36 (March 1975): 77-129.

____. "Life-Saving and Life-Taking: A Commentary." *Linacre Quarterly* 42 (May 1975): 110-115.

____. "Fetal Research, Morality, and Public Policy." *The Hastings Center Report* 5 (June 1975): 26-31.

____, and Leroy Walters. "Fetal Research and Public Policy." *America* 132 (June 21, 1975): 473-476.

____. "The Social Responsibility of the Christian." *The Australian Catholic Record* 52 (July 1975): 253-262; reprint, *Theology Digest* 24 (Spring 1976): 11-14.

____. "Life/Death Decisions: An Interview with Moral Theologian Fr. Richard McCormick, S.J." *St. Anthony Messenger* 83 (August 1975): 33-35.

____. "A Proposal for 'Quality of Life' Criteria for Sustaining Life." *Hospital Progress* 56 (September 1975): 503-509.

____. "Transplantation of Organs: A Commentary on Paul Ramsey." *Theological Studies* 36 (September 1975): 76-79.

____. "Indissolubility and the Right to the Eucharist: Separate Issues or One?" *Canon Law Society of America Proceedings of the 37th Annual Convention* (October 6-9, 1975): 26-37.

____. "Divorce and Remarriage." *Catholic Mind* 73 ((November 1975): 42-57; reprinted as *Scheidung Und Wiederverheiratung. Theologie Der Gegenwart* 18 (1975): 210- 220.

____. "The Karen Ann Quinlan Case: Editorial." *Journal of the American Medical Association* 234 (December 8, 1975): 1057.

____. "Experimentation on the Fetus: Policy Proposals." Chap. in *Appendix: Research on the Fetus.* Washington, DC: U.S. Department of Health, Education, and Welfare Publication, 1975.

____. "The Insights of the Judeo-Christian Tradition and the Development of an Ethical Code." Chap. in *Human Rights and Psychological Research: A Debate on Psychology and Ethics,* ed. Eugene Kennedy, 23-36. New York: Thomas Y. Crowell, 1975.

____. "Sexual Ethics—An Opinion." *National Catholic Reporter* 12 (January 30, 1976): 9.

____. "Notes on Moral Theology: April-September, 1975." *Theological Studies* 37 (March 1976): 70-119.

____. "The Preservation of Life." *Linacre Quarterly* 43 (May 1976): 94-100.

____. "Experimental Subjects: Who Should They Be?" *Journal of the American Medical Association* 235 (May 17, 1976): 2197.

____. "The Social Responsibility of the Christian." *Theology Digest* 24 (Spring 1976): 11-14.

____. "When the Neonate is Defective." *Contemporary Ob/Gyn* 7 (June 1976): 90, 92, 95-96, 99, 103, 107, 109, 111-112.

____. "The Moral Right of Privacy." *Hospital Progress* 57 (August 1976): 38-42.

____. "Sterilization and Theological Method." *Theological Studies* 37 (September 1977): 471-477.

____. "Experimentation in Children: Sharing in Sociality." *Hastings Center Report* 6 (December 1976): 41-46.

____. "The Principle of Double Effect." *Concilium* 120 (December 1976): 105-120.

____. "*Römische Erklärung Zur Sexualethik.*" *Theologie der Gegenwart* 19 (1976): 72- 76.

____. "Morality of War." *New Catholic Encyclopedia* 14 (1976): 802-807.

____. "Maker of Heaven and Earth." Chap. in *Christian Theology: A Case Method Approach*, eds. Robert A. Evans and Thomas E. Parker, 88-93. New York: Harper and Row, 1976.

____, and Andre Hellegers. "Legislation and the Living Will." *America* 136 (March 12, 1977): 210-213.

____. "Notes on Moral Theology: 1976." *Theological Studies* 38 (March 1977): 54-114.

____. "'Sleeper' on DNA." *National Catholic Reporter* (July 15, 1977): 9.

____. "Man's Moral Responsibility For Health." *Catholic Hospital* 5 (July-August 1977): 6-9.

____, et al. "A. C.& C. Symposium: Paying for Abortion: Is the Court Wrong?" *Christianity and Crisis* 37 (September 19, 1977): 202-207.

____. "Christianity and Morality." *Catholic Mind* 75 (October 1977): 17-29.

____. "*Sterilisation und Theologische Methode.*" *Theologie der Gegenwart* 20 (1977): 110-114.

____. "The Quality of Life, The Sanctity of Life." *Hastings Center Report* 8 (February 1978): 30-36.

____. "Notes on Moral Theology: 1977." *Theological Studies* 39 (March 1978): 76-138.

____. "Abortion: Rules for Debate." *America* 139 (July15-22, 1978): 26-30.

_____, and Andre Hellegers. "Unanswered Questions on Test Tube Life." *America* 139 (August12-19, 1978): 74-78

_____. "Some Neglected Aspects of Responsibility for Health." *Perspectives in Biology and Medicine* 22 (1978): 31-43.

_____. "Moral Norms and Their Meaning." *Lectureship* (Mt. Angel Seminary, 1978): 31- 47.

_____. "The Contemporary Moral Magisterium." *Lectureship* (Mt. Angel Seminary, 1978): 48-60.

_____, and Paul Ramsey, eds. *Doing Evil to Achieve Good: Moral Choice in Conflict Situations.* Chicago, IL: Loyola University Press, 1978.

_____. "Reproductive Technologies." In Vol. 4, *Encyclopedia of Bioethics.* Ed. Warren Reich. New York: Free Press, 1978, 1454-1464.

_____. "Freedman on the Rights of the Voiceless." *Journal of Medicine and Philosophy* 3 (1978): 211-221.

_____. "Abortion: A Changing Morality and Policy." *Hospital Progress* 60 (February 1979): 36-44.

_____. "Bioethical Issues and the Moral Matrix of U. S. Health Care." *ospital Progress* 60 (May 1979): 42-45.

_____, and Charles E. Curran, eds. *Readings in Moral Theology No. 1: Moral Norms and Catholic Tradition.* Mahwah, NJ: Paulist Press, 1979.

_____. "Notes on Moral Theology: 1978." *Theological Studies* 40 (1979): 59-112.

_____. "Restatement on Tubal Ligation Confuses Policy with Normative Ethics." *Hospital Progress* 61 (September 1980): 40.

_____. "The Fox Case." *Journal of the American Medical Association* 244 (November 14, 1980): 2165-2166.

_____, and Charles E. Curran, eds. *Readings in Moral Theology No. 2: The Distinctiveness of Christian Ethics.* Mahwah, NJ: Paulist Press, 1980.

_____, and Corrine Bayley. "Sterilization: The Dilemma of Catholic Hospitals." *America* 143 (1980): 222-225.

_____. *Notes on Moral Theology: 1965 through 1980* Washington, DC: University Press of America, 1980.

_____. "The Preservation of Life and Self-Determination." *Theological Studies* 41 (1980): 390-396.

_____, Barbara Gastel *et al,* eds. *Maternal Serum Alpha-Fetoprotein: Issues in the Prenatal Screening and Diagnosis of Neural Tube Defects.* Washington, DC: Government Printing Office, 1980, 128-129.

____. "No Short Cuts to Making Public Policy on Abortion." *Washington Star*, 23 March 1981.

____. "Marriage, Morality and Sex-Change Surgery: Four Traditions in Case Ethics." *Hastings Center Report* 11 (August 1981): 10-11.

____. "The Fifth Synod of Bishops." *Catholic Mind* 79 (September 1981): 46-57.

____, and William Barclay *et al.* "The Ethics of In Utero Surgery." *Journal of the American Medical Association* 246 (October 2, 1981): 1550-1555.

____. "Guidelines for the Treatment of the Mentally Retarded." *Catholic Mind* 79 (November 1981): 44-51.

____. "Theology as a Dangerous Discipline." *Georgetown Graduate Review* 1 (1981): 2-3.

____. *How Brave a New World?: Dilemmas in Bioethics.* Garden City, NY: Doubleday, 1981.

____, and Charles E. Curran, eds. *Readings in Moral Theology No. 3: Morality and the Magisterium.* Mahwah, NJ: Paulist Press, 1981.

____. "Notes on Moral Theology: 1980." *Theological Studies* 42 (1981): 74-121.

____. *"Kernenergie und Kernwaffen."* *Theologie der Gegenwart* 24 (1981): 147-156.

____. *"Scheidung und Wiederverheiratung als Pastorales Problem."* *Theologie der Gegenwart* 24 (1981): 21-32.

____. "Living Will Legislation, Reconsidered." *America* 145 (1981): 86-89.

____. "Infant Doe: Where to Draw the Line." *Washington Post*, 27 July 1982, 15 (A).

____. *"Les Sions Intensifs aux Nouveau-Nés Handicapés."* *Études* (November 1982): 493-502.

____. "Ethical Issues: A Look at the Issues." *Contemporary Ob/Gyn* 20 (November 1982): 227-232.

____. "1973-1983: Value Impacts of a Decade." *Hospital Progress* 63 (December 1982): 38-41.

____. "Pastoral Guidelines for Facing the Ambiguous Eighties." *The Future of Ministry* (Milwaukee, WI: St. Francis Seminary, 1982): 41-44.

____. *"Neuere Überlegungen zur Unveränderlichkeit Sittlicher Normen."* In *Sittliche Normen.* Edited by Walter Kerber, S.J. Düsseldorf: Patmos, 1982, 46-57.

____. "Notes on Moral Theology: 1981." *Theological Studies* 43 (1982): 69-124.

____. "Theology and Biomedical Ethics." *Église et Theologie* 13 (1982): 311-332.

____. "Theological Dimensions of Bioethics." *Logos* 3 (1982): 25-46.

____. "Notes on Moral Theology: 1982." *Theological Studies* 44 (1983): 71-122.

____. "Bioethics in the Public Forum." *Milbank Memorial Fund Quarterly* 61 (1983): 113-126.

____, and John Paris, S.J. "Saving Defective Infants: Options for Life or Death." *America* 148 (1983): 313-317.

____. "Nuclear Deterrence and the Problem of Intention: A Review of Positions." In *Catholics and Nuclear War*. Edited by Philip Murnion. New York: Crossroad, 1983, 168-182.

____, and Charles E. Curran, eds. *Readings in Moral Theology No. 4: The Use of Scripture in Moral Theology*. Mahwah, NJ: Paulist Press, 1984.

____. *Health and Medicine in the Catholic Tradition*. New York: Crossroad, 1984.

____. "Notes on Moral Theology: 1983." *Theological Studies* 45 (1984): 80-138.

____. "The Chill Factor: Recent Roman Interventions." *America* 150 (1984): 475-481.

____. *Notes on Moral Theology: 1981 through 1984*. Lanham, MD: University Press of America, 1984.

____. "Medicaid and Abortion." *Theological Studies* 45 (1984): 715-721.

____. "Was There Real Hope for Baby Fae." *Hastings Center Report* 15 (February 1985): 12-13.

____. "Genetic Technology and Our Common Future." *America* 152 (1985): 337-342.

____. "Caring or Starving? The Case of Clare Conroy." *America* 152 (1985): 269-273.

____. "Theology and Bioethics." In *Theology and Bioethics*. Edited by Earl Shelp. Dordrecht, Netherlands: Reidel, 1985, 95-114.

____. "Moral Argument in Christian Ethics." *Journal of Contemporary Health Law and Policy* 1 (1985): 3-23.

____. "Notes on Moral Theology: Moral Norms—an Update." *Theological Studies* 46 (1985): 50-64.

____. "Therapy or Tampering?: The Ethics of Reproductive Technology." *America* 153 (1985): 396-403.

____. "Gustafson's God: Who? What? Where? (etc.)." *Journal of Religious Ethics* 13 (1985): 53-70.

____. "The Past, Present, and Future of Moral Theology." *Proceedings of 1984 Theological Symposium*. Villanova, PA: Villanova University Press, 1985.

____. "The Magisterium." In *Authority, Community and Conflict*. Edited by Madonna Kolbenschlag. Kansas City, KS: Sheed and Ward, 1986, 34-37.

____. "*Gaudium et Spes* and the Biological Times." In *Questions of Special Urgency*. Edited by Judith Dwyer. Washington, DC: Georgetown University Press, 1986, 79- 95.

____. "Health and Medicine in the Catholic Tradition." *Ephemerides Theologicae Lovanienses* 62 (1986): 207-215.

____. "Symposium: Bioethical Issues in Organ Transplantation." *Southern Medical Journal* 79 (1986): 1471-1479.

____. "The Best Interests of the Baby." *Second Opinion* 2 (1986): 18-25.

____. "Biomedical Advances and the Catholic Perspective." In *Contemporary Ethical Issues in the Jewish and Christian Traditions*. Edited by Frederick Greenspahn. Hoboken, NJ: Ktav Publishing House, 1986, 30-52.

____. "The Search for Truth in the Catholic Context." *America* 155 (1986): 276-281.

____. "*L'Affaire Curran*." *America* 154 (1986): 261-267.

____, and Charles E. Curran, eds. *Readings in Moral Theology No. 5: Official Catholic Social Teaching*. Mahwah, NJ: Paulist Press, 1986.

____. "Notes on Moral Theology: 1985." *Theological Studies* 47 (1986): 69-88.

____. "Bishops as Teachers and Jesuits as Listeners." *Studies in the Spirituality of Jesuits* 18 (1986): 1-22.

____. Review of *Selective Nontreatment of Handicapped Newborns*, by Robert Weir. In *Perspectives in Biology and Medicine* 29 (Winter 1986): 327-329.

____. "Finality," "Double Effect," "Magisterium." In *Dictionary of Christian Ethics*. Edited by James Childress and John Macquarrie. Philadelphia, PA: Westminister, 1986.

____. "Ethics of Reproductive Technology: A. F. S. Recommendations, Dissent." *Health Progress* 68 (March 1987): 33-37.

____. "Document Is Unpersuasive." *Health Progress* 68 (July/August 1987): 53-55.

____. "Notes on Moral Theology: Dissent in Moral Theology and Its Implications." *Theological Studies* 48 (1987): 87-105.

____. "Surrogate Motherhood: A Stillborn Idea." *Second Opinion* 5 (1987): 128-132.

____. "Self-Assessment and Self-Indictment." *Religious Studies Review* 13 (1987): 37- 39.

____. "The Vatican Document on Bioethics." *America* 156 (1987): 24-28.

____. "The Vatican Document on Bioethics: A Response." *America* 156 (1987): 247- 248.

____, and John Paris, S.J. "The Catholic Tradition on the Use of Nutrition and Fluids." *America* 156 (1987): 356-361.

____. "Begotten, Not Made." *Notre Dame Magazine* 15 (1987): 22-25.

____. "Bishops' AIDS Letter 'Splendie' Theology." *National Catholic Reporter* 24 (January 22, 1988): 1, 5-6.

____. "Searching for the Consistent Ethic of Life." In *Personalist Morals*. Edited by J. A. Selling. Leuven: Leuven University Press, 1988, 135-146.

____. "A Moral Magisterium in Ecumenical Perspective?" *Studies in Christian Ethics* 1 (1988): 20-29.

____. "AIDS: The Shape of the Ethical Challenge." *America* 158 (1988): 147-154.

____. "The Shape of Moral Evasion in Catholicism." *America* 159 (1988): 183-188.

____, and Charles E. Curran, eds. *Readings in Moral Theology No. 6: Dissent in the Church*. Mahwah, NJ: Paulist Press, 1988.

____. "The Cost-Factor in Health Care." *Notre Dame Journal of Law, Ethics and Public Policy* 3 (1988): 161-167.

____. "Abortion: The Unexpected Middle Ground." *Second Opinion* 10 (March 1989): 41-50.

____. "Theology and Bioethics." *Hastings Center Report* 19 (March/April 1989): 5-10.

____. *The Critical Calling: Moral Dilemmas Since Vatican II*. Washington, DC: Georgetown University Press, 1989.

____. "Moral Theology 1940-1989: An Overview." *Theological Studies* 50 (1989): 3-24.

____. "Pluralism Within the Church." In *Catholic Perspectives on Medical Morals*. Edited by Edmund D. Pellegrino, John P. Langan, and John Harvey Collins. Dordrecht: Kluwer Academic Publishers, 1989, 147-167.

____. "Foreword." In *Why You Can Disagree and Remain a Faithful Catholic*, by Philip S. Kaufman. Bloomington, IN: Meyer-Stone Books, 1989, xi-xii.

____. "Sterilization: The Dilemma of Catholic Hospitals." In *History and Conscience*. Edited by R. Gallagher and Brendan McConvery. Southampton: Camelot Press, 1989, 105-122.

____. "Technology and Morality: An Example of Medicine." *New Theology Review* 2 (November 1989): 20-34.

____. "The Cruzon Decision: Missouri's Contribution." *Midwest Medical Ethics* 5 (1989): 3-6.

____. "Why Moral Decisions Should Not Be Left to Chance: An Interview." *U.S. Catholic* 55 (Fall 1990): 6-13.

____. "The First 14 Days." *The Tablet* 201 (March 10, 1990): 301-304.

____. "Clear and Convincing Evidence: The Case of Nancy Cruzon." *Midwest Medical Ethics* 6 (Fall 1990): 10-12.

____. "Changing My Mind About the Changeable Church." *The Christian Century* 107 (August 8-15, 1990): 732-736.

____. "*L'Affaire Curran II*." *America* 163 (1990): 127-132.

____. "Who or What Is the Pre-embryo?" *Kennedy Institute of Ethics Journal* 1 (March 1991): 1-15.

____. "The Pre-embryo as Potential: A Reply to John A. Robertson." *Kennedy Institute of Ethics Journal* 4 (December 1991): 303-305.

____. "Theology as Public Responsibility." *America* 165 (September 28, 1991): 184- 189.

____, and Charles E. Curran, eds. *Readings in Moral Theology No. 7: Natural Law and Theology*. Mahwah, NJ: Paulist Press, 1991.

____, and Sanford Leikin. "Terminal Illness and Suicide." *Ethics and Behavior* 1 (1991): 63-68.

____. "Henry the Unknown." *Ethics and Behavior* 1 (1991): 66-68.

____. "Physician-Assisted Suicide: Flight from Compassion." *Christian Century* 108 (December 4, 1991): 1132-1134.

____. "Behind the Scenes: Some Underlying Issues in Bioethics." *Catholic Library World* 63 (January-June 1992): 156-162.

____. "Moral Considerations: Ill-Considered." *America* 166 (March 14, 1992): 210-214.

____. "Moral Theology in the Year 2000: Tradition in Transition." *America* 166 (April 18, 1992): 312-318.

____. "Surrogacy: A Catholic View." *Creighton Law Review* 25 (1992): 1617-1634.

____. "Document Begets Many Legitimate Moral Questions." *National Catholic Reporter* 29 (October 15, 1993): 17.

____. "*Veritatis Splendor*." *Commentary* 12 (1993): 10-15.

____. "*Humanae Vitae*: 25 Years Later." *America* 169 (July 17-14, 1993): 6-8.

____. "Value Variables in Health Care Reform Debate." *America* 168 (May 29, 1993): 7- 13.

____. *"Veritatis Splendor* and Moral Theology." *America* 169 (October 30, 1993): 8-11.

____. "Killing the Patient." *The Tablet* 247 (October 30, 1993): 1410-1411.

____. "Hidden Persuaders: Value Variables in Bioethics." *America* 168 (1993): 7-13.

____, and Charles E. Curran, eds. *Readings in Moral Theology No. 8: Dialogue About Catholic Sexual Teaching.* Mahwah, NJ: Paulist Press, 1993.

____. "Should We Clone Humans? Wholeness, Individuality, Reverence." *Christian Century* 110 (November 17-24, 1993): 1148-1149.

____. *Corrective Vision: Explorations in Moral Theology.* Kansas City, KS: Sheed and Ward, 1994.

____. "Beyond Principlism Is Not Enough: A Theologian Reflects on the Real Challenge for U.S. Biomedical Ethics." In *A Matter of Principlism?: Ferment in U.S. Bioethics.* Edited by Edwin R. DuBose, Ron Hamel, and Laurence J. O'Connell. Valley Forge, PA: Trinity Press, 1994, 344-361.

____. "Blastomere Separation: Some Concerns." *Hastings Center Report* 24 (March/April 1994): 14-16.

____. "An Unusual Request: Lesbian Motherhood and Genetic Choices." *Ethics Behavior* 3 (1994): 217-219.

____. "Some Early Reactions to *Veritatis Splendor." Theological Studies* 55 (September 1994): 481-506.

SECONDARY SOURCES

Abbattista, A.D. F. Vigevano, G. Catena, and F. Parisi. "Anencephalic Neonates and Diagnosis of Death." *Transplant Process* 8 (December 29, 1997): 3634-3635

Abbott, S. J., Walter M., ed. *The Documents of Vatican II.* Piscataway, NJ: New Century Publishers, 1966.

Ackerman, Terrence. "Meningomyelocele and Parental Commitment: A Policy Proposal Regarding Selection for Treatment." *Man and Medicine* 5 (Fall 1980): 295-300.

Allen, William. "Severely Deformed Babies in Crisis." *Priest* 31 (January 1975): 31-33.

Allsopp, Michael, E. "Deontic and Epistemic Authority in Roman Catholic Ethics: The Case of Richard McCormick." *Christian Bioethics* 2 (1996): 97-113.

American Academy of Pediatrics. "Guidelines for Infant Bioethics Review Committees." *Pediatrics* 74 (1984): 306-310.

Anderson, D. and R. M. Kliegman. "The Relationship of Neonatal Alimentation Practices to the Occurence of Endemic Necrotizing Enterocolitis." *American Journal of Perinatology* 8 (1991).

Aquilino, John D. "Life or Death?: A Parent's Plea for Civility and Reason." *Chicago Tribune*, 26 July 1995, 15.

Aquinas, Thomas. *Summa Theologica.*   Volumes I-V. Westminister, MD: Christian Classics, 1984.

____. *Quaestiones Quodlibetales.* Rome: Italy, Marelli Publishers, 1956.

____. *De Veritate.* Translated by Mulligan-McGlynn Schmidt. Chicago, IL: Regency, 1952-54.

Arras, John D. *et al.* "The Effect of New Pediatric Capabilities and the Problem of Uncertainty." *Hastings Center Report* 17 (December 1987): 10-15.

____. "Toward an Ethic of Ambiguity." *Hastings Center Report* 14 (April 1984): 26-28.

Atkinson, David. Review of *How Brave a New World?: Dilemmas in*

Bioethics, by Richard McCormick. In *The Expository Times* 93 (March 1982): 188.

Avery, Gordon B., Mary Ann Fletcher, and Mhairi G. MacDonald, eds. *Neonatology: Pathophysiology and Management of the Newborn.* Philadelphia, PA: J. B. Lippincott Company, 1994.

Bailey, M.D., Leonard L. *et al.* "Cardiac Allotransplantation in Newborns as Therapy for Hypoplastic Left Heart Syndrome." *The New England Journal of Medicine* 315 (October 1986): 949-951.

____. "Role of Cardiac Transplantation in the Neonate." *Journal of Heart Transplant* 4 (1985): 502-507.

Baird, P. A. and A. D. Sadovnick. "Survival in Infants with Anencephaly." *Clinical Pediatrics* 23 (1984): 268-271.

Ballance, W. A. *et al.* "Pathology of Neonatal NEC: A Ten Year Experience." *Journal of Pediatric Medicine, Supplement 1, Pt. 2.* 117 (1990).

Barton, L, J.E. Hodgman, and Z. Pavlova. "Causes of Death in the Extremely Low Birth Weight Infant." *Pediatrics* 103 (February 1999): 446-451

Beauchamp, Thomas L. and James F. Childress. *Principles of Biomedical Ethics.* 3rd ed. New York: Oxford University Press, 1989.

Beller, F. and J. Reeve. "Brain Life and Brain Death—The Anencephalic as an Explanatory Example—A Contribution to Transplantation." *Journal of Medicine and Philosophy* 14 (1989): 5-23.

____, and G. Zlatnik. "The Beginning of Human Life—Medical Observations and Ethical Reflections." *Clinical Obstetrics and Gynecology* 35 (1992): 720-728.

Benner, Patricia. "The Role of Experience, Narrative, and Community in Skilled Ethical Comportment." *Advances in Nursing Science* 14 (1991): 1-21.

Bergsma, Daniel and Ann E. Pulver, eds. *Developmental Disabilities: Psychological and Social Implications.* New York: Alan R. Liss, 1976.

Berkow, M. D., Robert, ed. *The Merck Manual.* Rahway, NJ: Merck Research Laboratories, 1992.

Biddle, Celestine. *Reality and the Mind.* Milwaukee, WI: Bruce Publishing Company, 1936.

Birsch, Douglas. "Virtue Ethics." *Ethical Insights.* Mountain View, CA: Mayfield Publishing, 1999.

Blankinship, Jerome. Review of *Health and Medicine in the Catholic Tradition,* by Richard McCormick. In *Christian Century* 102 (July 3-10, 1985): 656-657.

Boff, Leonardo. *Trinity and Society.* New York: Orbis Books, 1988.

Boone, C. Keith. "Theology and Bioethics: A Marriage Not Made in Heaven." *Hastings Center Report* 16 (October 1986): 41-43.

Brady, Bernard. Review of *The Critical Calling: Reflections on Moral Dilemmas Since Vatican II,* by Richard McCormick. In *Journal of Religion* 72 (April 1992): 291-292.

Bresnahan, James, F. "Rahner's Christian Ethics." *America* 123 (1970): 351-354.

Bridge, Paul and Maryls Bridge. "The Brief Life and Death of Christopher Bridge." *Hastings Center Report* 11 (December 1981).

Brody, Baruch A. and Amir Halevy. "Is Futility A Futile Concept." *Journal of Medicine and Philosophy* 20 (April 1995): 123-144.

Bonano, Mark A. "The Case of Baby K: Exploring The Concept of Medical Futility." *Annals of Health Care* 4 (1995): 151-153.

Cahill, Lisa Sowle. "On Richard McCormick: Reason and Faith in Post-Vatican II Catholic Ethics." In *Theological Voices in Medical Ethics.* Edited by Allen Verhey and Stephen E. Lammers. Grand Rapids, MI: William B. Eerdmans Publishing Company, 1993. 78-105.

____. "Teleology, Utilitarianism, and Christian Ethics." *Theological Studies* 42 (1981): 601-629.

____. Review of *How Brave a New World?: Dilemmas in Bioethics*, by Richard A. McCormick, S.J. In *Anglican Theological Review* 63 (1981): 351-352.

____. "Within Shouting Distance: Paul Ramsey and Richard McCormick on Method." *Journal of Medicine and Philosophy* 4 (December 1979): 398-417.

Callahan, Daniel. "Living with the New Biology." *Center Magazine* 5 (1972): 4-12.

Campbell, A. "Children in a Persistent Vegetative State." *British Medical Journal* 289 (1984): 1022-1023.

____. "The Right to be Allowed to Die." *Journal of Medical Ethics* 9 (1983): 136- 140.

Caplan, A. and Cohen C. "Imperiled Newborns." *The Hastings Center* 17 (December 1987): 5-3.

Capron, Alexander, Tom Regan, Keith Reemtsma, Richard Sheldon, Richard McCormick, Albert Gore. "The Subject Is Baby Fae." *Hastings Center Report* 15 (February 1985): 8-13.

Castelli, James. "Life/Death Decisions." *St. Anthony Messenger* 83 (1975): 33-35.

Childress, James F. "Two by McCormick." *Hastings Center Report* 12 (January 1982): 40-42.

____. *Who Should Decide?* New York: Oxford Press, 1982.

Christiansen, Drew. "The Elderly and their Families: The Problems of Dependence." *New Catholic World* 223 (1980): 100-104.

Clark, Mary T. *An Aquinas Reader.* Garden City, NY: Image Books, 1972.

Clark, Peter A., S.J., "Building a Policy in Pediatrics for Medical Futility," *Pediatric Nursing* 27 (March-April, 2001): 180-184.

Clark, Peter A., S.J., "Medical Futility in Pediatrics: Is it Time for a Public Policy?" *Journal of Public Health Policy* 23 (2002): 66-89.

Clark, S.J., Peter A. & Catherine Mikus. "Time for a Formalized Medical Futility Policy." *Health Progress* 81 (July-August, 2000): 24-32

Clarke, Thomas. *Above Every Name.* Mahwah, NJ: Paulist Press, 1980.

Cohn, Victor. "Let Deformed Babies Die, GU Jesuit Says." *Washington Post* 7 July 1974, A6.

Congregation for the Doctrine of the Faith. "Declaration on Euthanasia." *Origins* 10 (August 1980): 257-267.

Connery, John R. "Quality of Life." *Linacre Quarterly* 53 (February 1986): 26-33.

____. "Prolongation of Life: A Duty and Its Limits." *Linacre Quarterly* 47 (May 1980): 151-165.

Cooper, M. Wayne. "Is Medicine Hermeneutics All the Way Down?" *Theoretical Medicine* 15 (June 1994): 149-180.

Copleston, F. C. *Aquinas.* New York: Penguin Books, 1955.

Coulter, M.D., David L. "Neurologic Uncertainty in Newborn Intensive Care." *The New England Journal of Medicine* 316 (April 2, 1986): 840-844.

Council of Ethical and Judicial Affairs of the American Medical Association. "The Use of Anencephalic Neonates as Organ Donors." *Journal of the American Medical Association* 273 (May 24-31, 1995): 1614-1618.

Covert, R. *et al.* "Factors Associated with Age of Onset of Necrotizing Enterocolitis." *American Journal of Perinatology* 6 (1989).

Cox, Harvey. "Evolutionary Progress and Christian Promise." *Concilium* 26. New York: Paulist Press, 1967.

Curran, Charles E., ed. *Moral Theology: Challenges for the Future—Essays in Honor of Richard A. McCormick, S.J.* New York: Paulist Press, 1990.

____. *Politics, Medicine, and Christian Ethics: A Dialogue with Paul Ramsey.* Philadelphia, PA: Fortress Press, 1973.

____. *Contemporary Problems in Moral Theology.* Notre Dame, IN: Fides Publishers, 1970.

____. *Absolutes in Moral Theology?* Washington, DC: Corpus Books, 1968.

Daniel, Stephen L. "Hermeneutical Clinical Ethics: A Commentary." *Theoretical Medicine* 15 (June 1994): 133-140.

Department of Health and Human Services. "Child Abuse and Neglect: Prevention and Treatment." *Federal Register* 50 (April 15, 1985): 14887-14892.

____. "Nondiscrimination on the Basis of Handicap Relating to Health Care of Infants: Proposed Rules." *Federal Register* 48 (1983): 9630-9632.

____. "Nondiscrimination on the Basis of Handicap Relating to Health Care of Infants: Proposed Rules." *Federal Register* 48 (1983): 30846-30852.

Diamond, Eugene F. "'Quality' vs. 'Sanctity' of Life in the Nursery." *America* 135 (1976): 396-398.

Doyle, James J. Review of *How Brave a New World?: Dilemmas in Bioethics,* by Richard A. McCormick, S.J. In *Theological Studies* 42 (September 1981): 498-499.

Drane, James F., and John Coulehan. "The Concept of Futility: Patients Do Not Have a Right to Demand Medically Useless Treatment." *Health Progress* 74 (December 1993): 28-32.

_____. *Becoming a Good Doctor: The Place of Virtue and Character in Medical Ethics*. Kansas City, MO: Sheed and Ward, 1988.

_____. *Religion and Ethics*. New York: Paulist Press, 1976.

DuBose, Edwin R., Ronald Hamel, and Laurence J. O'Connell, eds. *A Matter of Principles?: Ferment in U. S. Bioethics*. Valley Forge, PA: Trinity Press International, 1994.

Duff, M. D., Raymond S. and A. G. M. Campbell, M. D., "Moral and Ethical Dilemmas in the Special-Care Nursery." *The New England Journal of Medicine* 289 (October 25, 1973): 890-894.

_____. "Moral and Ethical Dilemmas: Seven Years Into the Debate and Human Ambiguity." *Annals of the American Academy of Political and Social Science* 447 (January 1977): 19-28.

_____. "On Deciding the Care for Severely Handicapped or Dying Persons: With Particular Reference to Infants." *Pediatrics* 57 (April 1976): 487-493.

Dunagan, M.D., William and Michael L. Ridner, M.D., eds. *Manual of Medical Therapeutics*, 26th ed. Boston, MA: Little, Brown and Company, 1986.

Dunn, Peter M. "Appropriate Care of the Newborn: Ethical Dilemmas." *Journal of Medical Ethics* 19 (1993): 82-84.

Dwyer, Judith, ed. *The New Dictionary of Catholic Social Thought*. Wilmington, DE: Glazier, 1994.

Dyck, Arthur J. *On Human Care: An Introduction to Ethics*. Nashville, TN: Abingdon, 1977.

Edel, Abraham. *Method in Ethical Theory*. London: Transaction Publishers, 1944.

Editorial Staff. "When the Neonate Is Defective." *Contemporary Ob/Gyn* 7 (June 1976): 90-112.

Eigo, Francis, ed. *Called to Love: Toward a Contemporary Christian Ethic*. Villanova, PA: Villanova University Press, 1985.

Engelhardt, H. Tristram. "Bioethics and the Process of Embodiment." *Perspectives in Biology and Medicine* 18 (Summer 1975): 486-500.

_____. "Euthanasia and Children: The Inquiry of Continued Existence." *Journal of Pediatrics* 83 (July 1973): 170-171.

Erde, E. "Studies in the Explanation of Issues in Biomedical Ethics—On Playing God." *Journal of Medicine and Philosophy* 14 (1989): 593-615.

Evans, Donald. "Paul Ramsey and Exceptionless Moral Rules." *American Journal of Jurisprudence* 16 (1970): 184-214.

Evans, Robert A. and Thomas Parker, eds. *Christians Theology: A Case Study Approach*. New York: Harper and Row, 1976.

Finnis, John M. *Natural Law and Natural Rights*. Oxford: Clarendon Press, 1980.

_____. "Natural Law and Unnatural Acts." *Heythrop Journal* 11 (1970): 365-387.

Firth, Roderick. "Ethical Absolutism and the Ideal Observer." *Philosophy and Phenomenological Research* 12 (March 1952): 326.

Fleischman, A. "Ethical Issues in Neonatology—A United States Perspective." *Annals of The New York Academy of Sciences* 530 (1988): 83-91.

Fletcher, Joseph. "The 'Right' to Live and the 'Right' to Die." *The Humanist* 34 (July-August 1974): 3-7.

_____. "Four Indicators of Humanhood—The Enquiry Matures." *Hastings Center Report* 4 (December 1974): 6-7.

_____. "Ethics and Euthanasia." *American Journal of Nursing* 73 (April 1973): 670-675.

_____. "Indicators of Humanhood: A Tentative Profile of Man." *Hastings Center Report* 2 (1972): 1-4.

Fost, M.D., Norman. "Passive Euthanasia of Patients with Down's Syndrome." *Archives of Internal Medicine* 142 (December 1982): 2295-2296.

_____. "Ethical Issues in the Treatment of Critically Ill Newborns." *Pediatric Annals* 10 (1981): 383-387.

_____. "Ethical Problems in Pediatrics." *Current Problems in Pediatrics* 6 (October 1976): 13-17.

Freedman, Benjamin. "Five Red Herrings and an Issue: Response to McCormick." *Journal of Medicine and Philosophy* 3 (September 1978): 222-225.

Freeman, J. "Early Management and Decision-Making for the Treatment of Myelomeningocele—A Critique." *Pediatrics* 73 (1984): 564-566.

Fuchs, Josef. *Personal Responsibility and Christian Morality*. Washington, DC: Georgetown University Press, 1983.

Gaffney, James. Review of *The Critical Calling: Reflections on Moral Dilemmas Since Vatican II*, by Richard McCormick. In *Theological Studies* 51 (Spring 1990): 547- 549.

Garland, Michael J. "Care of the Newborn: The Decision Not to Treat." *Perinatology/Neonatology* 1 (September-October 1977):10-17.

Gehk, Mary Beth and Judith A. Erlen. "An Ethical Dilemma in the Neonatal Intensive Care Unit: Providing Due Care." *Journal of Perinatology* XIII (1993): 50-54.

Gillon, R. "Philosophical Medical Ethics—Ordinary and Extraordinary Means." *British Medical Journal* 292 (1986): 259-261.

Glover, Jonathan. *Causing Death and Saving Lives*. New York: Penguin Books, 1977.

Gomella, Tricia Lacy., M. Douglas Cunningham, Fabien Eyal and Karin Zent. *Neonatology* 4 th Ed. (Stamford, CT: Appleton & Lange, 1999), 462.

Gostin, L. "A Moment in Human Development—Legal Protection, Ethical Standards and Social Policy on the Selective Non-Treatment of Handicapped Newborns." *American Journal of Law and Medicine* 11 (1985): 31-78.

Grecco, Richard. *Theology of Compromise: A Study of the Ethics of Charles E. Curran*. New York: Peter Lang Publishers, 1991.

Greenspahn, Frederick, E., ed. *Contemporary Ethical Issues in the Jewish and Christian Traditions*. Hoboken, NJ: Ktav Publishing House, 1986.

Griener, Glenn G. "The Physician's Authority to Withhold Futile Treatment." *Journal of Medicine and Philosophy* 20 (April 1995): 207-223.

Gula, Richard. *Reason Informed by Faith: Foundations of Catholic Morality*. New York: Paulist Press, 1989.

Gustafson, James M. *The Contributions of Theology to Medical Ethics*. Milwaukee, WI: Marquette University Press, 1975.

_____. Review of *Ambiguity in Moral Choice*, by Richard A. McCormick, S.J. In *Religious Studies* 10 (June 1974): 252-253.

_____. "Mongolism, Parental Desires and the Right to Life." *Perspectives in Biology and Medicine* XVI (1973): 529-559.

Guzzetta, M.D., F. *et al.* "Periventricular Intraparenchymal Echodensities in the Premature Newborn: Critical Determinant of Neurological Outcome." *Pediatrics* 78 (1986): 993-996.

Halac, E. *et al.* "Prenatal and Postnatal Corticosteroid Therapy to Prevent Neonatal Necrotizing Enterocolitis: A Controlled Trial." *Journal of Pediatrics* 117 (1990): 132- 138.

Hallett, Garth L. *Christian Moral Reasoning: An Analytic Guide*. Notre Dame, IN: University of Notre Dame Press, 1983.

Halevy, A. R.C. Neal and B.A. Brody, "The Low Frequency of Futility in an Adult Intensive Care Unit Setting," *Archives of Internal Medicine* 156 (1996): 100-104.

Hamlyn, D. W. *The Theory of Knowledge*. Garden City, NY: Doubleday and Co., 1970.

Happel, Stephen and James J. Walter. *Conversion and Discipleship: A Christian Foundation for Ethics and Doctrine*. Philadelphia, PA: Fortress Press, 1986.

Hastings Center Report. "On the Care of Imperiled Newborns (Symposium)." *The Hastings Center* 14 (April 1984): 24-42.

Hauerwas, Stanley. *Character and Christian Life: A Study in Theological Ethics*. San Antonio, TX: Trinity University Press, 1974.

_____. *Vision and Virtue*. Notre Dame, IN: Fides Publishers, 1974.

Haughey, John, ed. *Personal Values and Public Policy*. Mahwah, NJ: Paulist Press, 1979.

Heaney, Stephen J. "Aquinas and the Presence of the Human Rational Soul in the Early Embryo." *The Thomist* 56 (January 1992): 19-48.

Hesselink, I. John. Review of *Notes on Moral Theology 1965 through 1980*, by Richard McCormick. In *Christian Century* 98 (September 23, 1981): 941.

Higginson, Richard. "Life, Death and the Handicapped Newborn: A Review of the Ethical Issues." *Ethics and Medicine* 3 (1987): 45-48.

Hill, A. "Intraventricular Hemorrhage: Emphasis on Prevention." *Seminar in Pediatric Neurology* 5 (September 1998): 152-160.

Hodges, Louis W., ed. *Social Responsibility: Journalism, Law, and Medicine*. Lexington, VA: Washington and Lee University Press, 1973.

Holman, R.C., B.J. Stoll, M.J. Clark *et al.* "The Epidemiology of Necrotizing Enterocolitis Infant Mortality in the United States." *American Journal of Public Health* 87 (December 1997): 2026-2031.

Horan, Dennis J. and David Mall, eds. *Death, Dying, and Euthanasia*. Washington, DC: University Publications of America, 1977.

Howsepian, A. A. "Who or What We Are?" *Review of Metaphysics* 45 (March 1992): 483-502.

Infant Bioethics Task Force and Consultants. "Guidelines for Infant Bioethics Committees." *Pediatrics* 74 (August 1984): 306-310.

Janssens, Louis. "Ontic Good and Evil: Premoral Values and Disvalues." *Louvain Studies* 12 (1987): 62-82.

_____. "Artificial Insemination: Ethical Considerations." *Louvain Studies* 8 (Spring 1980): 3-29.

Jonsen, Albert R. and Toulmin, Stephen. *The Abuse of Casuistry*. Berkeley, CA: University of California Press, 1988.

_____, and Michael Garland, eds. *Ethics of Newborn Intensive Care*. Berkeley, CA: University of California Press, 1976.

Judicial Council of the American Medical Association. "Current Opinions of the Judicial Council of the American Medical Association." Chicago, IL: American Medical Association, 1982, 9.

Kamitsuka, M.D., M.K. Horton, and M.A. Williams. "The Incidence of Necrotizing Enterocolitis After Introducing Standardized Feeding Schedules for Infants Between 1250 and 2500 Grams and Less Than 35 Weeks of Gestation." *Pediatrics* 105 (February 2000): 379-384.

Keane, Philip S. "The Objective Moral Order: Reflections on Recent Research." *Theological Studies* 43 (1982): 260-278.

Keenan, James. "Virtue Ethics." In *Christian Ethics*, ed. Bernard Hoose. Collegeville, MN: Liturgical Press, 1998.

Keeton, W. Page *et al. Prosser and Keeton on the Law of Torts*. 5th ed. Minneapolis, MN: West, 1984.

Kelly, Gerald. *Medico-Moral Problems*. St. Louis, MO: The Catholic Health Association of the United States and Canada, 1958.

Kipnis, Kenneth and Gailynn Williamson. "Nontreatment Decisions for Severely Compromised Newborns." *Ethics* 95 (October 1984): 90-111.

Kirsten, Denise. "Patent Ductus Arteriosus in the Preterm Infant." *Neonatal Network* 15 (March 1996): 19-26.

Knauer, Peter. *"Überlegungen zur moraltheologischen Prinzippenlehre der Enzyklika 'Humanae Vitae.'"* *Theologie und Philosophie* 45 (1970): 60-74.

____. "The Hermeneutic Function of the Principle of Double Effect." *Natural Law Forum* 12 (1967): 132-162.

____. *"La détermination du bien et du mal moral par le principe du double effet."* *Nouvelle Revue Théologique*. 87 (1965): 356-376.

Kohl, Marvin, ed. *Beneficent Euthanasia*. Buffalo, NY: Prometheus Books, 1975.

____, ed. *Infanticide and the Value of Life*. Buffalo, NY: Prometheus Books, 1978.

Koop, M.D., C. Everett. "The Handicapped Child and His Family." *Linacre Quarterly* 48 (February 1981).

Kuhse, H. "Death by Non-Feeding: Not in the Baby's Best Interests." *Journal of Medical Humanities and Bioethics* 7 (Fall/Winter 1986): 79-90.

____, and G. Hughes. "Extraordinary Means and Sanctity of Life." *Journal of Medical Ethics* 7 (1981): 74-82.

____. "Debate: Extraordinary Means and Sanctity of Life." *Journal of Medical Ethics* 7 (1981): 74-82.

Jellinek, M.D., Michael S. *et al.* "Facing Tragic Decisions with Parents in the Neonatal Intensive Care Unit: Clinical Perspectives." *Pediatrics* 89 (January 1992): 119-122.

Johnson, James and David Smith, eds. *Love and Society: Essays in the Ethics of Paul Ramsey*. Missoula, MT: University of Montana Press, 1974.

Johnson, Paul R. "Selective Nontreatment and Spina Bifida: A Case Study in Ethical Theory and Application." *Bioethics Quarterly* 3 (Summer 1981): 91-111.

____. "Selective Nontreatment of Defective Newborns: An Ethical Analysis." *Linacre Quarterly* 47 (February 1980): 39-53.

Jonsen, A. R. *et al.* "Critical Issues in Newborn Intensive Care: A Conference Report and Policy Proposal. *Pediatrics* 55 (1975): 756-768.

Jonsen, Albert R. and Michael J. Garland, eds. *Ethics of Newborn Intensive Care*. Berkeley, CA: Health Policy Program, 1976.

Ladd, John, ed. *Ethical Issues Relating to Life and Death*. New York: Oxford University Press, 1979.

Landwirth, M.D., Julius. "Should Anencephalic Infants Be Used as Organ Donors?" *Pediatrics* 82 (August 1988): 257-260.

Langan, John. "Augustine on the Unity and the Interconnection of the Virtues." *Harvard Theological Review* 72 (January-April 1979): 81-95.

____. "Beatitude and Moral Law in St. Thomas." *The Journal of Religious Ethics* 5 (Fall 1977): 183-195

Lantos, J. "The Hastings Center Project on Imperiled Newborns—Supreme Court, Jury, or Greek Chorus." *Pediatrics* 83 (1989): 615-616.

Lantz, C. "The Anencephalic Infant as Organ Donor." *Health Law Journal* 4 (1996): 179- 195.

Levine, Malcolm and David Tudehope. *Essentials of Neonatal Medicine*. Oxford: Blackwell Scientific Publications, 1993.

Levy, Sanford S. "Richard McCormick and Proportionate Reason." *Journal of Religious Ethics* 13 (1985): 258-278.

Lisson, Edward L. Review of *Readings in Moral Theology No. 7: Natural Law and Theology*, eds. Richard McCormick and Charles E. Curran. In *Horizons* 20 (Spring 1993): 182.

Lister, D. "Ethical Issues in Infanticide of Severely Defective Infants." *Canadian Medical Association Journal* 135, (1986): 1401-1404.

Lonergan, Bernard. *Method in Theology*. New York: Herder and Herder, 1972.

____. *Insight: A Study of Human Understanding*. London: Longmans, Green and Co., 1957.

Long, W. A. *Fetal and Neonatal Cardiology*. Philadelphia, PA: W. B. Sanders, 1990.

Longwood, Merle. "Ethical Reflections on the Meaning of Death." *Dialogue* 11 (1972): 195-201.

Lorber, M.D., J. "Spina Bifida: To Treat or Not To Treat?" *Nursing Mirror* 47 (September 14, 1978): 13-19.

____. "Selective Treatment of Myelomeningocele: To Treat or Not To Treat?" *Pediatrics* 53 (1974): 307-310.

_____. "Spina Bifida Cystica: Results of the Treatment of 270 Consecutive Cases with Criteria for Selection for the Future." *Archives of Disease in Childhood* 47 (1972).

_____. "Results of Treatment of Myelomeningocele." *Developmental Medical Child Neurology* 13 (1971): 279-303.

Louisell, David, W. "Euthanasia and Bianthanasia: On Dying and Killing." *Linacre Quarterly* 10 (1974): 14-22.

Lusthaus, Evelyn W. "Involuntary Euthanasia and Current Attempts to Define Persons with Mental Retardation as Less Than Human." *Mental Retardation* 23 (1995): 148- 154.

MacIntyre, Alasdair. *After Virtue*. Notre Dame, IN: University of Notre Dame Press, 1984.

_____. "Theological Ethics and the Ethics of Medicine and Health Care." *Journal of Medicine and Philosophy* 4 (1979): 430-439.

Mackler, Aaron L. "Neonatal Intensive Care." *Scope Notes* 11 (1993): 1-12.

Maglalang, M.D., Apollo, Professor of Pediatrics and Director of Neonatology. Interview by author, 28 December 1995, Atlantic City, New Jersey. Atlantic City Medical Center.

Magnet, Joseph E. and Eike-Henner W. Kluge. *Withholding Treatment from Defective Newborn Children*. Quebec: Brown Legal Publications, 1985.

Maguire, Daniel. *"Recta Ratio* and the Intellectualistic Fallacy." *Journal of Religious Ethics* 10 (1982): 22-39.

_____. Review of *Notes on Moral Theology 1965 through 1980*, by Richard McCormick. In *Theological Studies* 43 (March 1982): 164-167.

Maguire, Marjorie R. Review of *How Brave a New World?: Dilemmas in Bioethics*, by Richard A. McCormick, S.J. In *Horizons* 9 (Fall 1992): 397-398.

Mason, J. K. "Parental Choice and Selective Non-Treatment of Deformed Newborns: A View from Mid-Atlantic." *Journal of Medical Ethics* 12 (1986): 67-71.

McBrien, Richard P., ed. *The Harper-Collins Encyclopedia of Catholicism*. San Francisco, CA: Harper-Collins Publishers, 1995.

McCarthy, Donald G. "Treating Defective Newborns: Who Judges Extraordinary Means?" *Hospital Progress* 62 (December 1981): 45-50.

McKinney, Ronald H. "The Quest for an Adequate Proportionalist Theory of Value." *The Thomist* 53 (January, 1989): 56-73.

McMahon, Kevin T. "What the Pennsylvania Bishops Really Said (A Reply to Richard A. McCormick, S.J.)." *Linacre Quarterly* 59 (August 1992): 6-10.

Medawar, Peter, B. *The Hope of Progress*. New York: Doubleday and Company, 1972.

Meilaender, Gilbert. "If This Baby Could Choose . . ." *Linacre Quarterly* 49 (November 1982): 313-321.

Melchin, Kenneth R. Review of *Readings in Moral Theology No. 7:*

Natural Law and Theology, eds. Richard McCormick and Charles E. Curran. In *Église et Théologie* 24 (1993): 453-454.

Merenstein, M.D., Gerald B. "Individualized Developmental Care: An

Emerging New Standard for Neonatal Intensive Care Units?" *Journal of the American Medical Association* 272 (September 2, 1994): 890-891.

Meyers, Christopher. "Intended Goals and Appropriate Treatment—An

Alternative to the Ordinary Extraordinary Distinction." *Journal of Medical Ethics* 10 (1984): 128- 130.

Mitchell, S. C. *et al.* "Congenital Heart Disease in 56,109 Births." *Circulation* 43 (1971): 323-335.

Modras, Ronald. "The Implications of Rahner's Anthropology for Fundamental Moral Theology." *Horizons* 12 (1985): 70-90.

Moller, J. H. and W. A. Neal. *Fetal, Neonatal, and Infant Cardiac Disease*. Norfolk, CT: Appleton and Lang, 1989.

Moltmann, Jurgen. *History of the Triune God: Contributions to Trinitarian Theology*. London, SCM, 1991.

_____. *The Trinity and the Kingdom: The Doctrine of God*. San Francisco, CA: Harper and Row, 1981.

Moskop, J. C. and L. Kopelman, eds. *Ethics and Critical Care Medicine*. Dordrecht, Netherlands: D. Reidel, 1985.

Mueller, J. J. *What is Theology?* Collegeville, MN: Liturgical Press, 1988.

_____. *What Are They Saying About Theological Method?* New York: Paulist Press, 1984.

Muraskas, M.D., Jonathan, Associate Professor of Pediatrics and Assistant Clinical Director of Neonatology. Interview by author, 8 December 1995, Maywood, Illinois. Loyola University Medical Center.

Murray, Thomas H. and Arthur L. Caplan. *Which Babies Shall Live? Humanistic Dimensions of the Care of Imperiled Newborns*. Clifton, NJ: Humana Press, 1985.

Natowicz, M.D., Marvin *et al.* "Genetic Disorders and Major Extracardiac Anomalies Associated with the Hypoplastic Left Heart Syndrome." *Pediatrics* 82 (November 1988): 698-706.

Nelin, Leif and George Hoffman. "The Use of Inhaled Nitric Oxide in a Wide Variety of Clinical Problems." *Pediatric Clinics of North America* 45 (June 1998): 531-548.

Nelson, James S. Review of *How Brave a New World?: Dilemmas in Bioethics*, by Richard A. McCormick, S.J. In *Journal of the American Academy of Religion* 50 (June 1982): 324-325.

____. Review of *Doing Evil to Achieve Good: Moral Choice in Conflict Situations*, by Richard McCormick and Paul Ramsey. In *Christian Scholar's Review* 10 (1980): 73- 74.

Neu, J., and M.D. Weiss. "Necrotizing Enterocolitis: Pathophysiology and Prevention." *Journal of Parenteral Enteral Nutrition* 23 (September-October 1999): Supplement 1 3-7.

Nolan, Kathleen. "Imperiled Newborns." *Hastings Center Report* 17 (December 1987): 5-7.

O'Connell, Timothy. *Principles for a Catholic Morality*. San Francisco, CA: Harper and Row, 1978.

O'Connor, June. Review of *Ambiguity in Moral Choice*, by Richard McCormick. In *Horizons* 1 (Autumn 1974): 137-138.

Odozor, Paulinus Ikechukwu. *Richard A. McCormick and the Renewal of Moral Theology*. Notre Dame, IN: Notre Dame Press, 1995.

O'Grady, John F. *Christian Anthropology: A Meaning for Human Life*. New York: Paulist Press, 1976.

O'Neil, R. "Determining Proxy Consent." *Journal of Medicine and Philosophy* 8 (1983): 389-403.

Oskandy, David L. *Severely Defective Newborns: The Catholic Physician's Dilemma*. St. Louis, MO: The Catholic Health Association of the United States, 1985. 8-14.

Paris, John J. "Terminating Treatment for Newborns: A Theological Perspective." In *Quality of Life: The New Medical Dilemma*. Edited by James J. Walter and Thomas A. Shannon. New York: Paulist Press, 1990. 151-160.

____, and Kevin J. O'Connell. "Withdrawal of Nutrition and Fluids from a Neurologically Devastated Infant: The Case of Baby T." *Journal of Perinatology* XI (1991): 372-373.

Parker, Leslie A. "Necrotizing Enterocolitis." *Neonatal Network* 14 (September 1995): 17-26.

Pellegrino, Edmund. "Decisions at the End of Life: The Use and Abuse of the Concept of Futility." In *The Dignity of the Dying Person: Proceedings of the Fifth Assembly of the Pontifical Academy of Life*. Vatican City, Italy: 2000, 219-241.

Pence, Gregory E., *Classic Cases in Medical Ethics*. 3rd edition. New York: McGraw- Hill, Inc., 2000.

Perlin, Seymour and Thomas Beauchamp, eds. *Ethical Issues in Death and Dying*. Englewood Cliffs, NJ: Prentice-Hall, 1978.

Phan, Peter C. "Contemporary Contexts and Issues in Eschatology." *Theological Studies* 55 (September 1994): 507-536.

Pius XII. "The Prolongation of Life." *Acta Apostolicae Sedis* 49 (1957): 1,031-1,032.

Pohlson, E. C., R. Schaller and D. Trapper. "Improved Survival with Primary Anastomosis in the Low-Birth-Weight Neonate with Esophageal Atresia and Tracheoesophageal Fistula." *Journal of Pediatric Surgery* 24 (1988): 415-420.

Popper, K. R. *Conjectures and Refutations*. New York: Harper and Row, 1968.

Post, Stephen G. "History, Infanticide, and Imperiled Newborns." *The Hastings Center* 18 (August/September 1988): 14-17.

Powell, T. and A. Hecimovic. "Baby Doe and the Search for a Quality of Life." *Exceptional Children* 51 (1985): 315-323.

President's Commission for the Study of Ethical Problems in Medicine and Biomedical and Behavioral Research. *Deciding to Forego Life-Sustaining Treatment: Ethical, Medical and Legal Issues in Treatment Decisions*. Washington, DC: United States Government Printing Office, 1983. 197-228.

Rahner, Karl. *Foundations of Christian Faith*. New York: Seabury Press, 1978.

_____. "The Problem of Genetic Manipulation." *Theological Investigations*. Vol. 9. New York: Herder and Herder, 1972, 225-252.

_____. "Reflections on the Unity of the Love of Neighbor and the Love of God." *Theological Investigations*. Vol. 6. Baltimore, MD: Helion, 1969, 231-249.

_____. "The Fundamental Option." *Theological Investigations*. Vol. 6. Baltimore, MD: Helicon, 1969.

Randolph, J. G., K. Newman, and K. D. Anderson. "Current Results and Repair of Esophageal Atresia with Tracheoesophageal Fistula Using Physiologic Status as a Guide to Therapy." *Annals of Surgery* 209 (1989): 520-526.

Ramsey, Paul. *Ethics at the Edges of Life: Moral and Legal Intersections*. New Haven: Yale University Press, 1978. 189-227.

_____. "Euthanasia and Dying Well." *Linacre Quarterly* 44 (1977): 37-46.

_____. "Prolonged Dying: Not Medically Indicated." *Hastings Center Report* 6 (February 1976): 14-17.

____. "The Enforcement of Morals: Nontherapeutic Research on Children—A Reply to Richard McCormick." *Hastings Center Report* 6 (August 1976): 21-30.

____. *The Patient as Person: Explorations in Medical Ethics*. New Haven: Yale University Press, 1970.

Reich, Warren T. "The Word 'Bioethics': The Struggle Over Its Earliest Meaning." *Kennedy Institute of Ethics Journal* 5 (March 1995): 19-34.

____, ed. *Encyclopedia of Bioethics*. Rev. Ed., Volumes 1-5. New York: Simon, Schuster, and MacMillan, 1995.

____. "The Word 'Bioethics': Its Birth and the Legacies of Those Who Shaped Its Meaning." *Kennedy Institute of Ethics Journal* 4 (December 1994): 319-335.

____. "Quality of Life and Defective Newborn Children: An Ethical Analysis." In *Quality of Life: The New Medical Dilemma*. Edited by James J. Walter and Thomas A. Shannon. New York: Paulist Press, 1990. 161-175.

____, ed. *Encyclopedia of Bioethics*. Volumes 1-4. New York: Free Press, 1978.

____. "On the Birth of a Severely Handicapped Infant." *Hastings Center Report* 3 (September 1973): 10-13.

____, and Richard A. McCormick. "Theologians View the Directives: Replies by Dr. Reich and Father McCormick to Dr. Diamond." *Hospital Progress* 54 (February 1973): 73-76.

Reiser, Stanley J., Arthur J. Dyck and William J. Curran, eds. *Ethics in Medicine*. Cambridge, MA: The MIT Press, 1982.

Rendtorff, Trutz. *Ethics: Basic Elements and Methodology in an Ethical Theology*. Philadelphia, PA: Fortress Press, 1986.

Rhoden, N. "Treatment Dilemmas for Imperiled Newborns." *Southern California Law Review* 58 (1985): 1283-1347.

Rigali, Norbert J. Review of *Notes on Moral Theology 1965 through 1980*, by Richard McCormick. In *Horizons* 9 (Spring 1982): 163-164.

Robertson, John A. "What We May Do with Pre-embryos: A Response to Richard A. McCormick." *Kennedy Institute of Ethics Journal* 1 (December 1991): 293-302.

____, and Norman Fost, M.D. "Passive Euthanasia of Defective Newborn Infants: Legal Considerations." *Journal of Pediatrics* 88 (1976).

Rossi, Philip. Review of *The Critical Calling: Reflections on Moral Dilemmas Since Vatican II*, by Richard McCormick. In *Horizons* 18 (Fall 1991): 348-349.

Roy, David J., ed. *Medical Wisdom and Ethics in the Treatment of Severely Defective Newborn and Young Children*. Montreal: Eden Press, 1978.

Sachdeva, R.C. *et al.* "Resource Consumption in a Pediatric Intensive Care Unit Setting." *Journal of Pediatrics* 128 (1996): 742-747.

Santurri, Edmund N. and William Werpehowski. "Substituted Judgment and the Terminally-Ill Incompetent." *Thought* 57 (December 1982): 484-501.

Schüller, Bruno. *"Zur Problematik allegemein verbindlicher ethischer Grundsätze." Theologie und Philosophie* 45 (1970): 1-23.

Selling, Joseph A. Review of *Readings in Moral Theology No. 7: Natural Law and Theology*, eds. Richard McCormick and Charles E. Curran. In *Louvain Studies* 17 (Winter 1992): 420.

Shaw, Anthony G. Randolph, and B. Manard. "Ethical Issues in Pediatric Surgery: A Nationwide Survey of Pediatricians and Pediatric Surgeons." *Pediatric* 59 (1977): 588-599.

Shelp, Earl E. *Born to Die? Deciding the Fate of Critically Ill Newborns.* New York: The Free Press, 1986.

____, ed. *Virtue and Medicine: Explorations in the Character of Medicine.* Dordrecht, Netherlands: D. Reidel, 1985.

____, ed. *Theology and Bioethics: Exploring the Foundations and Frontiers.* Dordrecht, Netherlands: D. Reidel, 1985.

____. "Courage and Tragedy in Clinical Medicine." *Journal of Medicine and Philosophy* 8 (November 1983): 417-429.

____, ed. *Beneficence and Health Care.* Dordrecht, Netherlands: D. Reidel Publishers, 1982.

Sheth,R. D. "Trends in Incidence and Severity of Intraventricular Hemorrhage." *Journal of Child Neurology* 13 (June 1998): 261-264.

Shewmon, D. A. "Anencephaly: Selected Medical Aspects." *Hastings Center Report* 18 (1988): 11-19.

Silverman, M.D., William A. "Overtreatment of Neonates?: A Personal Retrospective." *Pediatrics* 90 (December 1992): 971-976.

Singer, Peter. Review of *Doing Evil to Achieve Good: Moral Choices in Conflict Situations*, by Richard McCormick and Paul Ramsey. In *Hastings Center Report* 10 (February 1980): 42-44.

____. *Practical Ethics.* New York: Cambridge University Press, 1979.

Sittler, Joseph. *Grace Notes and Other Fragments.* Philadelphia, PA: Fortune Press, 1981.

____. *The Structure of Christian Ethics.* New Orleans, LA: Louisiana State University Press, 1958.

Smith, Barbara. "Narrative Versions, Narrative Theories." In *On Narrative.* Edited by W. J. T. Mitchell. Chicago, IL: University of Chicago Press, 1983.

Smith, David H. "On Letting Some Babies Die." *Hastings Center Studies* 2 (May 1974): 37-46.

Snyder, C.L., G.K. Gittes, J.P. Murphy *et al.* "Survival After Necrotizing Enterocolitis in Infants Weighing Less than 1,000 Grams: 25 Years' Experience at a Single Institution." *Journal of Pediatric Surgery* 32 (March 1997): 434-437.

Sontag, J. M.H. Wagner, J. Waldschmidt *et al.*, "Multisystem Organ Failure and Capillary Leak Syndrome in Severe Necrotizing Enterocolitis of Very Low Birth Weight Infants." *Journal of Pediatric Surgery* 33 (March 1998): 484-494.

Sparks, Richard C. *To Treat or Not To Treat?: Bioethics and the Handicapped Newborn.* New York: Paulist Press, 1988.

Spitz, L., E. Keily and R. J. Brereton. "Esophageal Atresia: A Five Year Experience with 148 Cases." *Journal of Pediatric Surgery* 22 (1987): 103-106.

Stanley, J. M. "The Appleton Consensus: Suggested International Guidelines for Decisions to Forego Medical Treatment." *Journal of Medical Ethics* 15 (September 1989): 129-136.

_____. "The Appleton International Conference: Developing Guidelines for Decisions to Forego Life-Prolonging Medical Treatment." *Journal of Medical Ethics* 18 Supplement (September 1992): 1-23.

Stoll, B. J. *et al.* "Epidemiology of Necrotizing Enterocolitis: A Case Control Study." *Journal of Pediatrics* 96 (1980): 447-451.

Strong, Carson. "The Tiniest Newborns." *The Hastings Center* 13 (February 1983): 14-19.

_____. "Decision Making in the NICU: The Neonatologist as Patient Advocate." *Hastings Center Report* 25 (1984).

Stumpf, M.D., David A. *et al.* "The Infant with Anencephaly." *New England Journal of Medicine* 322 (March 8, 1990): 669-673.

Swinyard, Chester A., ed. *Decision Making and the Defective Newborn.* Springfield, IL: Charles C. Thomas, 1978.

Tallo-Martinez, E., N. Claure and E. Bancalari. "Necrotizing Enterocolitis in Full-Term and Near-Term Infants: Risk Factors." *Biological Neonate* 71 ((1997): 292-298.

Thilo, M.D., Elizabeth, Paul A. Lazarte, M.D. and Jacinto A. Hernandez, M.D. "Necrotizing Enterocolitis in the First 24 Hours of Life." *Pediatrics* 73 (April 1984): 476-480.

Thomasma, David C. "Clinical Ethics as Medical Hermeneutics." *Theoretical Medicine* 15 (June 1994): 93-112.

Toohey, Timothy, J. Review of *Health and Medicine in the Catholic Tradition-Tradition in Transition*, by Richard A. McCormick, S. J. In *Journal of Pastoral Care* 39 (Spring 1985): 278.

Tooley, Michael. "Abortion and Infanticide." *Philosophy and Public Affairs* 2 (Fall 1972): 1-10.

____. "A Defense of Abortion and Infanticide." In *The Problem of Abortion*. Edited by Joel Feinberg. Belmont, CA: Wadsworth Publishing Company, 1973, 51-91.

Truog, Robert. "Futility in Pediatrics: From Case to Policy." *The Journal of Clinical Ethics* 11 (Summer 2000): 136-141.

Tubbs, James. "Moral Epistemology in Richard McCormick's Ethics." *Christian Bioethics* 2 (1996): 114-126.

Uauy, R. D. *et al.* "Necrotizing Enterocolitis in Very Low Birth Weight Infants: Biodemographic and Clinical Correlates." *Journal of Pediatrics* 119 (1991): 628-636.

Vacek, S. J., Edward, Collins. Review of *The Critical Calling: Reflections on Moral Dilemmas Since Vatican II*, by Richard A. McCormick, S. J. In *Journal of Religious Ethics* 20 (Spring 1992): 209.

____. "Proportionalism: One View of the Debate." *Theological Studies* 46 (1985): 287- 314.

Vaux, Kenneth. Review of *How Brave a New World?: Dilemmas in Bioethics*, by Richard McCormick. In *Theology Today* 38 (June 1982): 517-518.

____. Review of *How Brave a New World?: Dilemmas in Bioethics*, by Richard A. McCormick, S.J. In *Christian Century* 98 (April 8, 1981): 393-394.

Veatch, Robert, and C. Spicer, "Futile Care: Physicians Should Not Be Allowed to Refuse to Treat." *Health Progress* 10 (December 1993): 22-27.

____. "Medically Futile Care—The Role of the Physician in Setting Limits." *American Journal of Law and Medicine* 18 (1992): 15-36.

____. *A Theory of Medical Ethics*. New York: Basic Books, Inc., 1981.

____. *Death, Dying and the Biological Revolution*. New Haven, CT: Yale University Press, 1976.

____, Willard Gaylin, and Councilman Morgan, eds. *The Teaching of Medical Ethics*. New York: Institute of Society, Ethics and the Life Sciences, 1973.

Vohr, B., W.C. Allan, D.T. Scott *et al.* "Early-Onset Intraventricular Hemorrhage in Preterm Neonates: Incidence of Neurodevelopmental Handicap." *Perinatology* 23 (June 1999): 212-217;

Volpe, Joseph J. "Intraventricular Hemorrhage and Brain Injury in Premature Infants: Diagnosis, Prognosis, and Prevention." *Clinics in Perinatology* 16 (June 1989): 387- 411.

Walton, John, Jeremiah Barondess and Stephen Lock, eds. *The Oxford Medical Companion*. Oxford: Oxford University Press, 1994.

Walter, James J. "Termination of Medical Treatment: The Setting of Moral Limits from Infancy to Old Age." *Religious Studies Review* 16 (October 1990): 302-307.

____, and Thomas A. Shannon, eds. *Quality of Life: The New Medical Dilemma*. New York: Paulist Press, 1990.

____. "The Meaning and Validity of Quality of Life Judgments in Contemporary Roman Catholic Medical Ethics." *Louvain Studies* (Fall 1988): 195-208.

____. "A Public-Policy Option on the Treatment of Severely Handicapped Newborns." *Laval Theologique et Philosophique* 41 (1985): 239-250.

____. "Proportionate Reason and Its Three Levels of Inquiry: Structuring the Ongoing Debate." *Louvain Studies* 10 (Spring 1984): 30-40.

Walters, James, W. "Proximate Personhood As a Standard for Making Difficult Treatment Decisions: Imperiled Newborns as a Case Study." *Bioethics* 6 (January 1992): 12-22.

Warren, Mary Anne. "On the Moral and Legal Status of Abortion." *The Monist* 57 (January 1973): 43-61.

____. "Do Potential People Have Moral Rights?" *Canadian Journal of Philosophy* 7 (June 1977): 270-275.

Weber, Leonard J. *Who Shall Live?: The Dilemma of Severely Handicapped Children and Its Meaning for Other Moral Questions*. New York: Paulist Press, 1976.

Weinstein, S., G.W. Gaynor, N.D. Bridges *et al.*, "Early Survival of Infants Weighing 2.5 Kilograms or Less Undergoing First-Stage Reconstruction for Hypoplastic Left Heart Syndrome," *Circulation* 100 (November 9, 1999): Supplement III: 167-170.

Weir, Robert. and L. Gostin. "Decisions to Abate Life-Sustaining Treatment for Nonautonomous Patients—Ethical Standards and Legal Liability for Physicians After Cruzan." *Journal of the American Medical Association* 264 (1990): 1846-1853.

____. Abating Treatment with Critically Ill Patients. New York: Oxford Press, 1989.

____. "Selective Nontreatment—One Year Later—Reflections and Response." *Social Science and Medicine* 20 (1985): 1109-1117.

____. *Selective Nontreatment of Handicapped Newborns*. New York: Oxford University Press, 1984.

Wildes, S.J., Kevin, Francesc Abel, S.J., John C. Harvey. *Birth, Suffering and Death:Catholic Perspectives at the Edges of Life.* Boston, MA: Kluwer Academic Publishers, 1992.

Williams, D.L., A.C. Gelijns, A.J. Moskowicz *et al.* "Hypoplastic Left Heart Syndrome: Valuing the Survival." *Journal of Thorascic Cardiovascular Surgery* 19 (April 2000): 720-731

Williams, Robert H., ed. *To Live and To Let Die.* New York: Spinger-Verlag, 1973.

Zachary, M.D., R. B. "Ethical and Social Aspects of Treatment of Spina Bifida." *The Lancet* 2 (1969): 270-276.

Zalba, M. *Theologia Moralis Summa.* Vol. 3. Madrid: *La Editorial Catolica,* 1957.

Zaner, Richard, M. *Ethics and the Clinical Encounter.* Englewood, NJ: Prentice Hall, 1988.

_____, and Mary Rawlinson. "Medicine's Discourse and the Practice of Medicine." In *The Humanity of the Ill: Phenomenological Perspectives.* Edited by V. Kestenbaum. Knoxville, TN: University of Tennessee Press, 1982, 69-85.

_____. *The Context of Self: A Phenomenological Inquiry Using Medicine as a Clue.* Athens, OH: Ohio University Press, 1981.